Infections of the Liver and Biliary System

Editor

K. RAJENDER REDDY

GASTROENTEROLOGY CLINICS OF NORTH AMERICA

www.gastro.theclinics.com

Consulting Editor
ALAN L. BUCHMAN

June 2020 • Volume 49 • Number 2

ELSEVIER

1600 John F. Kennedy Boulevard • Suite 1800 • Philadelphia, Pennsylvania, 19103-2899
http://www.theclinics.com

GASTROENTEROLOGY CLINICS OF NORTH AMERICA Volume 49, Number 2
June 2020 ISSN 0889-8553, ISBN-13: 978-0-323-69565-7

Editor: Kerry Holland
Developmental Editor: Julia McKenzie

Gastroenterology Clinics of North America (ISSN 0889-8553) is published quarterly by Elsevier Inc., 360 Park Avenue South, New York, New York, NY 10010-1710. Months of issue are March, June, September, and December. Business and Editorial Offices: 1600 John F. Kennedy Blvd., Suite 1800, Philadelphia, PA 19103-2899. Customer Service Office: 6277 Sea Harbor Drive, Orlando, FL 32887-4800. Periodicals postage paid at New York, NY and additional mailing offices. Subscription prices are $365.00 per year (US individuals), $100.00 per year (US students), $730.00 per year (US institutions), $387.00 per year (Canadian individuals), $100.00 per year (Canadian students), $896.00 per year (Canadian institutions), $463.00 per year (international individuals), $220.00 per year (international students), and $896.00 per year (international institutions). Foreign air speed delivery is included in all *Clinics* subscription prices. All prices are subject to change without notice. **POSTMASTER:** Send address changes to *Gastroenterology Clinics of North America*, Elsevier Health Sciences Division, Subscription Customer Service, 3251 Riverport Lane, Maryland Heights, MO 63043. **Telephone: 1-800-654-2452 (U.S. and Canada); 314-447-8871 (outside U.S. and Canada). Fax: 314-447-8029. E-mail: journalscustomerservice-usa@elsevier.com (for print support); journalsonlinesupport-usa@elsevier.com (for online support).**

Reprints. For copies of 100 or more, of articles in this publication, please contact the Commercial Reprints Department, Elsevier Inc., 360 Part Avenue South, New York, New York 10010-1710. Tel. 212-633-3874, Fax: 212-633-3820, E-mail: reprints@elsevier.com.

Gastroenterology Clinics of North America is also published in Italian by Il Pensiero Scientifico Editore, Rome, Italy; and in Portuguese by Interlivros Edicoes Ltda., Rua Commandante Coelho 1085, 21250 Cordovil, Rio de Janeiro, Brazil.

Gastroenterology Clinics of North America is covered in *MEDLINE/PubMed (Index Medicus), Excerpta Medica, Current Contents/Clinical Medicine, Science Citation Index, ISI/BIOMED*, and *BIOSIS*.

Contributors

CONSULTING EDITOR

ALAN L. BUCHMAN, MD, MSPH, FACP, FACN, FACG, AGAF
Professor of Clinical Surgery, Medical Director, Intestinal Rehabilitation and Transplant Center, The University of Illinois at Chicago/UI Health, Chicago, Illinois, USA

EDITOR

K. RAJENDER REDDY, MD, FACP, FACG, FRCP, FAASLD
Ruimy Family President's Distinguished Professor of Medicine, Professor of Medicine in Surgery, Director of Hepatology, Medical Director of Liver Transplantation, Division of Gastroenterology and Hepatology, University of Pennsylvania, Philadelphia, Pennsylvania, USA

AUTHORS

AMEER ABUTALEB, MD
Division of Clinical Care and Research, Institute of Human Virology, Gastroenterology Fellow, Division of Gastroenterology and Hepatology, University of Maryland, Baltimore, Maryland, USA

RAKESH AGGARWAL, MD, DM
Professor, Department of Gastroenterology, Jawaharlal Institute of Postgraduate Medical Education and Research, Puducherry, India

SAHAR BAJIS, BPharm, MPH, PhD
Viral Hepatitis Clinical Research Program, The Kirby Institute, UNSW Sydney, Sydney, Australia

CHALERMRAT BUNCHORNTAVAKUL, MD
Division of Gastroenterology and Hepatology, Associate Professor, Department of Medicine, Rajavithi Hospital, College of Medicine, Rangsit University, Bangkok, Thailand

ANTONIO CRAXÌ, MD
Sezione di Gastroenterologia e Epatologia, PROMISE, Università di Palermo, Italia

GREGORY J. DORE, BSc, MBBS, MPH, FRACP, PhD
Professor, Viral Hepatitis Clinical Research Program, The Kirby Institute, UNSW Sydney, Sydney, Australia

SIRINA EKPANYAPONG, MD
Department of Medicine, Division of Gastroenterology and Hepatology, University of Pennsylvania, Philadelphia, Pennsylvania, USA

MARC G. GHANY, MD, MHSc
Liver Diseases Branch, National Institute of Diabetes, Digestive and Kidney Diseases, National Institutes of Health, Bethesda, Maryland, USA

AMIT GOEL, MD, DM
Additional Professor, Department of Gastroenterology, Sanjay Gandhi Postgraduate
Institute of Medical Sciences, Lucknow, India

HUMBERTO C. GONZALEZ, MD
Associate Professor of Medicine, Department of Gastroenterology and Hepatology,
Henry Ford Hospital, Wayne State University School of Medicine, Detroit, Michigan, USA

STUART C. GORDON, MD
Professor of Medicine, Department of Gastroenterology and Hepatology, Henry Ford
Hospital, Wayne State University School of Medicine, Detroit, Michigan, USA

THEO HELLER, MD
Liver Diseases Branch, National Institute of Diabetes and Digestive and Kidney Diseases,
National Institutes of Health, Bethesda, Maryland, USA

JULIAN HERCUN, MD
Liver Diseases Branch, National Institute of Diabetes and Digestive and Kidney Diseases,
National Institutes of Health, Bethesda, Maryland, USA

JIA-HORNG KAO, MD, PhD
Chair Professor, Graduate Institute of Clinical Medicine, National Taiwan University
College of Medicine, Department of Internal Medicine, Hepatitis Research Center,
Department of Medical Research, National Taiwan University, National Taiwan University
Hospital, Taipei, Taiwan

CHRISTOPHER KOH, MD, MHSc
Liver Diseases Branch, National Institute of Diabetes and Digestive and Kidney Diseases,
National Institutes of Health, Bethesda, Maryland, USA

SHYAM KOTTILIL, MBBS, PhD
Professor of Medicine, Division of Clinical Care and Research, Institute of Human
Virology, University of Maryland, Baltimore, Maryland, USA

JOSEPH K. LIM, MD
Professor of Medicine, Section of Digestive Diseases, Yale Liver Center, Professor of
Medicine, Director, Yale Viral Hepatitis Program, Yale University School of Medicine, New
Haven, Connecticut, USA

CHIH-LIN LIN, MD
Director, Department of Gastroenterology, Renai Branch, Taipei City Hospital,
Department of Psychology, National Chengchi University, Taipei, Taiwan

MAURICIO LISKER-MELMAN, MD, FAASLD
Professor of Medicine, Division of Gastroenterology, Hepatology Program, Washington
University School of Medicine, St Louis, Missouri, USA

MARIANNE MARTINELLO, MBBS, FRACP, PhD
Viral Hepatitis Clinical Research Program, The Kirby Institute, UNSW Sydney, Sydney,
Australia

SALVATORE PETTA, MD, PhD
Sezione di Gastroenterologia e Epatologia, PROMISE, Università di Palermo, Italia

HOMIE RAZAVI, PhD, MBA
Center for Disease Analysis Foundation, Lafayette, Colorado, USA

K. RAJENDER REDDY, MD, FACP, FACG, FRCP, FAASLD
Ruimy Family President's Distinguished Professor of Medicine, Professor of Medicine in Surgery, Director of Hepatology, Medical Director of Liver Transplantation, Division of Gastroenterology and Hepatology, University of Pennsylvania, Philadelphia, Pennsylvania, USA

REBECCA ROEDIGER, MD
Gastroenterology Fellow, Division of Gastroenterology, Hepatology Program, Washington University School of Medicine, St Louis, Missouri, USA

COLEMAN I. SMITH, MD
MedStar Georgetown Transplant Institute, MedStar Georgetown University Hospital, Washington, DC, USA

ELIAS SPYROU, MD, PhD
MedStar Georgetown Transplant Institute, MedStar Georgetown University Hospital, Washington, DC, USA; Nazih Zuhdi Transplant Institute, INTEGRIS Baptist Medical Center, Oklahoma City, Oklahoma, USA

ASHLEY N. TRAN, MD
Gastroenterology Fellow, Section of Digestive Diseases, Yale Liver Center, Yale University School of Medicine, New Haven, Connecticut, USA

Contents

> Viral hepatitis (A, B, C, D, and E) is the leading cause of inflammation of liver tissue (hepatitis). The disease burden associated with hepatitis A and E occurs shortly after infection; it is more severe among adults. With hepatitis A and E, the number of incident cases (new acute infections) is important from a public health perspective. Long-term hepatitis has been shown to cause cirrhosis and hepatocellular carcinoma in patients. The disease burden associated with hepatitis B, C, and D appears 10 to 20 years after infection. Thus, the prevalence of these infections is important from a public health perspective.

> Hepatitis A virus (HAV) is a positive-strand RNA virus that is transmitted feco-orally through person-to-person contact. Outbreaks are often linked to poor sanitation, overcrowding, or food and water contamination. Infection is often asymptomatic in children, but adults present with jaundice, abdominal pain, hepatitis, and hyperbilirubinemia. Diagnosis is through detection of immunoglobulin M antibodies against HAV, and treatment is supportive. Vaccination is the mainstay of prevention and should be given before exposure whenever possible.

> Enhancing host immunity by vaccination to prevent hepatitis B virus (HBV) infection remains the most important strategy for global control of hepatitis B. Currently, 187 countries have in place infant hepatitis B vaccination programs. Hepatitis B surface antigen prevalence has decreased to less than 1% in children after successful implementation of universal HBV vaccination in newborns. The incidence of primary liver cancer in children, adolescents, and young adults has drastically decreased to near zero in birth cohorts receiving hepatitis B vaccination. Elimination of chronic hepatitis B by 2030 is not a mission impossible.

Despite the availability of a protective vaccine for over 3 decades, the number of persons with chronic hepatitis B virus (HBV) infection remains high. These persons are at risk for cirrhosis and hepatocellular carcinoma. Current treatment is effective at inhibiting viral replication and reducing complications of chronic HBV infection, but is not curative. There is a need for novel, finite therapy that can cure chronic HBV infection. Several agents are in early-phase development and can be broadly viewed as agents that target the virus directly or indirectly or the host immune response. This article highlights key developments in antiviral/immuno-modulatory therapy, the rationale for these approaches, and possible therapeutic regimens.

Half a century after its discovery, hepatitis delta remains a pertinent global health issue with a major clinical impact in endemic regions and an underestimated prevalence worldwide. Hepatitis delta virus infection follows a challenging clinical course and is responsible for significant liver-related morbidity. Although the only currently available treatment (pegylated interferon) does not provide consistent results, emerging therapeutic options are promising. This article explores the epidemiology, natural history, as well as current and potential therapeutic options for hepatitis delta virus infection.

The World Health Organization has called for the elimination of hepatitis C virus (HCV) as a public health threat by 2030. Highly effective direct-acting antiviral agents provide the therapeutic tools required for elimination. In the absence of a vaccine, HCV elimination will require enhanced primary prevention and an increase in the proportions of people diagnosed and treated. Given that globally only 20% of people with chronic HCV are diagnosed, and around 5% have initiated HCV treatment, the task ahead is enormous. But, global public health needs optimism, and countries currently on track for HCV elimination provide a pathway forward.

Chronic hepatitis C virus infection remains a national and global public health burden and is associated with significant morbidity and mortality. Oral direct-acting antiviral combination regimens have excellent tolerability and efficacy with rates exceeding 90%. Sustained virologic response is associated with significant improvements in clinical outcomes. However, translation of sustained virologic response rates from trials to community settings has been poor with interferon-based regimens. We review and summarize key datasets from major real-world observational cohort studies. We review preliminary data from oral generic direct-acting antiviral formulations. Future real-world studies are needed to further clarify optimal treatment strategies for difficult-to-treat populations.

Humberto C. Gonzalez and Stuart C. Gordon

The cure of chronic hepatitis C infection has a major impact on the morbidity and mortality of infected patients. It is now clear that sustained virologic response improves overall survival and significantly reduces the risk of liver failure, fibrosis progression, need of liver transplantation, and incidence of hepatocellular carcinoma. Moreover, hepatitis C eradication improves a broad range of extrahepatic manifestations, such as dermatologic, neoplastic, cardiovascular, and endocrine, and improves quality of life.

Amit Goel and Rakesh Aggarwal

Hepatitis E virus is a common cause of acute hepatitis and acute liver failure in resource-constrained parts of the world. The disease is particularly severe when the infection occurs during pregnancy. In developed countries, human infections occur primarily through zoonotic transmission from animal reservoirs; however, clinical disease is less frequent than in the developing world. The virus strains prevalent in these areas also cause chronic infection in immunocompromised persons, which, if untreated, can progress to cirrhosis; such infection responds well to oral ribavirin. A safe and highly effective recombinant vaccine is available in China, but is not available elsewhere.

Chalermrat Bunchorntavakul and K. Rajender Reddy

Epstein-Barr virus (EBV) and cytomegalovirus (CMV) infections are common and are associated with a variety of liver manifestations. EBV and CMV infections, in immunocompetent hosts, commonly manifest as acute hepatitis, with severity varying from asymptomatic, self-limited icteric hepatitis to acute liver failure. Atypical manifestations, such as cholestasis, chronic hepatitis, precipitation of acute-on-chronic liver failure, and autoimmune hepatitis, are reported with EBV infection, whereas cholestasis, portal vein thrombosis, and Budd-Chiari syndrome are reported with CMV infection. In the setting of liver transplantation, CMV is the most common infectious complication and carries significant morbidity; EBV is the major cause of post-transplant lymphoproliferative disorders.

Salvatore Petta and Antonio Craxì

Hepatits C virus (HCV) infection has been largely associated with extrahepatic comorbidities such as diseases related to dysregulation of the immune system, neuropsychiatric disorders, and cardiometabolic alterations. These clinical consequences, together with experimental evidence, suggest a potential (in)direct effect of HCV, contributing to the pathogenesis of these diseases. Various studies have reported a positive effect of viral eradication on occurrence and outcomes of extrahepatic diseases. These observations and the availability of safe and effective direct antiviral agents further underline the need to search for virological eradication in all infected individuals independent of the severity of the liver disease.

Pyogenic liver abscesses are classified by the bacteria that have caused the abscess because this guides treatment and can point to the underlying cause. The most common cause is biliary disease. The diagnosis is made by imaging. Treatment is a combination of antibiotics and percutaneous drainage. Amebic liver abscess is caused by extraintestinal spread of Entamoeba histolytica. E histolytica is spread by fecal-oral transmission and typically colonizes the gastrointestinal tract. It is diagnosed based on imaging and the mainstay of treatment is metronidazole. Only about 15% of cases require percutaneous drainage. The prognosis is good, with almost universal recovery.

Hepatosplenic candidiasis and other fungal infections of the liver are uncommon in healthy individuals; however, high index of suspicion is essential in immunocompromised patients with prolonged fever. Parasitic infections are protozoan or helminthic; their distribution and epidemiology are variable among different world regions. Clonorchiasis, opisthorchiasis, fascioliasis, and ascariasis are helminthic infections that commonly involve the biliary systems. Signs and symptoms of cholangitis require prompt management to relieve biliary obstruction; addition of antihelminthic agents is essential. Parasitic infections are mostly transmitted to humans by fecally contaminated food and water. Proper hand and food sanitation measures are essential in preventing disease transmission.

GASTROENTEROLOGY
CLINICS OF NORTH AMERICA

SERIES OF RELATED INTEREST

Gastrointestinal Endoscopy Clinics of North America
(Available at: https://www.giendo.theclinics.com)
Clinics in Liver Disease
(Available at: https://www.liver.theclinics.com)

THE CLINICS ARE AVAILABLE ONLINE!
Access your subscription at:
www.theclinics.com

Foreword

Hepatitis and Other Liver Infections in the New Millennium

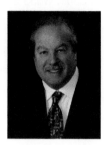

Alan L. Buchman, MD, MSPH
Consulting Editor

Historians may one day be able to explain why one refers to the "heart," or center of a problem or issue, rather than the "liver" of the issue: an equally important organ, albeit infinitely more complex. As with the heart and other organs, the liver is a target for various infectious organisms. Resultant infections in the liver may give rise to the eventual development of cirrhosis, hepatocellular carcinoma, death, or a need for liver transplantation; as such, viral hepatitis has been a major scourge in gastrointestinal illness. In addition, the effects of infectious hepatitis may not be limited to the liver, but may trigger systemic disease manifestations.

Beginning with the identification of the hepatitis C virus prior to the turn of the century, and subsequent screening of blood products, and then later, effective treatments for those afflicted, this scourge has largely been concurred, at least in North America. Although the development of a preventative vaccine has been elusive, disease eradication is no longer a wild dream. Hepatitis B actually followed an earlier and similar course and has become an uncommon disease in the United States, with less than 3000 new cases annually; successful vaccination has played a significant role. There are of course other viruses that still continue to affect the liver, including hepatitis A and E as well as cytomegalovirus, Epstein-Barr virus, and herpes simplex virus. In various parts of the world, fungal and parasitic organisms continue to wreak havoc on local populations, although in places such as Egypt, for example, public health measures have led to a substantial decrease in cases of schistosomiasis.

In this issue of *Gastroenterology Clinics of North America*, Dr Reddy and his team of authors have put together a concise review of infections of the liver and biliary system

Gastroenterol Clin N Am 49 (2020) xiii–xiv
https://doi.org/10.1016/j.gtc.2020.01.014
0889-8553/20/© 2020 Published by Elsevier Inc.

gastro.theclinics.com

wherein they discuss changes in the natural history of these diseases as well as contemporary epidemiology, prevention, and treatment.

Alan L. Buchman, MD, MSPH
Intestinal Rehabilitation and Transplant Center
Department of Surgery/UI Health
University of Illinois at Chicago
840 South Wood Street
Suite 402 (MC958)
Chicago, IL 60612, USA

E-mail address:
buchman@uic.edu

Preface

Infections of the Liver and Biliary System

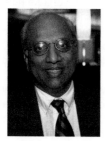

K. Rajender Reddy, MD, FACP, FACG, FRCP, FAASLD
Editor

Infections of the liver and biliary system are not uncommon as most of the infections are viral in nature. Globally, viral hepatitis is a major public health problem, parallels infections such as human immunodeficiency virus (HIV), malaria, and tuberculosis, and is associated with significant morbidity and mortality. More recent data, alarmingly, project the global mortality from hepatitis B and C to exceed that from tuberculosis, HIV, and malaria by 2040. Rapid advances have been made with hepatitis C virus therapy at a time when the focus has shifted toward global elimination, although the progress toward this goal has been slow. Similarly, hepatitis B vaccination has been available for over 3 decades while universal vaccination strategies have been variable across several countries and hepatitis B continues to be a problem. Thus, most countries are not on track to meet the World Health Organization threshold of elimination goals of decreasing new infections by 90% and mortality by 65% by 2030.

This issue of *Gastroenterology Clinics of North America* highlights some of the areas of considerable advances and challenges in viral hepatitis. Several experts and authoritative authors in their respective domains address various unique topics that include global epidemiology of viral hepatitis, hepatitis A, impact of hepatitis B vaccination on hepatocellular carcinoma, future therapies for hepatitis B, and status of delta infection, a challenging infection often overlooked. The readers are also presented an overview on the current status of efforts toward global elimination of hepatitis C and real-world data on the safety and efficacy of directly acting antiviral agents, including generics, in treating hepatitis C. Furthermore, expert authors address comorbidities due to hepatitis C and the impact of therapy on the spectrum of extrahepatic manifestations. Hepatitis E is resurfacing as an infection of significance, particularly in the western world where there is a prevalence of chronic infections. To that end, this issue addresses hepatitis E and its consequences, preventive strategies, and the global differences in this infection, a topic very relevant to our current day practice.

Gastroenterol Clin N Am 49 (2020) xv–xvi
https://doi.org/10.1016/j.gtc.2020.01.015
0889-8553/20/© 2020 Published by Elsevier Inc.

Cytomegalovirus (CMV) and Epstein-Barr virus (EBV) are not uncommon viral infections affecting the liver and have unique manifestations and consequences, and recognition of their importance is a reason for having these infections addressed as well.

While gastroenterologists and hepatologists often readily think of viral hepatitis as the sole cause of hepatic infections, there are other infections due to bacteria, fungi, and parasites that afflict the hepatobiliary system, and this issue endeavors to highlight them in addition. Endemicity of parasitic infections is variable across the world and more often are encountered in resource-constrained areas. These infections present a huge public health challenge and require awareness and expertise in recognition, diagnosis, and treatment of a spectrum of parasitic infections. To that end, there are comprehensive contributions on pyogenic and amebic abscesses, and fungal and parasitic infections of the liver and biliary tree.

In summary, a team of globally recognized investigators and clinicians have been assembled in this issue to address a broad spectrum of clinically relevant topics in viral hepatitis A through E while it also tackles CMV and EBV infections and bacterial, fungal, and parasitic infections of the liver. I hope you enjoy reading and learning from the various contributions, as I certainly have through the process of assembling them.

K. Rajender Reddy, MD, FACP, FACG, FRCP, FAASLD
Division of Gastroenterology
and Hepatology
University of Pennsylvania
2 Dulles, 3400 Spruce Street, HUP
Liver Transplant Office
Philadelphia, PA 19104, USA

E-mail address:
reddyr@pennmedicine.upenn.edu

Global Epidemiology of Viral Hepatitis

Homie Razavi, PhD, MBA

KEYWORDS

- Viral hepatitis • Epidemiology • HCV • HBV • Global • Hepatitis C • Hepatitis B

KEY POINTS

- Viral hepatitis (hepatitis A, B, C, D, and E) is the leading cause of inflammation of liver tissue (hepatitis).
- The disease burden associated with hepatitis A and E occurs shortly after infection, and it is more severe among adults. With hepatitis A and E, the number of incident cases (new acute infections) is important from a public health perspective.
- Long-term hepatitis can cause cirrhosis and hepatocellular carcinoma in patients. The disease burden associated with hepatitis B, C, and D appears 10 to 20 years after infection. Thus, the prevalence of these infections is important from a public health perspective.
- There were an estimated 3.4 (0.5–6.5) million symptomatic hepatitis A cases in 2005, 292 (251–341) million chronic hepatitis B in 2016, 71.1 (62.5–79.4) million chronic hepatitis C in 2015, 23.9 (10.4–27.6) million chronic hepatitis D in 2016, and 69,622 (12,400–132,732) new cases of hepatitis E in 2005.
- The annual deaths associated with viral hepatitis infections are 35,245 for hepatitis A in 2005, 884,000 for hepatitis B in 2015, 400,000 for hepatitis C in 2015, and 69,622 for hepatitis E in 2005.

INTRODUCTION

Hepatitis is defined as the inflammation of the liver tissue. Long-term (chronic) inflammation can lead to scarring of the tissues (fibrosis), irreversible scaring (cirrhosis), and hepatocellular carcinoma (HCC). Inflammation of the liver can be caused by several different factors: alcohol consumption, certain drugs, autoimmune disease, fatty liver disease, and viral infection. The focus of this analysis is viral hepatitis, which is also the leading cause of hepatitis globally. Viral hepatitis can be acute or chronic, and it can be diagnosed using serology tests (antibody) or molecular (presence of viral RNA or DNA) diagnostics. The latter provides a more accurate diagnosis, but it is also more expensive. Thus, most epidemiology studies use serology tests. There are 5 common types of viral hepatitis: A, B, C, D, and E, as summarized in **Table 1**.

Center for Disease Analysis Foundation, 1120 West South Boulder Road, Suite 102, Lafayette, CO 80026, USA
E-mail address: hrazavi@cdafound.org

Gastroenterol Clin N Am 49 (2020) 179–189
https://doi.org/10.1016/j.gtc.2020.01.001
gastro.theclinics.com

Table 1
Summary of common types of viral hepatitis

	Hepatitis A	Hepatitis B	Hepatitis C	Hepatitis D	Hepatitis E
Major sources of transmission	Contaminated food & water, inadequate sanitation, poor personal hygiene, behaviors associated with injection drug use	Mother to child, contact with blood and body fluids, sexual transmission	Contact with blood (injection of drugs, contaminated blood transfusion, sexual practices that lead to blood exposure)	Requires hepatitis B infection; contact with blood and body fluids, sexual transmission	Fecal-oral routes due to contaminated drinking water
Acute infection	✓	✓	✓	✓	✓
Chronic infection		✓	✓	✓	
Vaccine	✓	✓			✓ (China only)
Treatment		✓ (chronic)	✓ (2–3 mo)		

The disease burden and mortality associated with hepatitis A and E occur shortly after infection in the acute stage. There are biomarkers that can indicate if an individual has ever been infected with the hepatitis A or E virus, but there is minimal disease burden after the acute phase. Thus, for the purpose of this review, only annual acute cases are reported. The number of acute infections and the corresponding epidemiology are impacted by outbreaks caused by poor sanitary practices, social factors (poverty and increase in the homeless population), political factors (wars, conflicts), humanitarian emergencies, and vaccination campaigns in the case of hepatitis A.

On the other hand, most of the disease burden and mortality associated with hepatitis B, C, and D infections occur long after the initial infection. There are cases of fulminant hepatitis (acute liver failure) that can develop shortly after the initial infection, and a high rate of mortality is associated with it. However, fulminant hepatitis accounts for significantly fewer deaths as compared with deaths from HCC and cirrhosis, which can develop 10 to 20 years after the initial infections. Because the acute phase of hepatitis B, C, and D is often asymptomatic, it is difficult to estimate the number of new infections. In this review, the author focuses on the number of people with a chronic infection (prevalence) for these infections.

To understand the epidemiology of hepatitis B, C, and D over time, it is important to consider the inflow and outflow of infections that result in a change in the total number of infections over time. For example, the fall of the Soviet Union led to a large increase in injection drug use in former states and a rapid increase in new hepatitis C infections, which resulted in an increase in prevalence in these countries.[1–3] On the other hand, hepatitis B vaccination has resulted in a significant reduction in new infections among the vaccinated cohorts and a reduction of hepatitis B prevalence in countries with a high vaccination rate.[4,5] With both acute and chronic viral hepatitis infections, it is important to consider the year of the estimate because the numbers will change each year. In many cases, multiple studies that seem to contradict one another are actually both correct and are reporting data on a changing epidemiology over time.[6,7]

HEPATITIS A

Hepatitis A is an acute infection that occurs only in the susceptible population: those not vaccinated or infected previously. Historically, the number of new (acute) hepatitis A virus (HAV) infections were very low in high-income countries where there is almost no circulation of the virus despite the high proportion of adults susceptible to infection[8] and low-income countries where poor sanitary conditions resulted in a few susceptible adults (most were already infected as children when the symptoms are considerably less severe). However, the change in demographics is resulting in a new surge of HAV infections: uneven distribution of wealth, large-scale migration, globalization of food, and urbanization/population density. The increased homeless population and drug use in high-income countries have provided low-income settings within high-income countries.[9,10] On the other hand, better sanitation and an increasing middle-income class in low- and middle-income countries has resulted in larger susceptible populations. For example, the 1988 epidemic in Shanghai affected 292,000 people with HAV[11] after consumption of contaminated clams. Because of improved sanitation in the country, the infected population did not already have immunity to HAV as a result of infection at childhood that has minimal symptoms. The annual number of HAV infections and HAV-related deaths are shown in **Table 2**.[12]

Vaccines can prevent hepatitis A infection and provide long-term immunity. The current World Health Organization (WHO) recommendations are as follows: high endemicity countries, vaccination is not recommended; intermediate endemicity countries,

Table 2
Hepatitis A viral infection epidemiology

Year	HAV Acute Infections	HAV-Related Deaths	Death Rate, %
1990	117 million	30,283	0.026
2005	126 million	35,245	0.028

universal childhood vaccination; low endemicity countries, targeted vaccination in high-risk groups.[13]

HEPATITIS B

An estimated 292 (95% uncertainty interval of 251–341) million individuals were infected with chronic hepatitis B virus (HBV), corresponding to a prevalence of 3.9% (3.4%–4.6%) in 2016.[14] There are several indicators of past and present HBV infection and vaccination. Data relating to hepatitis B surface antigen positive (HBsAg) estimates, a good indicator of current infection, are described here. The global distribution of HBV is shown in **Fig. 1**. Only 3.5% of all HBV infections are in high-income countries with the remaining in low- and middle-income countries.[14] HBV infections are concentrated in sub-Saharan Africa and Asia, and the immigrant population from these regions accounts for most of the HBV infections in Northern America and Western Europe. Four countries (China, India, Nigeria, and Indonesia) account for 50% of all HBV infections.[14]

The largest risk factor for chronic HBV infection is perinatal transmission, which can be prevented with a birth and 3-dose vaccination, administration of hepatitis B immunoglobulin (HBIG) to infants, and antiviral treatment of high-viral-load mothers.[15–19] Horizontal transmission (sexual, exposure to contaminated blood, injection drug use) is also a risk factor, but most adults exposed to HBV spontaneously cure the infection.[20] The rates of HBV prophylaxis are shown in **Fig. 2** and .[14] The Gavi Vaccine Alliance provides 3-dose HBV vaccines, as part of the pentavalent vaccine, free of charge to low- and lower middle-income countries. As a result, HBV 3-dose vaccination rates are very high globally, but birth dose vaccination, use of HBIG, and peripartum treatment of infected mothers lag in low- and lower middle-income countries.

As the result of the above interventions, the prevalence of HBV among 5 year olds was 1.4% (1.2%–1.6%), corresponding to 1.8 (1.6–2.2) million infections in 2016 as shown in **Fig. 3**.[14] Three countries (Nigeria, India, and Indonesia), which have low HBV vaccination rates, account for more than 50% of all HBV infections

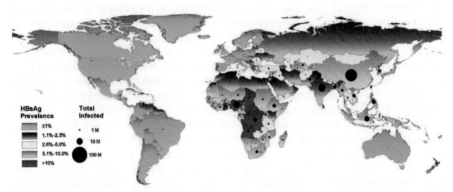

Fig. 1. Global distribution of HBV infection (adults and pediatric) in 2016.

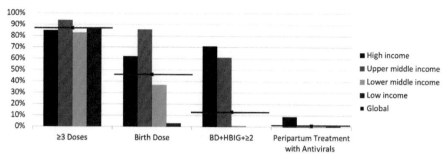

Fig. 2. HBV prophylaxis by country income in 2016.

among 5 year olds.[14] The lower prevalence is a good indicator of how the prophylaxis programs have been successful in reducing new infections in the younger age group.

However, hepatitis B remains the greatest failure of the global public health systems in the late twentieth century and highlights the important role that heuristics play in public health. The disease burden associated with infectious diseases typically follows the infection immediately (eg, HAV, hepatitis E virus [HEV], polio, malaria, small pox). The generally accepted strategy for elimination of infectious diseases and the associated disease burden is vaccination. However, the disease burden associated with HBV follows the infection after 20 years. The large global effort to increase HBV vaccination has been very successful in reducing new HBV infections[4,5] among the vaccinated cohorts, but the impact on disease burden (mortality, cirrhosis, and HCC) has been minimal. In 2015, an estimated 884,000 liver-related deaths were attributed to HBV, corresponding to 1 death every 36 seconds.[21] Current treatments can prevent disease progression, but globally, only 10% of all infections are diagnosed and 5% of the eligible population is treated.[14] To reduce the disease burden associated with HBV, the diagnosis and treatment of those already infected need to increase as outlined in the WHO elimination targets.[22]

HEPATITIS C

In 2015, an estimated 71.1 million (62.5–79.4) people had chronic (viremic) hepatitis C virus (HCV) infections corresponding to 1·0% (0.8%–1.1%).[23] This estimate is a decline from 2013, when an estimated 80.2 (64.4–102.9) million individuals had chronic HCV infections.[24] The decline is mainly due to an aging infected population that is dying of liver-related deaths and non-HCV-related causes as well as a

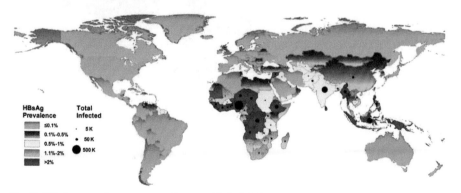

Fig. 3. HBsAg prevalence among 5 year olds in 2016.

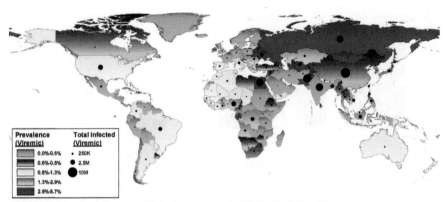

Fig. 4. Global distribution of HCV infection (adults and pediatric) in 2015.

ramp-up in curative therapies. All oral direct-acting antiviral (DAA) therapies with a high sustained viral response (>95%), pan-genotypic, short duration of treatment (8–12 week), and low side effects were launched in 2014 and thereafter. The increased treatment has led to a faster decline of HCV prevalence globally. This decline has been offset by an increasing injection drug use epidemic in Western countries, which has resulted in an increase in new HCV infections.[25–27] Overall, the total number of HCV infections continues to decline. The number of liver-related deaths associated with HCV infection was estimated at 400,000 in 2015.[21]

The global distribution of HCV infection is shown in **Fig. 4**.[23] Six countries (China, Pakistan, India, Egypt, Russia, and United States) accounted for more than 50% of all infections globally. As shown in the figure, although India's prevalence is low, the country's large population results in a large number of infections. On the other hand, the prevalence in Mongolia is high, but the country has a small population. Globally, 81% of all HCV infections were in low- and middle-income countries in 2015.

Historically, therapy response was highly dependent on the patient's genotype. This difference has narrowed with the new pan-genotypic therapies. The global distribution of HCV genotypes by the global burden of disease (GBD) regions is shown in **Fig. 5**.[23]

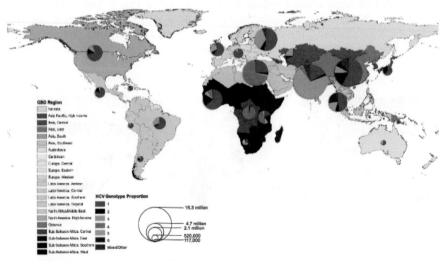

Fig. 5. HCV genotype and total infected by GBD region.

Approximately 44% of all HCV infections were genotype 1, 25% were genotype 3, 15% were genotype 4, with the remaining being genotypes 2, 5, and 6. In high-income countries, 60% of all HCV infections were genotype 1, whereas 36% of all infections in lower middle-income countries were genotype 3, and 45% of all HCV infections in low-income countries were genotype 4.[23]

The annual number of HCV patients initiating treatment has increased since the launch of DAAs (**Fig. 6**). However, as shown in the figure, most of this growth occurred in middle-income countries.[28] In fact, the number of patients initiating treatment in high-income countries has declined since its peak in 2015 because most countries focused on treating patients who were already diagnosed, without a robust screening strategy. In the early stages of HCV infection, liver damage is easier to reverse with treatment; however, HCV is largely asymptomatic, meaning most people are unaware that they should be tested. Without a screening strategy, patients are more likely to develop advanced disease before seeking care.

HEPATITIS D

Hepatitis D virus (HDV) only infects individuals already infected with HBV because it needs the HBV virus for replication. It is thought that HDV transmits from mother to child during delivery as well as through contact with blood and body fluids. Although

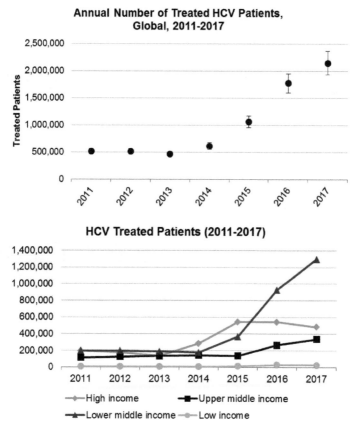

Fig. 6. Annual number of HCV-treated patients.

no good peer-reviewed global estimates are available, according to the Polaris Observatory, an estimated 8.0% (3.3%–10.5%) or 23.9 (10.4–27.6) million HBsAg-positive individuals were coinfected with HDV in 2016.[28] The global distribution of HDV prevalence among those already infected with HBV is shown in **Fig. 7**. HBV vaccination has resulted in a decrease in HBV prevalence and the corresponding reduction in HDV infections. Currently, except for 48 weeks of pegylated interferon, there are no other medications to successfully treat HDV infection, and those infected with HDV have the fastest progression to advanced liver disease and HCC as compared with all other viral hepatitis infections. Currently, the only way to prevent HDV infection is immunization against hepatitis B.

HEPATITIS E

The disease burden associated with HEV infection occurs in the acute phase. HEV virus is principally transmitted via the fecal-oral route or contaminated water, although animals can act as a reservoir for the virus, and transfusion with infected blood can also lead to infection. There are 4 common genotypes (1 through 4)[29,30]:

1. Genotypes 1 and 2 only in humans
2. Genotypes 2, 3, and 4 in humans, pigs, and other species

   Genotypes 1 and 2, which are most common in developing countries, with genotype 1 accounting for most infections. Genotype 3, common in Europe and the United States and typically caused by ingestion of undercooked animal meat (eg, pork liver). The infection typically resolves in 2 to 6 weeks but can cause fulminant hepatitis and death, especially in pregnant women.[31] The virus is excreted starting a few days before to 3 to 4 weeks after the onset of the disease. Similar to HAV infection, children infected with HAV have mild symptoms, whereas adults have much more severe symptoms: mild fever, nausea and vomiting, jaundice, and enlarged liver. Fulminant hepatitis can occur and accounts for nearly all the deaths associated with HEV infection.

   HEV infections are most common in Asia and Africa, where access to clean water and proper sanitation can be limited. Only a fraction of those infected with HEV infection develop any symptoms. The distribution of genotypes 1 and 2 HEV incident infections is shown in **Fig. 8**.[32] In 2005, there were an estimated 20.1 (2.8–37.0) million incident cases of genotypes 1 and 2 HEV globally, 3.4 (0.5–6.5) million symptomatic cases, 69,622 (12,400–132,732) deaths, and 3019 (1892–4424) stillbirths attributed

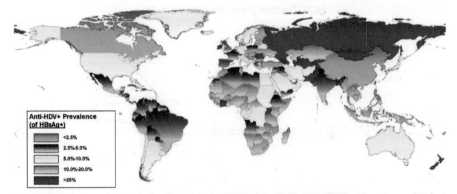

Fig. 7. Prevalence of HDV infection among HBsAg⁺ individuals (2016). (*Courtesy of* Polaris Observatory, Lafayette, CO; with permission.)

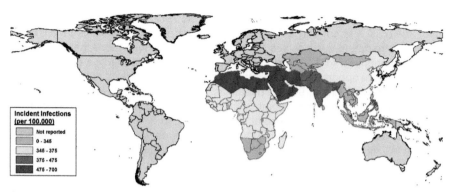

Fig. 8. Genotypes 1 and 2 HEV incident infections per 100,000 in 2005.

to HEV. In 2015, the WHO reported 44,000 deaths associated with HEV infection.[21] HEV is most common in developing countries, where contaminated water is a problem. Thus, these estimates account for most HEV infections. Currently, there is no treatment for HEV, and the only vaccine is available in China.[21]

SUMMARY

A summary of key epidemiology data for viral hepatitis is shown in **Table 3**. In 2015, the 69th World Health Assembly endorsed the global Health Sector strategy, which included the goal of eliminating hepatitis B and C.[33] The WHO followed by recommending global targets for elimination of HCV and HBV.[22] The WHO recommendations included targets for HBV vaccination, increase in harm reduction, screening of blood supply, diagnosing and treatment to achieve a 90% reduction in new infections, and a 65% reduction in liver-related mortality by 2030.

The justification for this strategy is that viral hepatitis is the leading cause of hepatitis globally and accounts for 1.34 million deaths annually.[21] Although the total number of HBV and HCV infections is declining as a result of HBV vaccination, HCV treatment and mortality (aging population) and the burden associated with HBV and HCV will increase as those already infected continue to age and progress to more advanced stages of liver disease.

Additional efforts will be needed to eliminate viral hepatitis. New and updated national strategies are needed to reduce new HAV and HEV infections, and new treatments are needed to reduce HDV disease burden among those already infected. The tools needed to eliminate HAV, HBV, and HCV exist today. There are vaccines for

Table 3 Viral hepatitis epidemiology summary					
	Hepatitis A	**Hepatitis B**	**Hepatitis C**	**Hepatitis D**	**Hepatitis E**
Acute infection	3.4 (0.5–6.5) million symptomatic cases (2005)				20.1 (2.8–37.0) million (2005)
Chronic infection		292 (251–341) million (2016)	71.1 (62.5–79.4) million (2015)	23.9 (10.4–27.6) million (2016)	
Annual deaths	35,245 (2005)	884,000 (2015)	400,000 (2015)	No data	69,622 (12,400–132,732) (2005)

hepatitis HAV and HBV. Vaccination of HBV will also prevent HDV because this virus needs the HBV virus to replicate. Today, there are treatments available for HBV and HCV. HCV treatment can achieve sustained viral response in more than 95% of all treated patients in 8 to 12 weeks, while HBV treatment needs to be taken lifelong. There is a unique opportunity to eliminate the disease burden associated with hepatitis B and C, which account for 96% of deaths associated with viral hepatitis infections.[21] However, national screening programs are needed to supplement the existing treatment strategy in order to find those already infected. In order to eliminate viral hepatitis, better data are also needed. As described here, understanding of viral hepatitis infection is limited by the available data and large uncertainty intervals.

DISCLOSURE

H. Razavi is a member of advisory boards for Gilead, AbbVie, and Merck. All proceeds go to the Center for Disease Analysis Foundation. He is the managing director of the Center for Disease Analysis (CDA) and the Center for Disease Analysis Foundation (CDAF). In the last 3 years, CDA has received research funding from Gilead, AbbVie, Pfizer, Intercept, and Vaccine Impact Modeling Consortium. CDAF has received grants from CDC Foundation, John Martin Foundation, ASTHO, Zeshan Foundation, and Private donors.

REFERENCES

1. Nemecek V, Health NIoP. Annual report of viral hepatitis 2012.
2. Castkova J, Benes C, Nemecek V. Virová hepatitida C v CR 2013.
3. Razavi H, Waked I, Sarrazin C, et al. The present and future disease burden of hepatitis C virus (HCV) infection with today's treatment paradigm. J Viral Hepat 2014;21(Suppl 1):34–59.
4. Cui F, Shen L, Li L, et al. Prevention of chronic hepatitis B after 3 decades of escalating vaccination policy, China. Emerg Infect Dis 2017;23(5):765–72.
5. Liang X, Bi S, Yang W, et al. Reprint of: epidemiological serosurvey of hepatitis B in China–declining HBV prevalence due to hepatitis B vaccination. Vaccine 2013; 31(S9):J21–8.
6. El-Zanaty F, Way A. Egypt demographic and health survey, 2008. Cairo (Egypt): Ministry of Health and Population; 2009. p. 431.
7. Ministry of Health and Population [Egypt], El-Zanaty and Associates [Egypt], and ICF International. 2015. Egypt Health Issues Survey 2015. Cairo, Egypt and Rockville, Maryland, USA: Ministry of Health and Population and ICF International.
8. Jacobsen KH, Wiersma ST. Hepatitis A virus seroprevalence by age and world region, 1990 and 2005. Vaccine 2010;28(41):6653–7.
9. Foster M, Ramachandran S, Myatt K, et al. Hepatitis A virus outbreaks associated with drug use and homelessness–California, Kentucky, Michigan, and Utah, 2017. MMWR Morb Mortal Wkly Rep 2018;67(43):1208–10.
10. Peak CM, Stous SS, Healy JM, et al. Homelessness and hepatitis A--San Diego County, 2016-2018. Clin Infect Dis 2019. [Epub ahead of print].
11. Halliday ML, Kang LY, Zhou TK, et al. An epidemic of hepatitis A attributable to the ingestion of raw clams in Shanghai, China. J Infect Dis 1991;164(5):852–9.
12. WHO. Evidence based recommendations for use of hepatitis A vaccines in immunization services: background paper for SAGE discussions: World Health Organization. 2011. Available at: https://www.who.int/immunization/sage/1_HepABackground_17Oct_final2_nov11.pdf. Accessed July 18, 2012.

13. Hepatitis A Vaccines. Releve epidemiologique hebdomadaire/Section d'hygiene du Secretariat de la Societe des Nations = Weekly epidemiological record/Health Section of the Secretariat of the League of Nations. 2000;75(5):38–44.
14. Razavi-Shearer D, Gamkrelidze I, Nguyen MH, et al. Global prevalence, treatment, and prevention of hepatitis B virus infection in 2016: a modelling study. Lancet Gastroenterol Hepatol 2018;3(6):383–403.
15. Poovorawan Y, Sanpavat S, Pongpunlert W, et al. Protective efficacy of a recombinant DNA hepatitis B vaccine in neonates of HBe antigen-positive mothers. JAMA 1989;261(22):3278–81.
16. Kang G, Ma F, Chen H, et al. Efficacy of antigen dosage on the hepatitis B vaccine response in infants born to hepatitis B-uninfected and hepatitis B-infected mothers. Vaccine 2015;33(33):4093–9.
17. Andre FE, Zuckerman AJ. Review: protective efficacy of hepatitis B vaccines in neonates. J Med Virol 1994;44(2):144–51.
18. Kubo A, Shlager L, Marks AR, et al. Prevention of vertical transmission of hepatitis B: an observational study. Ann Intern Med 2014;160(12):828–35.
19. Pan CQ, Duan Z, Dai E, et al. Tenofovir to prevent hepatitis B transmission in mothers with high viral load. N Engl J Med 2016;374(24):2324–34.
20. Edmunds WJ, Medley GF, Nokes DJ, et al. The influence of age on the development of the hepatitis B carrier state. Proc Biol Sci 1993;253(1337):197–201.
21. WHO. Global hepatitis report, 2017. Geneva (Switzerland): World Health Organization; 2017.
22. WHO. Combating Hepatitis B and C to reach elimination by 2030. Geneva (Switzerland): WHO; 2016.
23. Blach S, Zeuzem S, Manns M, et al. Global prevalence and genotype distribution of hepatitis C virus infection in 2015: a modelling study. Lancet Gastroenterol Hepatol 2016;2(3):161–76.
24. Gower E, Estes C, Blach S, et al. Global epidemiology and genotype distribution of the hepatitis C virus infection. J Hepatol 2014;61(1S):S45–57.
25. Dillon JF, Lazarus JV, Razavi HA. Urgent action to fight hepatitis C in people who inject drugs in Europe. Hepatology 2016;1:2.
26. Martin NK, Vickerman P, Hickman M. Mathematical modelling of hepatitis C treatment for injecting drug users. J Theor Biol 2011;274(1):58–66.
27. Friedland G. Infectious disease comorbidities adversely affecting substance users with HIV: hepatitis C and tuberculosis. J Acquir Immune Defic Syndr 2010;55(Suppl 1):S37–42.
28. Polaris observatory: CDA Foundation. 2017. Available at: www.polaris observatory.com. Accessed November 25, 2016.
29. Faramawi MF, Johnson E, Chen S, et al. The incidence of hepatitis E virus infection in the general population of the USA. Epidemiol Infect 2011;139(8):1145–50.
30. Shouval D. Focus. What is the significance of hepatitis E as a public health threat in the industrialized countries? Hepatitis E virus infection in Italy. J Hepatol 2011; 54(1):1–2.
31. Patra S, Kumar A, Trivedi SS, et al. Maternal and fetal outcomes in pregnant women with acute hepatitis E virus infection. Ann Saudi Med 2007;147(1):28–33.
32. Rein DB, Stevens GA, Theaker J, et al. The global burden of hepatitis E virus genotypes 1 and 2 in 2005. Hepatology 2012;55(4):988–97.
33. World Health Organization. Global health sector strategy on viral hepatitis, 2016–2021 towards ending viral hepatitis. World Health Organization; 2016.

Hepatitis A

Epidemiology, Natural History, Unusual Clinical Manifestations, and Prevention

Ameer Abutaleb, MD[a,b], Shyam Kottilil, MBBS, PhD[a],*

KEYWORDS

- Hepatitis A virus • Hepatitis A vaccine • Acute liver failure • Hepatitis A outbreak
- Hepatitis A prevention

KEY POINTS

- Hepatitis A occurs around the world and causes an acute hepatitis, which is typically subclinical.
- Clinical illness is not common in endemic areas because of early childhood exposures, but poses a large risk to travelers from nonendemic areas.
- Diagnosis of hepatitis A typically requires serologic testing.
- Jaundice, anorexia, right upper quadrant pain, and elevated alanine aminotransferase levels are classically described in acute hepatitis A.
- Hepatitis A is preventable through vaccination.

INTRODUCTION

Early studies in viral hepatitis noted 2 distinct patterns of infection, suggesting the involvement of multiple hepatitis viruses.[1] For several years, these 2 patterns of infection were dubbed "infectious hepatitis" for clinically apparent infection and "serum hepatitis" for clinically inapparent infection. After discovery of the Australia antigen, serum hepatitis was renamed hepatitis B, and infectious hepatitis was renamed hepatitis A.[2] The hepatitis A virus (HAV) was characterized in 1973 by Feinstone and colleagues.[3] It is transmitted by a fecal-oral route, causing a self-limited infectious hepatitis, but can also cause large epidemics through person-to-person contact.[4] HAV is a positive-sense RNA virus in the *Herpavirus* genus of the Picornaviridae family, with 4 genotypes characterized in humans. It is a nonenveloped small (27 nm) particle in an icosahedral shape.

---

[a] Division of Clinical Care and Research, Institute of Human Virology, University of Maryland, 725 West Lombard Street Suite, Baltimore, MD 21201, USA; [b] Division of Gastroenterology & Hepatology, Department of Medicine, University of Maryland, 22 South Greene Street, N3W156, Baltimore, MD 21201, USA
* Corresponding author.
E-mail address: skottilil@ihv.umaryland.edu

Gastroenterol Clin N Am 49 (2020) 191–199
https://doi.org/10.1016/j.gtc.2020.01.002
0889-8553/20/© 2020 Elsevier Inc. All rights reserved.

Most HAV infections that occur in developing countries are not clinically apparent and cause no symptoms, likely because of partial immunity in endemic areas. In contrast, infections in developed countries often are characterized by jaundice and an acute hepatitis, especially in adolescents and adults. HAV cannot cause chronic infection, unlike hepatitis B and C.[4] Diagnostic testing for HAV is readily available as is a commercial HAV vaccine[5] (**Table 1**).

EPIDEMIOLOGY

HAV infections are seen around the globe, with greater prevalence in developing countries and low-income regions.[6] HAV is hyperendemic in sub-Saharan Africa and South Asia, with nearly no at-risk adults because of the frequency of early childhood exposure. Intermediate endemicity is seen in Latin America, the Middle East, North Africa, Eastern Europe, and middle-income regions in Asia.[7] Countries with stronger economies, such as the United States and countries in Western Europe, have lower rates of HAV infection, but the susceptibility of their nonimmune adult population becoming ill from HAV is much higher than the lower-income countries.[8,9] There is a paradoxic effect with regards to HAV in countries that are demonstrating upward mobility in their economy. The first HAV exposure in their citizens occurs later in life when compared with lower-income countries, ultimately posing a difficult public health problem in their HAV epidemiologic transition.[10]

HAV is transmitted feco-orally between people in close contact with each other.[11] Transmission commonly occurs from children to their parents, one of the reasons that daycare centers are often implicated in HAV spread.[12] HAV from food and water contamination often involves a food service worker who did not appropriately wash hands and sanitize after defecation.[13] Fresh produce can be a culprit in spreading HAV infection, because the virus is difficult to wash off surfaces of fruits and vegetables.[14] Contaminated water, whether by inadequate chlorination or by poor irrigation infrastructure, leads to both contained and epidemic infections.[15] Transient viremia after initial acquisition is responsible for rarely seen parenteral transmission.[16] Risk factors in developed countries include men having sex with men (MSM), travel to an endemic

Table 1 Hepatitis A in a nutshell	
Epidemiology	Estimated 1.4 million cases per year globally Infections can be sporadic or epidemic
Transmission	Fecal-oral via 　Person-to-person contact 　Consumption of contaminated food or water
Diagnosis	Presence of IgM antibodies to HAV
Treatment	Supportive
Classical presentation	Children 　Asymptomatic Adults 　Jaundice, hyperbilirubinemia, RUQ pain, anorexia
Unusual presentations	Relapsing hepatitis Prolonged cholestasis Acute liver failure
Prevention	HAV vaccine
Postexposure prophylaxis	HAV vaccine HAV immune globulin

Abbreviation: RUQ, right upper quadrant.

country, and intravenous drug use.[17–19] Developed countries remain with locales where HAV is endemic, as seen in Native American tribes in the western United States.[20]

HAV outbreaks occur and commonly are associated with poor sanitary conditions. Outbreaks are often related to water contamination and inadequate sewage disposal in both developing and developed countries.[21] Outbreaks in higher-income nations are often linked to a source of contaminated food or water.[22] Shellfish are associated with HAV transmission because of their water filtration effect, which effectively concentrates the virus, and have been the cause of prior large epidemics.[23]

A recent HAV outbreak that reached international attention was the San Diego outbreak, with 590 confirmed cases between November 22, 2016 and June 21, 2018 of genotype 1b HAV in San Diego, California. Most cases were either boys or men, and major risk factors included homelessness, injection drug use, and MSM. Approximately 17% of cases were hepatitis C virus coinfected, and 5% of cases were hepatitis B virus (HBV) coinfected. The San Diego outbreak, and more recently, an outbreak in Michigan highlight that the epidemiology of HAV outbreaks may be shifting from contaminated food and water to poor sanitation revolving around homelessness, overcrowding, and injection drug use.[9] The same pattern is being seen in the now ongoing Kentucky outbreak, with more than four thousand infections and 43 deaths.[24] The outbreak is largely spread by patients using drugs and without stable housing, as was the case in San Diego. Challenges in hepatitis A vaccination in rural Kentucky and limited funding and resources to acquire vaccine were thought to be the major reasons this outbreak is now the largest and deadliest in the United States.[25]

NATURAL HISTORY

After a nonimmune subject acquires HAV, the virus is taken up through the enterohepatic circulation and enters the liver, where it replicates.[26,27] HAV has been shown to be able to infect enteric cells in culture,[28] but there seems to be no evidence of significant replication in the gut. Virions can be detected in stool and blood before onset of symptoms. Several days later, serum transaminases rise. Prodromal symptoms occur about a month following exposure and can consist of fever, malaise, nausea, vomiting, and anorexia. Prodromal symptoms are common in adult infections but not as much in children.[4] Adult infections will typically also be characterized by jaundice, diarrhea, and hyperbilirubinemia, peaking 7 to 10 days after the onset of jaundice. Jaundice will typically resolve much faster than the malaise and anorexia, which can last for months. Pediatric infections will often be asymptomatic or have very few symptoms.[29]

UNUSUAL CLINICAL MANIFESTATIONS

Acute liver failure from HAV is rare, occurring in about 1 in every 300 cases, and very infrequently results in death or the need for liver transplantation.[30] A relapsing hepatitis is infrequently seen in adult infections with recurrent symptoms typically occurring within 6 months of prior infection. Relapsing hepatitis is characterized by shedding of HAV in the stool and elevated transaminases. Occasionally, the elevation in transaminases will be asymptomatic.[31] Hepatitis A–associated prolonged cholestasis has also been reported after infection, for periods up to 1 year.[32,33] Extrahepatic manifestations previously reported include rash, kidney injury, myocarditis, and Guillain-Barre syndrome.[34]

DIAGNOSIS

Diagnosis of HAV infection is typically confirmed by serologic evidence of a recent infection, that is, detection of immunoglobulin M (IgM) antibodies against HAV. Concordance between assays is high, but there is about a 10% reported rate of discrepancy.[35] IgM antibodies typically peak about a month after exposure and can persist for up to a year. False negative results can be seen in early infection, while the patient is viremic and interval antibody retesting should be considered.[26,36] False positive results have been reported in a variety of scenarios, including patients with rheumatoid factor or other autoimmune disease.[37] IgM antibodies to HAV can be detected in the setting of recent HAV immunization or recent HAV vaccine boosting.[38,39] IgG response typically follows IgM response after 1 week, typically persists for life, and confers neutralizing activity to future HAV exposures. Durability of IgG response may be limited in immunosuppression, as previously demonstrated in human immunodeficiency virus (HIV) -infected persons with an absence of detectable HAV antibodies several years after vaccination[40] (**Fig. 1**).

Serum detection of HAV RNA can be technically done but rarely used in diagnosis of acute hepatitis A infection. Hepatitis A viremia is detectable in serum of immunocompetent hosts within a few days of infection and persists for 3 to 4 weeks.[41] Immunosuppressed patients may have persistent hepatitis A viremia beyond 4 weeks.[42] HAV RNA has also been detected in stool and saliva of infected hosts, but at much lower concentrations than serum.[43] RNA can be detected by real-time polymerase chain reaction (PCR) or nested PCR methods. Molecular characteristics of HAV, although not important in diagnosis, have been used in epidemiologic studies and can assist in phylogenetic analysis of early outbreaks and epidemics.[35]

TREATMENT

The treatment of acute hepatitis A is supportive.[44] Liver failure from hepatitis A is rare, but is estimated to occur in less than 5% of cases.[45] Immediate referral to a transplant center is critical for cases of HAV-associated fulminant liver failure.

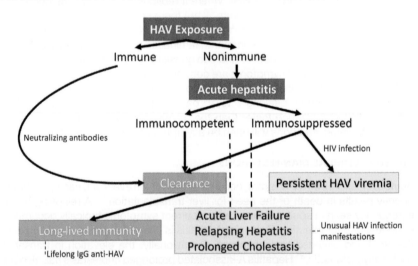

Fig. 1. Effects of HAV exposure in immunocompetent and immunosuppressed patients. Patients immunized against HAV before exposure can clear the virus via preformed neutralizing antibodies. Nonimmune patients who are immunocompetent typically clear the virus after the infectious hepatitis, whereas immunosuppressed patients may sustain a chronic viremia. In rare cases, both immunocompetent and immunosuppressed hosts may manifest an unusual presentation of HAV, including but not limited to liver failure, relapsing hepatitis, and prolonged cholestasis.

Therapeutics has been previously investigated for cases of HAV-associated liver failure. ALF-5755, a C-type lectin, was administered to 10 subjects with HAV-associated liver failure. There was no evidence of improvement in transplant-free survival rate.[46] N-acetylcysteine, although shown to be very effective for acetaminophen-induced liver failure, does not seem to confer any benefit for HAV-associated acute liver failure.[47]

Interferon (IFN) as a treatment of acute hepatitis A infection has been previously evaluated and shown to be effective in cell cultures.[48] Case reports of IFN treatment of acute hepatitis A are limited, and its utility is unclear.[49] Direct-acting antivirals have been evaluated in cell culture systems and shown to have potential effectiveness in inhibiting HAV replication and in antiviral activity.[50–52] Drug development and clinical trials are limited by difficulty in enrolling subjects before they resolve their infection to measure potential outcomes of intervention.

PREVENTION

Sanitation measures play an important role in HAV infection prevention, including but not limited to careful attention to hygiene, particularly in the food service industry.[53] Food service workers who are ill with jaundice of unclear cause should be restricted from work. Hospitalized patients with HAV should be on enteric precautions for 1 week after the onset of jaundice, when viral shedding in the stool is at its highest.[54]

Prevention of HAV by vaccine is the standard approach across much of the world, and many countries have adopted universal vaccination against HAV in their children[55] (Table 2). HAV vaccine is also a mainstay of postexposure prophylaxis.[56] The United States offers 2 commercially available hepatitis A vaccines and 1 combination HAV-HBV vaccine.[57] The HAV vaccine is typically administered in 2 doses, 6 months apart, whereas the HAV-HBV vaccine usually requires 3 doses.[58] Live-attenuated HAV vaccines are used in China with good success.[59]

The efficacy of both live-attenuated and inactivated vaccines has been well established in large trials across the globe collectively encompassing nearly 750,000 patients.[60] Both vaccines confer a protective effect against hepatitis A when given before exposure. Immunogenicity of the 2 HAV vaccines in the United States, when compared head to head, was equal.[61] An antibody titer greater than or equal to 20 mIU/mL is thought to be protective.[62] Lower protection rates following vaccination are observed in immunosuppressed persons, including HIV infection, inflammatory bowel disease, and organ transplant recipients.[63]

Nonvaccinated persons traveling to HAV endemic regions should have a single dose of vaccine before their departure.[64] Persons with chronic liver disease, the elderly, and the immunocompromised should receive both vaccine and immunoglobulin at 0.02 mL/kg at

Table 2			
Vaccine preparations in the United States and populations that are recommended to receive HAV vaccine			
Vaccine Name	**Protects Against**	**Dosing Schedule**	**Relevant Populations**
Havrix	HAV	Two doses 6 mo apart	Children 1–2 y old
Vaqta	HAV	Two doses 6 mo apart	Travel to endemic area
Twinrix	HAV, HBV	Three doses at 0, 1, and 6 mo	MSM
			PWID
			Chronic liver disease
			Health care workers

Abbreviation: PWID, people who inject drugs.

a separate injection site.[56,65] Postexposure prophylaxis for HAV is best achieved with either HAV vaccine or immunoglobulin, and both seem to be equally effective.[66,67]

SUMMARY

HAV continues to be a global health issue, with the highest rates in lower-income countries. Infections are typically linked with contaminated food or water and almost always tied to poor sanitary conditions. Treatment is supportive, and there are no drug therapies available for acute hepatitis A infection. Vaccination is the most effective form of prevention and is also used in postexposure prophylaxis. Universal vaccination for HAV in children should be adopted whenever possible and has been shown to reduce HAV burden around the globe.

DISCLOSURE

The authors have nothing to disclose.

REFERENCES

1. Krugman S, Ward R, Giles JP, et al. Infectious hepatitis: detection of virus during the incubation period and in clinically inapparent infection. N Engl J Med 1959; 261:729–34.
2. Blumberg BS, Gerstley BJ, Hungerford DA, et al. A serum antigen (Australia antigen) in Down's syndrome, leukemia, and hepatitis. Ann Intern Med 1967;66(5): 924–31.
3. Feinstone SM, Kapikian AZ, Purceli RH. Hepatitis A: detection by immune electron microscopy of a viruslike antigen associated with acute illness. Science 1973;182(4116):1026–8.
4. Martin A, Lemon SM. Hepatitis A virus: from discovery to vaccines. Hepatology 2006;43(2 Suppl 1):S164–72.
5. Innis BL, Snitbhan R, Kunasol P, et al. Protection against hepatitis A by an inactivated vaccine. JAMA 1994;271(17):1328–34.
6. Jacobsen KH. Globalization and the changing epidemiology of hepatitis A virus. Cold Spring Harb Perspect Med 2018;8(10). https://doi.org/10.1101/cshperspect. a031716.
7. Jacobsen KH, Wiersma ST. Hepatitis A virus seroprevalence by age and world region, 1990 and 2005. Vaccine 2010;28(41):6653–7.
8. Havelaar AH, Kirk MD, Torgerson PR, et al. World Health Organization global estimates and regional comparisons of the burden of foodborne disease in 2010. PLoS Med 2015;12(12):e1001923.
9. Wooten DA. Forgotten but not gone: learning from the hepatitis A outbreak and public health response in San Diego. Top Antivir Med 2019;26(4):117–21.
10. Zakaria S, Fouad R, Shaker O, et al. Changing patterns of acute viral hepatitis at a major urban referral center in Egypt. Clin Infect Dis 2007;44(4):e30–6.
11. Lemon SM. Type A viral hepatitis. New developments in an old disease. N Engl J Med 1985;313(17):1059–67.
12. Klevens RM, Miller JT, Iqbal K, et al. The evolving epidemiology of hepatitis A in the United States: incidence and molecular epidemiology from population-based surveillance, 2005-2007. Arch Intern Med 2010;170(20):1811–8.
13. Schwarz NG, Revillion M, Roque-Afonso AM, et al. A food-borne outbreak of hepatitis A virus (HAV) infection in a secondary school in Upper Normandy, France, in November 2006. Euro Surveill 2008;13(22). pii=18885.

14. Croci L, De Medici D, Scalfaro C, et al. The survival of hepatitis A virus in fresh produce. Int J Food Microbiol 2002;73(1):29–34.
15. Ahmad T, Adnan F, Nadeem M, et al. Assessment of the risk for human health of enterovirus and hepatitis A virus in clinical and water sources from three metropolitan cities of Pakistan. Ann Agric Environ Med 2018;25(4):708–13.
16. Hettmann A, Juhasz G, Dencs A, et al. Phylogenetic analysis of a transfusion-transmitted hepatitis A outbreak. Virus Genes 2017;53(1):15–20.
17. Tanaka S, Kishi T, Ishihara A, et al. Outbreak of hepatitis A linked to European outbreaks among men who have sex with men in Osaka, Japan, from March to July 2018. Hepatol Res 2019;49(6):705–10.
18. Aasheim ET, Seymour M, Balogun K, et al. Acute hepatitis A in an elderly patient after care worker travel to high endemicity country. Hum Vaccin Immunother 2013;9(11):2480–2.
19. Foster M, Ramachandran S, Myatt K, et al. Hepatitis A virus outbreaks associated with drug use and homelessness–California, Kentucky, Michigan, and Utah, 2017. MMWR Morb Mortal Wkly Rep 2018;67(43):1208–10.
20. Cheek JE, Hennessy TW, Redd JT, et al. Epidemic assistance from the Centers for Disease Control and Prevention involving American Indians and Alaska Natives, 1946-2005. Am J Epidemiol 2011;174(11 Suppl):S89–96.
21. Bizri AR, Fares J, Musharrafieh U. Infectious diseases in the era of refugees: hepatitis A outbreak in Lebanon. Avicenna J Med 2018;8(4):147–52.
22. Purpari G, Macaluso G, Di Bella S, et al. Molecular characterization of human enteric viruses in food, water samples, and surface swabs in Sicily. Int J Infect Dis 2019;80:66–72.
23. Xu ZY, Li ZH, Wang JX, et al. Ecology and prevention of a shellfish-associated hepatitis A epidemic in Shanghai, China. Vaccine 1992;10(Suppl 1):S67–8.
24. Kentucky's Hepatitis A outbreak surpasses 3,000 cases. 2018. Available at: https://www.wlky.com/article/kentuckys-hepatitis-a-outbreak-surpasses-3000-cases/25592667. Accessed March 8, 2019.
25. Kentucky's 'too low and too slow' response to nation's worst hepatitis A outbreak. 2019. Available at: https://www.courier-journal.com/story/news/investigations/2019/02/21/kentucky-hepatitis-response-too-slow-deadly-outbreak-worst-in-united-states/2453874002/. Accessed March 8, 2019.
26. Lemon SM, Walker CM. Hepatitis A virus and hepatitis E virus: emerging and re-emerging enterically transmitted hepatitis viruses. Cold Spring Harb Perspect Med 2018;9(6):a031823.
27. Walker CM. Adaptive immune responses in hepatitis A virus and hepatitis E virus infections. Cold Spring Harb Perspect Med 2018;9(9):a033472.
28. Mathiesen LR, Moller AM, Purcell RH, et al. Hepatitis A virus in the liver and intestine of marmosets after oral inoculation. Infect Immun 1980;28(1):45–8.
29. Shin EC, Jeong SH. Natural history, clinical manifestations, and pathogenesis of hepatitis A. Cold Spring Harb Perspect Med 2018;8(9). https://doi.org/10.1101/cshperspect.a031708.
30. Kim JD, Cho EJ, Ahn C, et al. A model to predict 1-month risk of transplant or death in hepatitis a-related acute liver failure. Hepatology 2019;70(2):621–9.
31. Cuthbert JA. Hepatitis A: old and new. Clin Microbiol Rev 2001;14(1):38–58.
32. Schiff ER. Atypical clinical manifestations of hepatitis A. Vaccine 1992;10(Suppl 1):S18–20.
33. Munoz-Martinez SG, Diaz-Hernandez HA, Suarez-Flores D, et al. Atypical manifestations of hepatitis A virus infection. Rev Gastroenterol Mex 2018;83(2):134–43.

34. Allen O, Edhi A, Hafeez A, et al. A very rare complication of hepatitis A infection: acute myocarditis–a case report with literature review. Case Rep Med 2018;2018: 3625139.

35. Park SH, Kim EJ, Lee JH, et al. Molecular characterization of hepatitis A virus isolated from acute gastroenteritis patients in the Seoul region of Korea. Eur J Clin Microbiol Infect Dis 2009;28(10):1177–82.

36. Lee HK, Kim KA, Lee JS, et al. Window period of anti-hepatitis A virus immunoglobulin M antibodies in diagnosing acute hepatitis A. Eur J Gastroenterol Hepatol 2013;25(6):665–8.

37. Tennant E, Post JJ. Production of false-positive immunoglobulin M antibodies to hepatitis A virus in autoimmune events. J Infect Dis 2016;213(2):324–5.

38. Fayol V, Ville G. Evaluation of automated enzyme immunoassays for several markers for hepatitis A and B using the Abbott IMx analyser. Eur J Clin Chem Clin Biochem 1991;29(1):67–70.

39. Castrodale L, Fiore A, Schmidt T. Detection of immunoglobulin M antibody to hepatitis A virus in Alaska residents without other evidence of hepatitis. Clin Infect Dis 2005;41(9):e86–8.

40. Crum-Cianflone NF, Wilkins K, Lee AW, et al. Long-term durability of immune responses after hepatitis A vaccination among HIV-infected adults. J Infect Dis 2011;203(12):1815–23.

41. Hughes JA, Fontaine MJ, Gonzalez CL, et al. Case report of a transfusion-associated hepatitis A infection. Transfusion 2014;54(9):2202–6.

42. Lin KY, Chen GJ, Lee YL, et al. Hepatitis A virus infection and hepatitis A vaccination in human immunodeficiency virus-positive patients: a review. World J Gastroenterol 2017;23(20):3589–606.

43. Joshi MS, Bhalla S, Kalrao VR, et al. Exploring the concurrent presence of hepatitis A virus genome in serum, stool, saliva, and urine samples of hepatitis A patients. Diagn Microbiol Infect Dis 2014;78(4):379–82.

44. Chalmers TC, Eckhardt RD, Reynolds WE, et al. The treatment of acute infectious hepatitis. Controlled studies of the effects of diet, rest, and physical reconditioning on the acute course of the disease and on the incidence of relapses and residual abnormalities. J Clin Invest 1955;34(7, Part II):1163–235.

45. Lee WM, Squires RH Jr, Nyberg SL, et al. Acute liver failure: summary of a workshop. Hepatology 2008;47(4):1401–15.

46. Nalpas B, Ichai P, Jamot L, et al. A proof of concept, phase II randomized European trial, on the efficacy of ALF-5755, a novel extracellular matrix-targeted antioxidant in patients with acute liver diseases. PLoS One 2016; 11(3):e0150733.

47. Gunduz H, Karabay O, Tamer A, et al. N-acetyl cysteine therapy in acute viral hepatitis. World J Gastroenterol 2003;9(12):2698–700.

48. Crance JM, Leveque F, Chousterman S, et al. Antiviral activity of recombinant interferon-alpha on hepatitis A virus replication in human liver cells. Antiviral Res 1995;28(1):69–80.

49. Yoshiba M, Inoue K, Sekiyama K. Interferon for hepatitis A. Lancet 1994; 343(8892):288–9.

50. Morris TS, Frormann S, Shechosky S, et al. In vitro and ex vivo inhibition of hepatitis A virus 3C proteinase by a peptidyl monofluoromethyl ketone. Bioorg Med Chem 1997;5(5):797–807.

51. Blaum BS, Wunsche W, Benie AJ, et al. Functional binding of hexanucleotides to 3C protease of hepatitis A virus. Nucleic Acids Res 2012;40(7):3042–55.

52. Jiang X, Kanda T, Nakamoto S, et al. The JAK2 inhibitor AZD1480 inhibits hepatitis A virus replication in Huh7 cells. Biochem Biophys Res Commun 2015;458(4): 908–12.
53. Trujillo-Ochoa JL, Viera-Segura O, Fierro NA. Challenges in management of hepatitis A virus epidemiological transition in Mexico. Ann Hepatol 2018;18(1):14–22.
54. Koenig KL, Shastry S, Burns MJ. Hepatitis A virus: essential knowledge and a novel identify-isolate-inform tool for frontline healthcare providers. West J Emerg Med 2017;18(6):1000–7.
55. Souto FJD, de Brito WI, Fontes CJF. Impact of the single-dose universal mass vaccination strategy against hepatitis A in Brazil. Vaccine 2019;37(6):771–5.
56. Nelson NP, Link-Gelles R, Hofmeister MG, et al. Update: recommendations of the advisory committee on immunization practices for use of hepatitis A vaccine for postexposure prophylaxis and for preexposure prophylaxis for international travel. MMWR Morb Mortal Wkly Rep 2018;67(43):1216–20.
57. O'Leary ST, Kimberlin DW. Update from the advisory committee on immunization practices. J Pediatric Infect Dis Soc 2018;7(3):181–7.
58. Beran J, Kervyn D, Wertzova V, et al. Comparison of long-term (10 years) immunogenicity of two- and three-dose regimens of a combined hepatitis A and B vaccine in adolescents. Vaccine 2010;28(37):5993–7.
59. World Health Organization. Global advisory committee on vaccine safety, 16-17 June 2010. Geneva, Switzerland: World Health Organization; 2010. Report No.: 85.
60. Irving GJ, Holden J, Yang R, et al. Hepatitis A immunisation in persons not previously exposed to hepatitis A. Cochrane Database Syst Rev 2012;(7):CD009051.
61. Braconier JH, Wennerholm S, Norrby SR. Comparative immunogenicity and tolerance of Vaqta and Havrix. Vaccine 1999;17(17):2181–4.
62. Lemon SM, Binn LN. Serum neutralizing antibody response to hepatitis A virus. J Infect Dis 1983;148(6):1033–9.
63. Garcia Garrido HM, Wieten RW, Grobusch MP, et al. Response to hepatitis A vaccination in immunocompromised travelers. J Infect Dis 2015;212(3):378–85.
64. Hepatitis A questions and answers for health professionals. 2018. Available at: http://www.cdc.gov/hepatitis/hav/havfaq.htm#c2. Accessed March 8, 2019.
65. Vento S, Garofano T, Renzini C, et al. Fulminant hepatitis associated with hepatitis A virus superinfection in patients with chronic hepatitis C. N Engl J Med 1998; 338(5):286–90.
66. Victor JC, Monto AS, Surdina TY, et al. Hepatitis A vaccine versus immune globulin for postexposure prophylaxis. N Engl J Med 2007;357(17):1685–94.
67. Betz TG. Hepatitis A vaccine versus immune globulin for postexposure prophylaxis. N Engl J Med 2008;358(5):531 [author reply: 532].

Hepatitis B

Immunization and Impact on Natural History and Cancer Incidence

Chih-Lin Lin, MD[a,b], Jia-Horng Kao, MD, PhD[c,d,e,f,*]

KEYWORDS

- Hepatitis B virus • Hepatitis B vaccination • Hepatocellular carcinoma

KEY POINTS

- Currently, 187 countries have in place infant hepatitis B vaccination programs.
- The hepatitis B vaccination coverage rate among infants has reached 75% worldwide.
- The timely implementation of hepatitis B virus (HBV) vaccination at birth is still a major issue in low-coverage areas, such as Africa, Southeast Asia, and Western Pacific Regions.
- The prevalence of hepatitis B surface antigen has decreased to less than 1% in children after successful implementation of universal HBV vaccination in newborns.
- The incidence of primary liver cancer in children, adolescents and young adults has drastically decreased to near zero in birth cohorts receiving hepatitis B vaccination.

INTRODUCTION

As a global health problem, there are more than 2 billion people infected with hepatitis B virus (HBV) worldwide. It is estimated that as many as 257 million of them have chronic HBV infection, and approximately 15% to 40% will die of HBV-related liver disease and its consequences.[1,2] The disease spectrum of chronic HBV infection includes inactive carrier state, chronic hepatitis, liver cirrhosis, and hepatocellular

Grant/Funding Support: This work was supported by grants from the National Taiwan University Hospital, the Ministry of Health and Welfare, and the Ministry of Science and Technology, Executive Yuan, Taiwan.

[a] Department of Gastroenterology, Renai Branch, Taipei City Hospital, No. 10, Sec. 4, Renai Rd, Taipei 10629, Taiwan; [b] Department of Psychology, National Chengchi University, Taipei, Taiwan; [c] Graduate Institute of Clinical Medicine, National Taiwan University College of Medicine, National Taiwan University, 1 Chang-Te Street, Taipei 10002, Taiwan; [d] Department of Internal Medicine, National Taiwan University Hospital, Taipei, Taiwan; [e] Hepatitis Research Center, National Taiwan University, National Taiwan University Hospital, Taipei, Taiwan; [f] Department of Medical Research, National Taiwan University, National Taiwan University Hospital, Taipei, Taiwan
* Corresponding author. Graduate Institute of Clinical Medicine, National Taiwan University College of Medicine, 1 Chang-Te Street, Taipei 10002, Taiwan.
E-mail address: kaojh@ntu.edu.tw

Gastroenterol Clin N Am 49 (2020) 201–214
https://doi.org/10.1016/j.gtc.2020.01.010

carcinoma (HCC). Recent advances in antiviral therapy have achieved the treatment goals of preventing disease progression and reducing HCC risk in patients with chronic HBV infection.[3] However, elimination of HBV is still a challenging task and only a small proportion of patients can have a functional cure.[4,5] Most patients require long-term or even lifelong treatment. Thus, enhancing host immunity through vaccination to prevent susceptible individuals from acute HBV infection remains the mainstay of global HBV control. In this review, the impact of HBV immunization on the global epidemiology of HBV and clinical outcomes, especially the incidence of HBV-related HCC, is summarized and discussed.

HEPATITIS B VIRUS VIROLOGY AND NATURAL HISTORY OF HEPATITIS B

HBV is a partially double-stranded circular DNA virus. HBV encodes 4 overlapping genes: S gene for the surface protein (HBsAg), C gene for the core protein (HBcAg), P gene for the DNA polymerase, and X gene for protein as a transcriptional transactivator.[6] Because of evolutionary changes in nucleotide sequences, several point mutations and deletions or insertions are observed in the HBV genome. The long-term evolution of HBV has been linked to the development of various genotypes, sub-genotypes, recombinants, and even quasispecies.[7]

In the natural history of HBV infection, the most common risk factor for developing chronic hepatitis B (CHB) infection is the age at which infection occurs. More than 90% of HBV-infected infants born to highly viremic carrier mothers will become chronic carriers. On the contrary, only 5% to 10% of healthy adults who are exposed to HBV progress to chronic infection. Patients with chronic HBV infection in endemic areas usually would have acquired HBV perinatally or in early childhood, leading to a high risk of chronicity.[8] The long-term outcomes of CHB vary widely. In treatment-naïve patients with CHB, the annual incidence of cirrhosis has been estimated to be 2% to 10%.[8] The annual incidence of HCC in cirrhotic patients exceeds 2%, whereas it is less than 1% for non-cirrhotic carriers.[9,10] We now recognize that in the era of antiviral therapy, through immune enhancement by pegylated interferon-α or long-term viral suppression by nucleos(t)ide analogues, liver disease progression from chronic hepatitis to cirrhosis and eventually HCC is preventable. Several meta-analyses have reported that interferon-based therapy reduces the risk of cirrhosis, cirrhotic complications, and HCC incidence in patients with CHB.[11–13] Long-term nucleos(t)ide analogue therapy also results in the improvement of biochemical, serologic, and histologic outcomes.[14] In particular, the yearly HCC incidence rate is significantly reduced in patients receiving nucleos(t)ide analogues with high potency and low drug resistance (such as entecavir and tenofovir disoproxil fumarate).[15–17]

Hepatitis B viral factors predictive of clinical outcomes have been identified in earlier cohort studies.[18] Among them, serum HBV DNA level is the strongest predictor of adverse outcomes in adults with chronic HBV infection. The risk of cirrhosis and HCC were increased significantly as the HBV-DNA level increased.[19,20] In parallel with HBV DNA levels, serum HBsAg levels were positively associated with HCC development in a dose-response relationship, especially in patients with low viral load (HBV DNA level <2000 IU/mL).[21] A recent study noted that hepatitis B core-related antigen (HBcrAg) may stratify HCC risk in patients with CHB with intermediate viral load (HBV DNA level of 2000–20,000 IU/mL).[22] In addition to quantitative viral factors, HBV genotypes C and D, basal core promoter mutant, and pre-S deletion mutant are qualitative viral factors associated with an increased risk of cirrhosis and HCC.[23] Integration of risk of hepatitis B viral factors for HCC are recommended to be considered in current HBV treatment guidelines to implement individualized management of CHB.[24]

HEPATITIS B VIRUS VACCINATION

The first hepatitis B vaccine, a plasma-derived vaccine, has been licensed and approved for the prevention of HBV infection since 1981. This vaccine was composed of harvesting antigen from the plasma of people with chronic HBV infection. The vaccine contains no live virus and is safe even for people with reduced immune function. Because of the safety concerns in using human serum with potential contamination risk, recombinant yeast-derived or mammalian-cell–derived vaccines were developed in 1986. Most yeast-produced vaccines prepared by inserting an HBV S gene into yeast cell, contain only the major HBsAg protein. However, mammalian-cell–derived vaccines containing the pre-S1, pre-S2 proteins and the major HBsAg protein may induce a faster and higher anti-HBs response.[25] Considering that maternal or vertical transmission during the perinatal period and horizontal transmission in early life are the major transmission routes,[8] hepatitis B vaccination, in infancy and early childhood, is the most cost-effective strategy for the prevention of HBV infection. The World Health Organization (WHO) thus recommended, in 1997, that hepatitis B vaccine be incorporated into routine infant and childhood Expanded Programs on Immunization.[26] Currently, 187 countries have introduced infant HBV vaccination programs.[27] Although a variety of hepatitis B vaccine schedules have been proposed, WHO recommends the administration of hepatitis B vaccines in 3 doses to infants. The schedules are first dose at birth, with the second dose given 1 month after the first dose. Finally, the third dose is to be administered 1 to 12 months later. By 2010, the hepatitis B vaccination coverage rate among infants had reached an estimate of 75% worldwide.[28] Hepatitis B immune globulin (HBIG) contains high concentrations of anti-HBs. HBIG provides protection against acute and chronic HBV infection when administered soon after HBV exposure. For the prevention of perinatal HBV transmission, WHO recommends HBIG as an additional agent to hepatitis B vaccine within 24 hours of birth.[29] However, due to the feasibility and cost issue, additional HBIG is recommended only for infants born to hepatitis B e-antigen (HBeAg)-positive carrier mothers.[30]

In addition to vertical transmission, it is well known that horizontal transmission is not unusual in HBV hyperendemic areas. Therefore, WHO recommends that persons at risk of HBV infection also receive hepatitis B vaccination. High-risk individuals include the following (**Box 1**)[29,31,32]:

1. Blood and/or blood products recipients
2. Hemodialysis or peritoneal dialysis patients
3. Recipients of solid organ transplantations
4. Persons with chronic disease (chronic hepatitis C, fatty liver disease, alcoholic liver disease, autoimmune hepatitis, human immunodeficiency virus infection, diabetes mellitus)
5. Persons detained in prisons
6. Injection-drug users
7. Sexual exposure to HBsAg-positive persons (heterosexual and men who have sex with men)
8. Health care workers
9. Unvaccinated travelers before leaving for endemic areas

Because postvaccination seroprotection is not achieved in all infants who received complete passive-active immunoprophylaxis, postvaccination serologic testing for HBsAg and anti-HBs in infants of age 9 to 12 months is recommended by the Centers for Disease Control and Prevention of the United States.[33] If HBsAg-negative infants

---

Box 1
Persons recommended to receive hepatitis B vaccination

All infants

Unvaccinated children

Persons at risk for horizontal infection
   Blood and/or blood products recipients
   Recipients of solid organ transplantations
   Sex partners of hepatitis B surface antigen (HBsAg)-positive persons
   Persons with more than one sex partner
   Men who have sex with men
   Persons at risk for infection by percutaneous or mucosal exposure to blood
   Injection-drug users
   Residents and staff of facilities for developmentally disabled persons
   Health care and public safety personnel with risk for exposure to blood or blood-
   contaminated body fluids
   Hemodialysis or peritoneal dialysis patients
   International travelers to high or intermediate levels of endemic area with hepatitis B virus
   infection (HBsAg prevalence of $\geq$2%)
   Persons with hepatitis C virus infection
   Persons with chronic liver disease
   Persons with human immunodeficiency virus infection
   Persons detained in prisons
   All other persons seeking protection from hepatitis B virus infection

From Sarah Schillie, Claudia Vellozzi, Arthur Reingold, et al. Prevention of Hepatitis B Virus Infection in the United States: Recommendations of the Advisory Committee on Immunization Practices. MMWR Recommendations and Reports 2018;67;1-31; with permission.

---

have anti-HBs less than 10 mIU/mL, revaccination with a single dose of hepatitis B vaccine is advised with postvaccination serologic testing 1 to 2 months later. If persistently low level of anti-HBs (<10 mIU/mL) is encountered, 2 additional doses of hepatitis B vaccine are suggested to complete the second vaccine series.[32]

THE DURATION OF POSTVACCINATION SEROPROTECTION

The duration of postvaccination seroprotection in infants is largely unknown. Although protective anti-HBs antibody levels ($\geq$10 mIU/mL) develop in 96% of infants at 6 months after 3 doses of vaccination,[34] the concentration of anti-HBs gradually declines after 1 year, with even loss of anti-HBs in teenagers. The earlier study in Taiwan showed that inadequate concentration of anti-HBs was found in nearly two-thirds of 15-year-old children who received complete primary neonatal immunization.[35] In particular, 33% of children who were born to HBeAg-positive mothers had anti-HBc seroconversion.[35] An observational cohort study of Alaska Native adults also revealed that only 51% of vaccine responders still had an anti-HBs level $\geq$10 mIU/mL at 30 years after receiving primary HBV vaccine series. Among vaccinees with low or undetectable anti-HBs levels, 88% responded to a booster dose.[36] A recent systematic review showed that the seroprotection rates were 96.4% at 1 year, 83.3% at 5 years and then decreased gradually to 75% at 20 years after a complete vaccination course.[37] Therefore, it is imperative to determine the risk of HBV breakthrough infection in vaccinated individuals and whether a booster vaccination is required.[38] In a recent meta-analysis, including 9356 individuals who received primary hepatitis B vaccination, the incidence of HBV breakthrough infection at 5 to 20 years after primary vaccination was quite low (0.7%).[39] In addition, most newly HBV-infected individuals developed only transient HBV viremia with subclinical hepatitis. A strong and rapid anamnestic response of anti-HBs antibody was also observed after HBV infection.[40] This anamnestic effect of protective immunity also can be triggered by booster vaccination. After booster vaccination, most vaccinees developed protective levels of anti-HBs within 1 month.[41,42] These observations indicated that individuals receiving primary vaccination could maintain the ability to generate protective immunity on subsequent exposure to HBV or booster vaccination. Thus, postvaccination breakthrough HBV infection is rare, and a booster dose should not be universally administered for immunocompetent individuals.[43]

THE OBSTACLES TO INCREASE HEPATITIS B VIRUS VACCINE COVERAGE RATE

Although 187 countries have introduced infant HBV vaccination programs since 1997, the global hepatitis B vaccination coverage rate among infants has been only approximately 75%.[28] Several challenges exist to in enhancing hepatitis B vaccine coverage rate worldwide. First, WHO reported that 3% of the countries in the whole world did not incorporate HBV vaccine as a part of nationwide infant vaccination program by the end of 2018.[27] Second, because perinatal transmission is the main route of chronic HBV infections, the first dose of HBV vaccine with or without HBIG within 24 hours of delivery is recommended; otherwise, the protective efficacy will decrease.[44] Furthermore, delaying the first vaccine dose to after 6 hours of birth may not decrease the risk of occult HBV infection of newborns.[45] Unfortunately though, only 105 countries introduced the first dose of HBV vaccine within 24 hours after delivery. Thus, timely vaccination is essential for the prevention of perinatal infection. Third, WHO reported that millions of newborns were still unvaccinated in the countries where universal HBV vaccination has been implemented.[46] A global analysis revealed that noninstitutional delivery (such as home-birth) was significantly correlated with hepatitis B vaccine coverage rate in African, Southeast Asian, and Western Pacific regions.[47] Therefore, promoting and increasing institutional deliveries is an important strategy to increase HBV vaccine coverage rate.

THE CHANGING HEPATITIS B VIRUS EPIDEMIOLOGY AFTER HEPATITIS B VIRUS VACCINATION

HBV infection is one of the more common viral infections worldwide. The prevalence of HBsAg ranges from 2% to 20%. In high endemic areas, such as Asia and Africa, the prevalence of HBsAg is more than 8%.[8] Universal hepatitis B vaccination in newborns is the most cost-effective way to reduce the global burden of chronic HBV infections. Hepatitis B vaccine induces a protective concentration of anti-HBs in approximately 90% to 95% of vaccinees after the 3-dose schedule has been completed. Taiwan is hyperendemic for HBV infection, and 40% of HBV carriers have been estimated to have been born to HBsAg-positive mothers. Moreover, 85% to 95% of newborns with HBV exposure evolved to chronic HBV infection.[48] After the successful implementation of nationwide universal hepatitis B vaccination program in 1984,[49] 97% of vaccination coverage rate was reached in 2004. The HBV infection rate (the prevalence of anti-HBc positivity) dramatically decreased from 38.0% to 4.6% in children. The prevalence rate of HBsAg also markedly decreased from 10.9% in children who were born before the implementation of vaccination program to 0.5% in children who were born after the implementation of the program.[50] Similarly, the tremendous impact of universal hepatitis B immunization on the change of HBsAg prevalence in children was also observed in other countries.[51] Compared with the high prevalence of HBsAg in adults, the prevalence of HBsAg among children decreased to 1.0% in

China,[52] 0.12% in South Korea,[53] 0.6% in Iran,[54] 0.5% in Colombia,[55] 0.6% in Italy,[56] 0.3% in Saudi Arabia,[57] and 0.3% in Canada[58] after the launch of universal hepatitis B immunization.

The implementation of universal hepatitis B immunization also reduced the incidence of acute fulminant hepatitis in infants. The nationwide studies from Taiwan showed that the mortality associated with fulminant hepatitis in newborns was markedly decreased after the launch of universal immunization program.[59,60]

VACCINE FAILURE

Despite effective HBV vaccines being available for more than 3 decades, there are still a portion of vaccinated individuals who fail to produce protective anti-HBs. Several reasons may lead to vaccine failure (**Box 2**). This problem still remains a challenge in the universal vaccination era. Maternal HBeAg positivity, as well as high viral load with incomplete passive-active immunization strategy, results in vaccine failure and may increase the risk of mother-to-child transmission (MTCT) of HBV.[60] HBIG administration is important for newborns of HBeAg-positive mothers. However, delay or failure of HBIG administration at birth has led to a high incidence of HBV infection.[48] Ideally, HBIG should be given within 12 hours after birth for infants born to HBeAg-positive mothers. The second challenge is with HBsAg-positive mothers with a high viral load. According to a prospective study, including 303 HBsAg-positive mother-infant pairs in Taiwan, maternal high viral load was an independent factor associated with risk of MTCT of HBV.[61] Antiviral therapy is thus complementary to HBV vaccination in preventing MTCT of HBV. Previous studies showed that HBV-infected mothers with high viral load receiving antiviral prophylaxis with tenofovir disoproxil fumarate in the third trimester of pregnancy had a significantly lower rate of infant HBsAg positivity than those highly viremic HBV-infected mothers who did not receive antiviral prophylaxis.[62,63]

Several reports have indicated that premature or low birth weight infants were risk factors associated with an inadequate immune response to on-time hepatitis B vaccine.[64–66] Therefore, the American Academy of Pediatrics and Centers for Disease

---

Box 2
Factors associated with hepatitis B vaccine failure

Hepatitis B viral factors for failure in infants
    Maternal hepatitis B e-antigen positivity[a]
    Maternal high hepatitis B viral load[a]
    Vaccine escape mutant (such exposure may not be protected by vaccination in infants and adults)

Host factors for failure in infants and adults
    Preterm or low birth weight infants[a]
    Alcoholism[b]
    End-stage renal disease[b]
    Status of immune suppression[b]
    Diabetes mellitus[b]
    Drug abuse[b]
    Genetic variants (HLA loci)[b]

Inappropriate passive-active immunization[a]

  [a] Infants.
  [b],Adults.

Control and Prevention advisory panel recommended delaying the initiation of hepatitis B vaccination in premature infants until they reach 2 kg weight to improve the immunogenicity.[67]

The universal hepatitis B vaccination, targeting at the major HBsAg protein, has increased the incidence of HBV S-gene mutants that may cause vaccine failure. Most of these mutations occur in and around the "a" determinant of the S gene, such as G145R, T126S, P120S, and P127S.[68,69] These mutations may cause infection in previously immunized (anti-HBs–positive) or naïve (anti-HBs–negative) individuals.[70] The molecular epidemiology of vaccine escape mutants remains largely unknown. In Taiwan, the prevalence of vaccine escape mutants in HBV DNA-positive children significantly increased from 7.8% in 1984 (before implementation of universal hepatitis B immunization) to 28.1% in 1994 (10 years after implementation of universal hepatitis B immunization in Taiwan).[71] Another prospective study, in Taiwan, showed that the well-immunized children born to mothers with genotype C infection had higher risk of HBV breakthrough infection than those children born to mothers with genotype B infection.[72] Further, a long-term follow-up study demonstrated that immunized children with vaccine escape mutant infection developed earlier HBeAg seroconversion and reached low viral load status than children with wild-type HBV infection.[73] In addition, vaccine escape mutants were detected in a small number of children with HCC development.[73] Another recent study from South America revealed that the emergence of vaccine escape mutants was closely associated with HBV genotype D infection.[74] For the detection of vaccine escape mutant or occult HBV infection, long-term surveillance is required.

Most of the children or adults receiving the complete series of hepatitis B vaccination acquire protective anti-HBs responses; however, 5% to 10% of vaccinees fail to produce protective anti-HBs concentration. The factors associated with vaccine failure include old age, alcoholism, end-stage renal disease, status of immune suppression, diabetes mellitus, drug abuse, and human immunodeficiency virus infection.[75] Host genetic variants of human leukocyte antigen (HLA) loci, including HLA-DP, HLA-DQ, HLA-DR, were also associated with nonresponse or low response to hepatitis B vaccine.[76]

PREVENTION OF HEPATITIS B VIRUS–RELATED HEPATOCELLULAR CARCINOMA

The causal relationship between chronic HBV infection and the development of HCC has been well established.[3] Preventive strategies of HBV infection can reduce the incidence of HCC as well as affect the contribution to morbidity and mortality from HCC, a malignancy with extremely poor prognosis. Through avoiding susceptible individuals from contracting HBV infection, neonatal immunization with hepatitis B vaccine is the most effective strategy of primary prevention of HBV-related HCC.[8] After 3 decades of hepatitis B vaccination, the incidence of primary liver cancer in children has been reduced in several countries.[51] One of the most successful stories is Taiwan, a hyperendemic area for HBV infection.[18] The nationwide universal hepatitis B vaccination program was launched in 1984 (**Table 1**). Before the 1980s, most newborns who were born to HBsAg-positive mothers became HBV carriers.[48] The annual incidence of liver cancer was 0.92 per 100,000 in children. After the implementation of universal hepatitis B vaccination program, the incidence of HCC dramatically decreased to 0.23 per 100,000 in the vaccinated children.[77] A population-based cancer registry in Taiwan also revealed that annual incidence had decreased (16.6%) in children but slightly increased (1.3%) in the adult population during 2003 to 2011. Of particular note, the incidence rate of primary liver cancer in children has decreased to zero since

Table 1
The achievements of the universal hepatitis B immunization program in Taiwan

| Achievements | Universal Hepatitis B Immunization Since 1984 | | Reference |
	Before 1984	After 1984~2019	
Vaccination coverage rate	0	97% in 2004	Ni et al,[50] 2007
The prevalence rate of HBsAg in children	10.9%	0.5%	Ni et al,[50] 2007
The prevalence rate of anti-HBc in children	38%	4.6%	Ni et al,[50] 2007
Mortality associated with fulminant hepatitis	0.733 per 100,000 person-years	0.174 per 100,000 person-years	Chien et al,[60] 2014
Incidence of HCC in children	0.92 per 100,000 person-years	0.23 per 100,000 person-years	Chang et al,[77] 2016

Abbreviations: HBc, hepatitis B core; HBsAg, hepatitis B surface antigen; HCC, hepatocellular carcinoma.

2011.[78] Nevertheless, incomplete HBV immunization at birth was recognized as the strongest risk predictor of HCC, with a hazard ratio of 2.52, in infancy to early adulthood.[60]

The impact of the hepatitis B vaccine on the incidence of HCC in children has also been confirmed in other countries. In a population-based, randomized, controlled trial in China, the HBV-vaccinated cohort had a significantly lower HCC incidence rate compared with the unvaccinated cohort with a hazard ratio of 0.16.[79] South Korea also gained great health benefit through the national immunization program against HBV since 1995. Compared with a period before the initiation of a national immunization program (1991–1994), the relative risk of liver cancer mortality in adolescents significantly reduced to 70% after implementation of national immunization program (2003–2006).[80] In Alaska, where the immunization program was implemented in 1984, the incidence of HCC in children (<20 years) decreased from 3 per 100,000 in 1984 to 1988, to zero in 1995 to 1999 and HCC has been eliminated in children since 1999.[81]

These lines of solid evidence from Taiwan and other countries indicate that neonatal hepatitis B vaccination significantly reduces HCC incidence in children, adolescents, and young adults. Nowadays, hepatitis B vaccine is considered as an anticancer vaccine by primarily preventing HBV-related HCC. Indeed, hepatitis B vaccine is the first "anticancer" vaccine in the human history.[51]

PERSPECTIVE

In 2016, World Health Assembly declared to combat viral hepatitis and eliminate HBV and hepatitis C virus (HCV) by 2030. Through the International Viral Hepatitis Elimination Meeting, the strategies of HBV and HCV prevention and elimination were proposed to reach these goals.[82] The introduction of direct-acting antiviral (DAA) agents in 2013 makes HCV elimination a realistic expectation; however, several challenges exist in the progress of HBV elimination. First, because of the lack of financial support, certain countries did not incorporate HBV vaccine as part of a nationwide infant vaccination program. Second, the timely HBV vaccination at birth is still a major

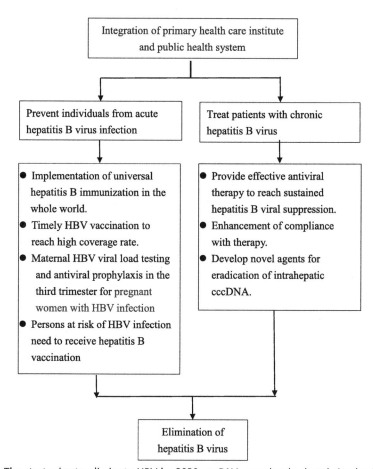

Fig. 1. The strategies to eliminate HBV by 2030. cccDNA, covalently closed circular DNA.

issue in low-coverage areas, such as Africa, Southeast Asia, and Western Pacific regions. Third, HBV viral load testing and antiviral prophylaxis in the third trimester of pregnancy to prevent MTCT in expectant mothers with HBV infection should be promoted. Fourth, the prevention strategy for HBV horizontal transmission is not satisfactory. It is important to raise the awareness in persons at risk of contracting HBV infection. In addition, hepatitis B vaccination for high-risk individuals should be implemented. Last but not least, compared with DAA agents for cure of HCV, HBV has been left behind in achieving curative therapies. Although effective anti-HBV therapy could maintain profound viral suppression, eradication of intrahepatic covalently closed circular DNA remains the holy grail for HBV cure.

SUMMARY

After the implementation of HBV vaccine into neonatal immunization programs, persistent HBV infection and HBV-related liver disease in children has dramatically declined over the past 3 decades. The successful experiences from several countries reveal that HBV-related HCC in children is almost eradicated after the introduction of hepatitis B vaccination in infants. To achieve the global goals of WHO to eliminate HBV by 2030, higher coverage rates of neonatal HBV vaccination, and better strategies against horizontal transmission, are urgently awaited to prevent new infections. Early antiviral therapy for patients with chronic HBV infection will reduce HBV reservoirs. The final challenge is in the development of new treatment strategies to cure HBV. Most importantly, a national HBV elimination program should be integrated into primary health care and public health systems and be proactively pursued across the world (**Fig. 1**).

DECLARATION OF INTEREST

All authors have no conflict of interest.

REFERENCES

1. Ott JJ, Stevens GA, Groeger J, et al. Global epidemiology of hepatitis B virus infection: new estimates of age-specific HBsAg seroprevalence and endemicity. Vaccine 2012;30:2212–9.
2. Thomas DL. Global elimination of chronic hepatitis. N Engl J Med 2019;380: 2041–50.
3. Lin CL, Kao JH. Review article: the prevention of hepatitis B-related hepatocellular carcinoma. Aliment Pharmacol Ther 2018;48:5–14.
4. Lin CL, Kao JH. Review article: novel therapies for hepatitis B virus cure - advances and perspectives. Aliment Pharmacol Ther 2016;44:213–22.
5. Revill PA, Chisari FV, Block JM, et al. Members of the ICE-HBV Working Groups; ICE-HBV Stakeholders Group Chairs; ICE-HBV Senior Advisors, Zoulim F. A global scientific strategy to cure hepatitis B. Lancet Gastroenterol Hepatol 2019;4:545–58.
6. Lau JY, Wright TL. Molecular virology and pathogenesis of hepatitis B. Lancet 1993;342:1335–40.
7. Kao JH, Chen DS. HBV genotypes: epidemiology and implications regarding natural history. Curr Hepat Rep 2006;5:5–13.
8. Kao JH, Chen DS. Global control of hepatitis B virus infection. Lancet Infect Dis 2002;2:395–403.
9. Fattovich G, Stroffolini T, Zagni I, et al. Hepatocellular carcinoma in cirrhosis: incidence and risk factors. Gastroenterology 2004;127:S35–50.
10. Kao JH. Hepatitis B virus genotypes and hepatocellular carcinoma in Taiwan. Intervirology 2003;46:400–7.
11. Miyake Y, Kobashi H, Yamamoto K. Meta-analysis: the effect of interferon on development of hepatocellular carcinoma in patients with chronic hepatitis B virus infection. J Gastroenterol 2009;44:470–5.
12. Yang YF, Zhao W, Zhong YD, et al. Interferon therapy in chronic hepatitis B reduces progression to cirrhosis and hepatocellular carcinoma: a meta-analysis. J Viral Hepat 2009;16:265–71.
13. Wong GL, Yiu KK, Wong VW, et al. Meta-analysis: reduction in hepatic events following interferon-alfa therapy of chronic hepatitis B. Aliment Pharmacol Ther 2010;32:1059–68.
14. Su TH, Kao JH. Improving clinical outcomes of chronic hepatitis B virus infection. Expert Rev Gastroenterol Hepatol 2015;9:141–54.
15. Wu CY, Lin JT, Ho HJ, et al. Association of nucleos(t)ide analogue therapy with reduced risk of hepatocellular carcinoma in patients with chronic hepatitis B: a nationwide cohort study. Gastroenterology 2014;147:143–51.

16. Su TH, Hu TH, Chen CY, et al, C-TEAM study group and the Taiwan Liver Diseases Consortium. Four-year entecavir therapy reduces hepatocellular carcinoma, cirrhotic events and mortality in chronic hepatitis B patients. Liver Int 2016;36:1755–64.

17. Papatheodoridis GV, Idilman R, Dalekos GN, et al. The risk of hepatocellular carcinoma decreases after the first 5 years of entecavir or tenofovir in Caucasians with chronic hepatitis B. Hepatology 2017;66:1444–53.

18. Lin CL, Kao JH. Perspectives and control of hepatitis B virus infection in Taiwan. J Formos Med Assoc 2015;114:901–9.

19. Iloeje UH, Yang HI, Su J, et al. Predicting liver cirrhosis risk based on the level of circulating hepatitis B viral load. Gastroenterology 2006;130:678–86.

20. Chen CJ, Yang HI, Su J, et al. REVEAL-HBV Study Group. Risk of hepatocellular carcinoma across a biological gradient of serum hepatitis B virus DNA level. JAMA 2006;295:65–73.

21. Tseng TC, Liu CJ, Yang HC, et al. High levels of hepatitis B surface antigen increase risk of hepatocellular carcinoma in patients with low HBV load. Gastroenterology 2012;142:1140–9.

22. Tseng TC, Liu CJ, Hsu CY, et al. High level of hepatitis B core-related antigen increases risks of hepatocellular carcinoma in chronic hepatitis B patients with intermediate viral load. Gastroenterology 2019;157:1518–29.

23. Lin CL, Kao JH. Natural history of acute and chronic hepatitis B: The role of HBV genotypes and mutants. Best Pract Res Clin Gastroenterol 2017;31:249–55.

24. Lin CL, Kao JH. Risk stratification for hepatitis B virus related hepatocellular carcinoma. J Gastroenterol Hepatol 2013;28:10–7.

25. Shouval D. Hepatitis B vaccines. J Hepatol 2003;39(suppl 1):S70–6.

26. McGregor A. WHO: world health assembly. Lancet 1992;339(8804):1287.

27. Available at: https://www.who.int/news-room/fact-sheets/detail/immunization-coverage. Accessed June 17, 2019.

28. Centers for Disease Control and Prevention (CDC). Global routine vaccination coverage, 2010. MMWR Morb Mortal Wkly Rep 2011;60:1520–2.

29. WHO position paper on hepatitis B vaccines - October 2009. Wkly Epidemiol Rec 2009;84:405–20.

30. Ni YH, Chang MH, Wu JF, et al. Minimization of hepatitis B infection by a 25-year universal vaccination program. J Hepatol 2012;57:730–5.

31. Chang MH, Chen DS. Prevention of hepatitis B. Cold Spring Harb Perspect Med 2015;5:a021493.

32. Schillie S, Vellozzi C, Arthur R, et al. Prevention of hepatitis B virus infection in the United States: recommendations of the Advisory Committee on Immunization Practices. MMWR Recomm Rep 2018;67:1–31.

33. Schillie S, Murphy TV, Fenlon N, et al. Update: Shortened interval for postvaccination serologic testing of infants born to hepatitis B-infected mothers. MMWR Morb Mortal Wkly Rep 2015;64:1118–20.

34. Hwang LY, Beasley RP, Stevens CE, et al. Immunogenicity of HBV vaccine in healthy Chinese children. Vaccine 1983;1:10–2.

35. Lu CY, Chiang BL, Chi WK, et al. Waning immunity to plasma-derived hepatitis B vaccine and the need for boosters 15 years after neonatal vaccination. Hepatology 2004;40:1415–20.

36. Bruce MG, Bruden D, Hurlburt D, et al. Antibody levels and protection after hepatitis B vaccine: results of a 30-year follow-up study and response to a booster dose. J Infect Dis 2016;214:16–22.

37. van den Ende C, Marano C, van Ahee A, et al. The immunogenicity of GSK's re-combinant hepatitis B vaccine in children: a systematic review of 30 years of experience. Expert Rev Vaccines 2017;16:789–809.

38. Su TH, Chen PJ. Emerging hepatitis B virus infection in vaccinated populations: a rising concern? Emerg Microbes Infect 2012;1:e27.

39. Poorolajal J, Mahmoodi M, Majdzadeh R, et al. Long-term protection provided by hepatitis B vaccine and need for booster dose: a meta-analysis. Vaccine 2010; 28:623–31.

40. Stramer SL, Wend U, Candotti D, et al. Nucleic acid testing to detect HBV infection in blood donors. N Engl J Med 2011;364:236–47.

41. Jan CF, Huang KC, Chien YC, et al. Determination of immune memory to hepatitis B vaccination through early booster response in college students. Hepatology 2010;51:1547–54.

42. Wang ZZ, Gao YH, Lu W, et al. Long-term persistence in protection and response to a hepatitis B vaccine booster among adolescents immunized in infancy in the western region of China. Hum Vaccin Immunother 2016;13:909–15.

43. Zhao H, Zhou YH. Revaccination against hepatitis B in late teenagers who received vaccination during infancy: yes or no? Hum Vaccin Immunother 2017; 14:456–63.

44. Marion SA, Tomm Pastore M, Pi DW, et al. Long-term follow-up of hepatitis B vaccine in infants of carrier mothers. Am J Epidemiol 1994;140:734–46.

45. Lu Y, Liu YL, Nie JJ, et al. Occult HBV infection in immunized neonates born to HBsAg-positive mothers: a prospective and follow-up study. PLoS One 2016; 11:e0166317.

46. World Health Organization. Global routine vaccination coverage, 2014. Wkly Epidemiol Rec 2015;46:617–32.

47. Allison RD, Patel MK, Tohme RA. Hepatitis B vaccine birth dose coverage correlates worldwide with rates of institutional deliveries and skilled attendance at birth. Vaccine 2017;35:4094–8.

48. Stevens CE, Toy P, Kamili S, et al. Eradicating hepatitis B virus: the critical role of preventing perinatal transmission. Biologicals 2017;50:3–19.

49. Chen DS, Hsu NHM, Sung JL, et al. A mass vaccination program in Taiwan against hepatitis B virus infection in infants of hepatitis B surface antigen-carrier mothers. JAMA 1987;257:2597–603.

50. Ni YH, Huang LM, Chang MH, et al. Two decades of universal hepatitis B vaccination in Taiwan: impact and implication for future strategies. Gastroenterology 2007;132:1287–93.

51. Kao JH. Hepatitis B vaccination and prevention of hepatocellular carcinoma. Best Pract Res Clin Gastroenterol 2015;29:907–17.

52. Luo Z, Li L, Ruan B. Impact of the implementation of a vaccination strategy on hepatitis B virus infections in China over a 20-year period. Int J Infect Dis 2012;16:e82–8.

53. Park NH, Chung YH, Lee HS. Impacts of vaccination on hepatitis B viral infections in Korea over a 25-year period. Intervirology 2010;53:20–8.

54. Mohaghegh Shelmani H, Karayiannis P, Ashtari S, et al. Demographic changes of hepatitis B virus infection in Iran for the last two decades. Gastroenterol Hepatol Bed Bench 2017;10(Suppl1):S38–43.

55. Garcia D, Porras A, Rico Mendoza A, et al. Hepatitis B infection control in Colombian Amazon after 15 years of hepatitis B vaccination. Effectiveness of birth dose and current prevalence. Vaccine 2018;36:2721–6.

56. Stroffolini T, Guadagnino V, Rapicetta M, et al, Sersale's Study Collaborating Group. The impact of a vaccination campaign against hepatitis B on the further decrease of hepatitis B virus infection in a southern Italian town over 14 years. Eur J Intern Med 2012;23:e190–2.

57. Al-Faleh FZ, Al-Jeffri M, Ramia S, et al. Seroepidemiology of hepatitis B virus infection in Saudi children 8 years after a mass hepatitis B vaccination programme. J Infect 1999;38:167–70.

58. Huynh C, Minuk GY, Uhanova J, et al. Serological and molecular epidemiological outcomes after two decades of universal infant hepatitis B virus (HBV) vaccination in Nunavut, Canada. Vaccine 2017;35(35 Pt B):4515–22.

59. Kao JH, Hsu HM, Shau WY, et al. Universal hepatitis B vaccination and the decreased mortality from fulminant hepatitis in infants in Taiwan. J Pediatr 2001;139:349–52.

60. Chien YC, Jan CF, Chiang CJ, et al. Incomplete hepatitis B immunization, maternal carrier status, and increased risk of liver diseases: a 20-year cohort study of 3.8 million vaccinees. Hepatology 2014;60:125–32.

61. Wen WH, Chang MH, Zhao LL, et al. Mother-to-infant transmission of hepatitis B virus infection: significance of maternal viral load and strategies for intervention. J Hepatol 2013;59:24–30.

62. Chen HL, Lee CN, Chang CH, et al, Taiwan Study Group for the Prevention of Mother-to-Infant Transmission of HBV (PreMIT study). Efficacy of maternal tenofovir disoproxil fumarate in interrupting mother-to-infant transmission of hepatitis B virus. Hepatology 2015;62:375–86.

63. Pan CQ, Duan Z, Dai E, et al. China Study Group for the Mother-to-Child Transmission of Hepatitis B. Tenofovir to prevent hepatitis B transmission in mothers with high viral load. N Engl J Med 2016;374:2324–34.

64. Losonsky GA, Wasserman SS, Stephens I, et al. Hepatitis B vaccination of premature infants: a reassessment of current recommendations for delayed immunization. Pediatrics 1999;103:E14.

65. Sood A, Singh D, Mehta S, et al. Response to hepatitis B vaccine in preterm babies. Indian J Gastroenterol 2002;21:52–4.

66. Freitas da Motta MS, Mussi-Pinhata MM, Jorge SM, et al. Immunogenicity of hepatitis B vaccine in preterm and full term infants vaccinated within the first week of life. Vaccine 2002;20:1557–62.

67. American Academy of Pediatrics, Committee on Infectious Diseases. Update on timing of hepatitis B vaccine for premature infants and children with lapsed immunization. Pediatrics 1994;94:403–4.

68. Carman WF, Zanetti AR, Karayiannis P, et al. Vaccine-induced escape mutant of hepatitis B virus. Lancet 1990;336:325–9.

69. Hsu HY, Chang MH, Ni YH, et al. Surface gene mutants of hepatitis B virus in infants who develop acute or chronic infections despite immunoprophylaxis. Hepatology 1997;26:786–91.

70. Qin Y, Liao P. Hepatitis B virus vaccine breakthrough infection: surveillance of S gene mutants of HBV. Acta Virol 2018;62:115–21.

71. Hsu HY, Chang MH, Ni YH, et al. Survey of hepatitis B surface variant infection in children 15 years after a nationwide vaccination programme in Taiwan. Gut 2004; 53:1499–503.

72. Wen WH, Chen HL, Ni YH, et al. Secular trend of the viral genotype distribution in children with chronic hepatitis B virus infection after universal infant immunization. Hepatology 2011;53:429–36.

73. Hsu HY, Chang MH, Ni YH, et al. Long-term follow-up of children with postnatal immunoprophylaxis failure who were infected with hepatitis B virus surface antigen gene mutant. J Infect Dis 2013;207:1047–57.

74. Di Lello FA, Ridruejo E, Martínez AP, et al. Molecular epidemiology of hepatitis B virus mutants associated with vaccine escape, drug resistance and diagnosis failure. J Viral Hepat 2019;26:552–60.

75. Chen DS. Hepatitis B vaccination: the key towards elimination and eradication of hepatitis B. J Hepatol 2009;50:805–16.

76. Wang L, Zou ZQ, Wang K. Clinical relevance of HLA gene variants in HBV infection. J Immunol Res 2016;2016:9069375.

77. Chang MH, You SL, Chen CJ, et al, Taiwan Hepatoma Study Group. Long-term effects of hepatitis B immunization of infants in preventing liver cancer. Gastroenterology 2016;151:472–80.

78. Hung GY, Horng JL, Yen HJ, et al. Changing incidence patterns of hepatocellular carcinoma among age groups in Taiwan. J Hepatol 2015;63:1390–6.

79. Qu C, Chen T, Fan C, et al. Efficacy of neonatal HBV vaccination on liver cancer and other liver diseases over 30-year follow-up of the Qidong Hepatitis B Intervention Study: a cluster randomized controlled trial. PLoS Med 2014;11: e1001774.

80. Yeo Y, Gwack J, Kang S, et al. Viral hepatitis and liver cancer in Korea: an epidemiological perspective. Asian Pac J Cancer Prev 2013;14:6227–31.

81. McMahon BJ, Bulkow LR, Singleton RJ, et al. Elimination of hepatocellular carcinoma and acute hepatitis B in children 25 years after a hepatitis B newborn and catch-up immunization program. Hepatology 2011;54:801–7.

82. Popping S, Bade D, Boucher C, et al. The global campaign to eliminate HBV and HCV infection: International Viral Hepatitis Elimination Meeting and core indicators for development towards the 2030 elimination goals. J Virus Erad 2019; 5:60–6.

Hepatitis B
Current Status of Therapy and Future Therapies

Elias Spyrou, MD, PhD[a,b], Coleman I. Smith, MD[a],
Marc G. Ghany, MD, MHSc[c],*

KEYWORDS

- Vaccines • Infection • Cirrhosis • Hepatocellular carcinoma
- Antiviral/immunomodulatory therapy

KEY POINTS

- The number of persons with chronic hepatitis B virus (HBV) infection is high.
- These persons are at risk for complications of cirrhosis and hepatocellular carcinoma.
- There is a need for novel, finite therapy that can cure chronic HBV infection.
- This article highlights key developments in antiviral/immunomodulatory therapy, the rationale for choosing these approaches, and possible therapeutic regimens.

INTRODUCTION

Chronic hepatitis B virus (HBV) infection is a substantial global public health problem. Despite the availability of a protective vaccine for more than 3 decades, the prevalence of infection remains high. Worldwide it is estimated there are 257 million persons with chronic HBV infection, which results in 887,000 deaths annually primarily from complications of cirrhosis and hepatocellular carcinoma (HCC).[1] Although currently approved treatments, peginterferon and nucleos(t)ide analogues, are effective at inhibiting viral replication and reducing complications of chronic HBV infection, they are not curative and, in the case of nucleos(t)ide analogues, must be administered long term, if not indefinitely, because of persistence of the covalently closed circular DNA (cccDNA) in the hepatocyte nucleus.[2] Therefore, there is a need for new treatments that could lead to sustained, off-treatment inhibition of viral replication and

Funding: This work was in part supported by the Intramural Research Program of NIDDK, NIH. M.G. Ghany is an employee of the NIH.
[a] MedStar Georgetown Transplant Institute, MedStar Georgetown University Hospital, Washington, DC, USA; [b] Nazih Zuhdi Transplant Institute, INTEGRIS Baptist Medical Center, Oklahoma City, OK, USA; [c] Liver Diseases Branch, National Institute of Diabetes, Digestive and Kidney Diseases, National Institutes of Health, Building 10, Room 9B-16, 10 Center Drive MSC 1800, Bethesda, MD 20892-1800, USA
* Corresponding author.
E-mail address: marcg@intra.niddk.nih.gov

loss of hepatitis B surface antigen (HBsAg). The search for new antiviral agents with activity against HBV has been hampered by the small and compact nature of the HBV genome with few druggable viral targets and a lack of experimental systems or animal models that faithfully recapitulate the viral life cycle in the presence of an intact immune system. Nevertheless, recent improvements in model systems have facilitated the identification of several novel therapeutic approaches against HBV, as shown in **Fig. 1**. There are now more than 30 agents under investigation that either directly or indirectly target the HBV.[3] This article highlights key developments in antiviral/immunomodulatory therapy, the rationale for choosing these approaches, and possible therapeutic regimens.

GOALS OF NOVEL THERAPY AND DEFINITIONS OF CURE

The goals of novel therapies for chronic hepatitis B are to cure the chronic infection and thereby prevent complications of chronic liver disease, cirrhosis, HCC, and liver-related death. It is important to appreciate that any definition of a cure should encompass eradication of the chronic viral infection as well as resolution of the underlying liver disease. It is expected that complete viral eradication should result in resolution of liver disease, but this may not be true for patients with cirrhosis. The optimal treatment end point would be eradication of intrahepatic cccDNA and integrated HBV DNA, loss of HBsAg, and undetectable HBV DNA, referred to as a complete sterilizing cure. This end point may not be a feasible one, because currently it is not possible to eradicate cccDNA and integrated HBV DNA. In addition, complete sterilizing cure may not be necessary to reduce complications of chronic HBV infection. Current efforts are focused on achieving loss of HBsAg and undetectable HBV DNA in serum with or without seroconversion to hepatitis B surface antibody (anti-HBs) after completion of a finite course of treatment, resolution of residual liver injury, and a reduced risk of cirrhosis and HCC, referred to as functional cure. This end point may still be challenging given the recent observation that HBsAg may originate from integrated HBV

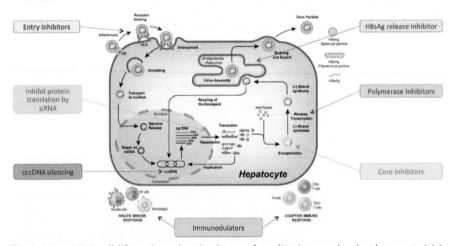

Fig. 1. Hepatitis B cell life cycle and main classes of medications under development. AAA, poly adenosine monophosphate; CD, cluster of differentiation; HBc, hepatitis B core/capsid protein; HBe, hepatitis B e; HBeAg, hepatitis B e antigen; HBs, hepatitis B surface protein; HBXs, HBV X proteins; HSP, heparan sulfate proteoglycans; NK, natural killer; NTCP, sodium taurocholate cotransporting polypeptide; pgDNA, pregenomic DNA; rcDNA, relaxed circular DNA; siRNA, small interfering RNA.

DNA.[4] An alternate and perhaps more attainable goal may be complete viral suppression but persistence of HBsAg in serum after completion of a finite course of treatment, referred to as a partial cure. This end point is observed in a proportion of patients, but, in the absence of HBsAg loss, is unlikely to be durable because there is a 15% to 40% lifetime risk of disease reactivation, and risk of HCC may be higher compared with patients who achieve HBsAg loss.[5]

NEW THERAPEUTIC APPROACHES FOR CHRONIC HEPATITIS B

A greater understanding of the HBV life cycle and the host immune response has led to the development of many new therapeutic approaches to treat chronic HBV infection. Broadly they can be viewed as agents that target the virus directly (direct-acting antiviral) or indirectly through modulation of a host factor (indirect-acting antiviral) or the host immune response (immunotherapy). These various strategies are discussed in more detail later.

HEPATITIS B VIRUS LIFE CYCLE

To better understand the mechanism of action of direct-acting antiviral agents under development, review of the viral life cycle is informative (see **Fig. 1**). HBV initiates infection by first loosely attaching to heparan sulfate proteoglycans on the hepatocyte membrane, then it binds to its entry receptor, the hepatocyte-specific bile acid transporter, sodium taurocholate, cotransporting polypeptide (NTCP) through an interaction with the pre-S1 lipopeptide of the large (L) envelope protein. This stage is followed by fusion of the HBV envelope with the endosomal membrane and endocytosis of the virus.[6–8] Next, there is uncoating with release of the double-stranded relaxed circular DNA genome (rcDNA) and its transport into the hepatocyte nucleus. In the nucleus, host cellular enzymes repair the rcDNA to form cccDNA.[2,9] The cccDNA serves as the transcriptional template for all messenger RNAs (mRNAs) as well as the pregenomic RNA (pgRNA), which is the template for viral replication.

Four viral transcripts (polymerase, core, surface, and X) are exported to the cytoplasm where they are translated into 7 viral proteins. In the cytoplasm, core proteins self-assemble into a viral nucleocapsid and the pgRNA and viral polymerase are packaged into the newly formed nucleocapsid through an encapsidation reaction. Viral replication is achieved using an RNA template, pgRNA, within the nucleocapsid. The mature viral capsids containing rcDNA are then enveloped with the small, medium, and large (S, M, L) surface proteins in the endoplasmic reticulum and secreted from the infected cell as intact virions or transported back to the nucleus to replenish the cccDNA pool.

ENTRY INHIBITORS

HBV entry into hepatocytes requires the coordinated binding of the virus to heparin sulfate proteoglycans, a low-affinity receptor that mediates hepatocyte attachment, followed by a high-affinity interaction with the NTCP receptor for viral internalization.[8,10] The NTCP receptor confers the species specificity to HBV.[11,12] Knowledge of this process has led to the development of several classes of specific and nonspecific inhibitors of viral entry (**Table 1**).[13–16] Entry inhibitors may lead to clearance of cccDNA by preventing de novo infection of uninfected hepatocytes.

Agents such as heparin, suramin, and synthetic antilipopolysaccharide peptides can bind to the virus or cellular heparan sulfate proteoglycans (poly-L-lysine) and

Table 1
Agents in the development pipeline for chronic hepatitis B

Target	Mechanism of Action	Class	Compounds in Development
Viral entry	Antibodies targeting pre-S1 or small surface protein	Monoclonal antibodies	GC1102
	Attachment inhibitors that block viral interaction with entry receptors	Heparin Poly-L-lysine Conjugated bile salts	— — —
	Reversibly/irreversibly block the NTCP receptor	Synthetic N-acylated pre-S1 Cyclosporine	Myrcludex B (Bulevirtide) —
cccDNA	Inactivate cccDNA	Zinc finger nucleases Transcription activator-like effector nuclease CRISPR/cas9 system	— — EBT106 HBV CRISPR-CAS-9 lipid nanoparticle
	Degrade cccDNA	Interferon α, γ TNF-α Lymphotoxin-β receptor agonists	— — —
	Functionally silence cccDNA	Epigenomic modifiers	
Viral transcripts	Degrade mRNA	siRNA	AB-729 ARB-1467 ARB-1740 DCR-HBVS Hepbarna (BB-HB-331) JNJ-3989 (ARO-HBV) Lunar-HBV Vir-2218 (ALN-HBV)
	Bind viral mRNA to prevent viral protein production	Antisense oligonucleotides	IONIS-HBVRx (GSK3228836) IONIS-HBVLRx (GSK33389404) RG6004 RO7062931
	Cause degradation of HBV RNA in the nucleus	DHQ	AB452 RG7834
	Downregulate viral mRNA	FXRα agonist	EYP001

Category	Description		
Core protein assembly modulators	Inhibit encapsidation of pregenomic RNA or nucleocapsid assembly	Heteroaryldihydropyrimidines	Morphothiadin (GLS4)
		Phenylpropenamide	AT-61; AT-130
		Pyridazinone derivatives	3711
		Sulfamoylbenzamide	AB-423, AB 506 JNJ-6379, JNJ-0440, NVR 3-778
		Isothiafludine	NZ-4
		2-amino-n-(2,6-dichloropyridin-3-yl) acetamide derivatives	BCM-599
		5,5'-bis[8-(phenylamino)-1-naphthalenesulfonate]	Bis-ANS
		—	ABI-H2158, ABI-H0731, ABI-H3733
		—	RG7907
		—	QL-007
		—	EDP-514
		—	CB-HBV-001
HBsAg release inhibitors	Synthetic oligonucleotides that bind HBsAg	Nucleic acid polymers	Rep 2139 Rep 2165
Targeting host pathways	Apoptosis	Apoptosis inducer	APG-1387
	Cyclophilin	Cyclophilin inhibitor	CRV 431 (CPI 431–32)
Boost innate immunity	Agonists of sensing arm of innate immune system	Toll-like receptor-7 agonist	AL-034 ANA773 RO6864018 (RG7795) RG7854
		Toll-like receptor-8 agonist	GS-9688
		RIG-I and NOD2 agonist	Inarigivir (SB9200)
		STING agonists	—
		TCR-like antibodies	—

(continued on next page)

Table 1
(continued)

Target	Mechanism of Action	Class	Compounds in Development
Boost humoral immunity	—	Anti-HBs	HBIg
	—	Anti-HBs monoclonal antibody	GC1102
Boost adaptive immunity	Checkpoint inhibitors	Anti–CTLA-4	—
		Anti–PD-1	Nivolumab
	Engineering new HBV-specific T cells	TCR gene transfer	LTCR-H2-1
		CAR-T cells	—
Therapeutic vaccines	Induction of HBV-specific B and T cells	T-cell vaccines	HepTcell
		DNA vaccines	HB-110
			INO-1800
			JNJ 64300535
		Viral vectors expressing HBV proteins	TG1050
			TomegaVax HBV
		Virus-like particle vaccine	VBI-2601
		Inactivated parapoxvirus nonspecific vaccine	AIC 649
		Antigen-antibody fusion vaccine	Chimigen HBV

Abbreviations: CAR-T, chimeric antigen receptor T; CRISPR/cas9, clustered regularly interspaced short palindromic repeats–associated nuclease 9; CTLA-4, cytotoxic T-lymphocyte–associated antigen 4; DHQ, dihydroquinolizinone; FXR, farnesoid X receptor alpha; PD-1; programmed cell death protein 1; STING, stimulator of IFN genes; TCR, T-cell receptor; TNF-α, tumor necrosis factor-α.

nonspecifically interrupt viral attachment to proteoglycans but none of them have been evaluated in the clinic.[10,17-19]

More specific agents are ones that either target the antigenic loop of the HBV S domain or N-terminal epitopes in the pre-S1 domain, such as neutralizing antibodies (Ma18/7, KR127, 17.1.41/19.79.5, hepatitis B immunoglobulin [HBIg]), or ones that reversibly (taurocholate and ezetimibe)[6,15] or irreversibly bind to NTCP (Myrcludex B, cyclosporin A, and its derivatives such as SCYX1454139).[10,20,21] HBIg, a mixture of antibodies that target HBsAg purified from the plasma of vaccinated individuals, is the only approved medication but requires parenteral administration and large doses to be effective. It has not been tested as a therapeutic agent in clinical studies.[22-25] Similarly, taurocholate and ezetimibe require high concentrations to be effective but their short half-lives at the receptor may limit their clinical application.

In contrast, Myrcludex B (Bulevirtide), an HBV large surface protein–derived synthetic lipopeptide, has a long half-life at the receptor and irreversibly blocks the NTCP receptor in nonsaturating concentrations.[26] Myrcludex was evaluated in a phase IIa proof-of-concept study in 40 patients with hepatitis B e antigen (HBeAg)–negative chronic hepatitis B without cirrhosis. Patients were randomized to receive Myrcludex B at one of 5 dosages: 0.5 mg, 1 mg, 2 mg, and 5 mg for 12 weeks, and 10 mg once daily for 24 weeks. HBV DNA declined greater than 1 log in 6 out of 8 patients in the 10-mg dosing group and in 7 out of 32 patients in the lower dosing groups; however, no patient experienced HBsAg loss.[27] Studies of Myrcludex either alone or in combination with pegylated interferon in patients with chronic delta hepatitis yielded more promising results. Among 60 patients with HBV/hepatitis D virus (HDV) coinfection who were randomized to receive pegylated interferon alone, pegylated interferon plus Myrcludex B 2 or 5 mg, or Myrcludex B 2 mg for 48 weeks, 3 out of 15 (20%) patients in the pegylated interferon plus 2 mg of Myrcludex B arm achieved HBsAg loss 24 weeks off therapy and this number increased to 4 out of 15 (27%) 48 weeks off therapy. No HBsAg loss was observed in any of the other treatment arms.[28] Thus, Myrcludex B in combination with other antiviral agents may be a promising treatment of chronic delta hepatitis.

TARGETING COVALENTLY CLOSED CIRCULAR DNA

cccDNA plays a key role in the viral life cycle, where it serves as the template for viral transcription and the pgRNA, the template for viral replication. Elimination of cccDNA is considered the Holy Grail of HBV treatment because its persistence in the nucleus of infected hepatocytes is the major reason why cure of HBV is currently not possible. Strategies to block cccDNA formation, enhance its destruction, silence its transcription, and stimulate cell division to promote its elimination are currently under investigation.

DNA cleavage enzymes, such as homing endonucleases or meganucleases, zinc finger nucleases, transcription activator–like effector nucleases, and clustered regularly interspaced short palindromic repeats–associated system 9 (CRISP/Cas-9) proteins, act by inducing targeted breaks in double-stranded DNA. The breaks in double-stranded DNA are repaired by homologous repair in the case of homologous template such as double-stranded DNA and single-stranded DNA or nonhomologous end repair in the absence of template and the mutated cccDNA is eventually lost. In vitro studies showing inhibition of HBV replication have provided evidence that such an approach can work; however, specificity for viral targets and efficient and safe delivery of the gene editing agent to eliminate cccDNA from all infected hepatocytes are major challenges that need to be overcome.[29-36]

Another approach being pursued is to use agents that upregulate apolipoprotein B mRNA editing enzyme catalytic subunit 3A and 3B (APOBEC3A/B) deaminases. Upregulation of APOBEC3A/B by interferon-α (IFN-α) and lymphotoxin-b has been shown to lead to noncytolytic degradation of cccDNA in vitro, but the degradation of the cccDNA pool is incomplete.[37] Other cytokines including IFN-γ, tumor necrosis factor-α (TNF-α), and interleukin (IL) 1β can also lead to cccDNA degradation via a similar mechanism.[38,39]

In the nucleus, the viral cccDNA is organized into a chromatinlike structure that makes it amenable to epigenetic manipulation.[40] Several compounds have been shown in vitro to silence cccDNA transcription. IFN-α inhibits transcription of genomic and subgenomic RNAs derived from cccDNA, both in HBV-replicating cells in culture and in HBV-infected chimeric urokinase-type plasminogen activator/severe combined immunodeficiency (uPA/SCID) mice repopulated with primary human hepatocytes.[41] The HBV X protein (HBX), which is essential for viral transcription, has been shown to act through degradation of the host structural maintenance of chromosomes (Smc) complex Smc5/6, which can selectively block extrachromosomal DNA transcription. HBX destroys the Smc5/6 complex, thereby removing the inhibition on transcription and permits HBV gene expression.[42,43] Thus, targeting the HBX might be a viable approach to silencing cccDNA. Pevonedistat, a neural-precursor-cell-expressed developmentally down-regulated 8 (NEDD-8)-activating enzyme inhibitor, restored Smc5/6 protein levels and suppressed viral transcription in cultured hepatocytes.[44] However, the observation that there is reactivation of cccDNA as soon as HBX becomes available again may be a major limitation to this approach.[45,46] At present, no cccDNA targeting strategies have been evaluated in clinical trials.

TARGETING VIRAL TRANSCRIPTS

It has been proposed that high levels of viral antigens may inhibit the host immune response and contribute to persistence of HBV, based mostly on evidence from host evasion strategies of other viruses. Thus, targeting the viral mRNA, through the use of molecular approaches such as RNA interference, antisense oligonucleotides, and ribozymes, may be an effective way to control HBV infection.[9]

Four viral genes are transcribed from the cccDNA template by host RNA polymerase II in the hepatocyte nucleus. All mRNA transcripts share a common 3′ terminus and encode the 7 viral proteins: core, e, polymerase, small surface, middle surface, large surface, and X. Therefore, targeting this region with a small interfering RNA (siRNA) that can induce the cell's RNA-induced silencing complex/argonaute 2 could lead to degradation of all viral transcripts and would allow simultaneous suppression of all viral proteins. Several siRNAs have been designed for this purpose, including ARB-1467, ARB-1740, ALN-HBV, Hepbarna (BB-HB-331), Lunar-HBV, ARC-520, and ARC-521.[47–50] In clinical trials, ARC-520 and ARC-521, in combination with entecavir, was well tolerated and showed a decrease of HBsAg, total HBV DNA, and cccDNA in both HBeAg-negative and HBeAg-positive patients.[51] An interesting observation from these studies was that the decline in HBsAg levels was lower among HBeAg-negative compared with HBeAg-positive patients. This reduced efficacy among HBeAg-negative patients was subsequently shown in a chimpanzee model to be caused by production of HBsAg from integrated HBV DNA and absence of binding sites for the siRNA on the 3′ end of the transcripts.[4] Use of a second siRNA targeting another region of preS/S was able to result in reduction of HBsAg levels in HBeAg-negative chimpanzees that was similar to that achieved in HBeAg-positive animals. However, studies with this compound were discontinued because of the possible fatal toxicity of the delivery vehicle in nonhuman primates.

An alternate approach to block viral protein expression is to use liver-directed antisense oligonucleotides that act through steric hindrance and/or RNA degradation by ribonuclease H cleavage. Two antisense molecules, IONIS-HBVRx (GSK3228836) and IONIS-HBVLRx (GSK33389404), linked to a trimer of N-acetyl-galactosamine (GalNAc) moieties, allows delivery of the antisense molecule to the liver via the hepatocyte-expressed asialoglycoprotein. Such an approach may reduce off-target toxicities associated with antisense oligonucleotides.[52] These agents are currently in phase I trials. Note that both siRNA and antisense oligonucleotides do not eliminate cccDNA, and rebound of HBsAg to pretreatment levels after treatment is stopped has been observed, leading to concerns about the durability of response. In addition, viral mutations and quasispecies may contribute to rebound and limit the applicability of this approach. Therefore, it is likely that repeated courses of therapy or use in combination with other approaches would most likely be required.[53]

RG7834 is a novel, small-molecule compound belonging to the dihydroquinolizinones chemical class that leads to selective degradation of HBV transcripts in infected hepatocytes and in the human liver chimeric uPA/SCID mouse model that acts similar to siRNA but through a different mechanism.[54]

TARGETING VIRAL NUCLEOCAPSID ASSEMBLY

The HBV core protein is not only a structural component of the viral nucleocapsid but is involved in nearly every stage of the HBV life cycle, including subcellular trafficking and release of the HBV genome, RNA metabolism, capsid assembly and transport, and reverse transcription,[55] and modulation of the host innate immune response, making the HBV core protein a promising target for HBV treatment.

Several compounds referred to as core protein assembly modulators (CpAMs) are under investigation. All the compounds bind to a hydrophobic pocket on the capsid formed at the interface between core protein dimers. These molecules inhibit nucleocapsid assembly, encapsidation of pgRNA, or both, leading to inhibition of rcDNA synthesis from pgRNA, as reverse transcription takes place only in the viral nucleocapsid.[56,57] Two classes of CpAMs have been identified based on their mechanism of action. Class I typified by heteroaryl dihyropyridines, increase the kinetics of capsid formation, and lead to the formation of misassembled capsids. Class 2 is typified by phenylpropenamides, which accelerate capsid assembly and form morphologically normal capsids that are empty and lack viral pgRNA and HBV polymerase. Some CpAMs may have additional effects, such as affecting the conversion of rcDNA to cccDNA. Importantly, CpAMs seem to be active against most HBV genotypes and some have shown activity against nucleos(t)ide analogue-resistant strains.[58–61] There are now several CpAMs in differing stages of clinical development (see **Table 1**).

NVR 3-778, a sulfamoyl benzamide derivative, was the first-in-class CpAM evaluated either alone or with peginterferon in a proof-of-concept phase 1b trial among HBeAg-positive patients without cirrhosis. Reductions in both HBV DNA and HBV RNA were observed and were greatest in the group that received NVR 3-778 plus peginterferon alfa ($\sim$2 $\log_{10}$ copies/mL for both respectively), compared with the groups given NVR 3-778 or peginterferon alfa alone (reduction in HBV DNA of 1.43 $\log_{10}$ copies/mL and 1.06 $\log_{10}$ copies/mL respectively and reduction in HBV RNA of 1.42 $\log_{10}$ copies/mL and 0.89 $\log_{10}$ copies/mL, respectively). NVR 3-778 dosed at 400 mg or lower was ineffective at suppressing HBV DNA and HBV RNA. Viral rebound was observed after treatment was stopped. Overall treatment was well tolerated.[62]

A novel CpAM, JNJ 56136379 (JNJ-6379), showed promise as an antiviral in treatment-naive patients with chronic hepatitis B without cirrhosis. Efficacy and safety of JNJ-6379 at 3 doses of 25 mg, 75 mg, and 150 mg administered for 28 days was evaluated in a randomized, double-blind, placebo-controlled phase 1b study among 36 HBeAg-positive and HBeAg-negative patients. Substantial dose-dependent reductions in HBV DNA and HBV RNA from baseline were observed, with up to 2.9 log IU/mL reduction in HBV DNA and 1.7 log reduction in HBV RNA observed with the 150-mg and 75-mg doses, respectively. The drug showed no dose-limiting toxicities, with exposure increasing in a dose-dependent manner.[63]

RO7049389 is a small-molecule, class I HBV CpAM that induces formation of abnormal HBV core aggregates, resulting in defective capsid assembly and thereby suppressing HBV replication. RO7049389 administered in single and multiple ascending doses among healthy volunteers was shown to be safe and well tolerated across all tested doses. RO7049389 was administered at 200 mg twice a day for 28 days to 6 patients with chronic HBV infection, and showed a median decline in HBV DNA of 2.7 $\log_{10}$ IU/mL from baseline and was less than the limit of detection in 3 out of 6 patients. These preliminary but promising results suggest that RO7049389 has excellent anti-HBV activity.[64]

Preliminary results from a phase 1b trial of AB-506, a potent, oral class II capsid inhibitor, evaluating multiple doses of AB-506, with or without a nucleos(t)ide analogue, once daily for 28 days among HBeAg-positive or HBeAg-negative subjects with chronic hepatitis B reported a mean decline in HBV DNA of −2.0 log (160-mg dose) and −2.8 log (400-mg dose) from baseline at day 28 and a mean decline in HBV RNA of −2.4 log from baseline at day 28 for both doses.[65] However, further development of AB-506 was discontinued because of the observation of 2 cases of acute hepatitis in the phase 1a 28-day clinical trial in healthy volunteers.

ABI-H0731 is a potent and selective oral HBV core protein inhibitor. Interim results are available from 2 randomized, double-blind, placebo-controlled phase 2a studies. In the first study (ABI-H0731-201), ABI-H0731, 300 mg once daily or placebo was administered to HBeAg-positive or HBeAg-negative individuals with chronic HBV infection already suppressed on standard-of-care nucleos(t)ide analogues (n = 73). In the second study (ABI-H0731-202), ABI-H0731, 300 mg plus entecavir or entecavir plus placebo daily was given to treatment-naive HBeAg-positive individuals (n = 25). In the nucleos(t)ide-suppressed HBeAg+ cohort (ABI-H0731-201), significant reductions in HBV RNA levels were observed in the group receiving nucleos(t)ide analogues plus ABI-H0731compared with the those receiving nucleos(t)ide analogues plus placebo at week 12 (2.34 $\log_{10}$ IU/mL vs 0.05 $\log_{10}$ IU/mL, $P<.001$). In the treatment-naive HBeAg+ cohort (ABI-H0731-202), significantly greater declines in HBV DNA levels were noted with the combination of ABI-H0731 and entecavir compared with entecavir plus placebo at week 12 (4.54 vs 3.29 $\log_{10}$ IU/mL, $P<.011$) and HBV RNA levels at week 12 (2.27 vs 0.44 U/mL, $P<.005$). No patient lost HBeAg or HBsAg, although decreases in HBeAg and HBsAg levels were noted in some individuals in both studies.[66] These encouraging early data suggest that capsid inhibitors can result in substantial reduction in HBV DNA and HBV RNA levels. Longer-term studies alone and in combination with other antiviral agents will be needed to determine whether CpAMs will result in loss of serum HBsAg, HBeAg, and cccDNA.

HEPATITIS B VIRUS POLYMERASE INHIBITORS

All currently approved nucleos(t)ide analogues target the DNA polymerase activity of the viral polymerase. The purpose of developing new HBV polymerase inhibitors is to augment their antiviral efficacy and improve oral bioavailability and safety compared with the current nucleos(t)ide analogues.[9] Besifovir, CMX-157, AGX-1009, and lagociclovir are newer HBV polymerase inhibitors in development.[53,67,68]

Besifovir has entered phase III trials and in doses of 90 mg or 150 mg has shown the same antiviral efficacy as 96 weeks of treatment with 0.5 mg of entecavir.[69] Besifovir had good antiviral activity against wild-type and drug-resistant mutant strains.[70] The drug was well tolerated, but dose-dependent carnitine depletion was observed in some patients and, as a result, these patients had to receive carnitine supplementation.[71]

Additional approaches are focused on targeting the ribonuclease H (RNase H) activity of the HBV polymerase, which is required for production of new virions. Abolishing RNase H activity results in the formation of defective HBV DNA. At present there are no compounds that inhibit RNase H activity in clinical trials.

TARGETING HEPATITIS B SURFACE ANTIGEN

Clearance of HBsAg is the primary focus of drug development. Therefore, compounds that can directly target HBsAg resulting in its clearance would be highly desirable. Nucleic acid polymers (NAPs) are synthetic oligonucleotides that bind HBsAg and block its release through a poorly understood mechanism.[72] It has been proposed that NAPs possibly interfere with the assembly/release of HBV subviral particles.[73,74] REP-2139 and REP-2165 are candidate NAPs in clinical development and, in combination with pegylated interferon 2a or thymosin alpha-1, showed significant decline of HBV DNA and HBsAg levels with anti-HBs seroconversion in some HBeAg-positive Asian patients.[75] REP 2139 and REP 2165 have been studied in combination with tenofovir and pegylated interferon 2a. All patients received lead-in tenofovir for 24 weeks, after which they were continued on tenofovir and randomized to receive pegylated interferon 2a plus REP 2139 or pegylated interferon 2a plus placebo for 24 weeks. Significant declines in HBsAg levels were noted in patients receiving REP 2139, with 9 out of 10 patients achieving greater than 4 log decline in HBsAg levels and 8 out of 10 experiencing HBsAg loss compared with only 1 out of 10 patients not receiving REP 2139 24 to 48 weeks off therapy.[76] Further follow-up is required to determine whether these interesting results are sustained.

MODULATING THE HOST IMMUNE RESPONSE

The immunologic response in patients with chronic HBV infection is characterized by a weak innate and HBV-specific cellular immune response. The focus of current immunologic approaches is to restore the host immune response to HBV that may lead to viral clearance.[77] Therapeutic strategies being pursued to induce innate immunity include the use of cytokines and pattern-recognition receptor agonists to stimulate production of interferon. Strategies to reconstitute functional HBV-specific immunity include nonspecific approaches, such as checkpoint inhibitors to reawaken the T-cell response, and more specific approaches using genetically engineered/modified T cells and therapeutic vaccines.

BOOSTING INNATE IMMUNITY

HBV is considered a stealth virus and is not associated with induction of a strong innate immune response.[78] However, several lines of evidence suggest that an adequate innate immune response can suppress HBV replication.[79] As an example, IFN-α, IFN-γ, TNF-α, and IL-1a, produced by nonparenchymal liver cells, can suppress or even eradicate HBV from infected hepatocytes through a noncytolytic mechanism.[41,80] In addition, lymphotoxin-b–mediated activation of APOBEC (apolipoprotein B mRNA editing enzyme, catalytic polypeptide–like) or activation of retinoic acid-inducible gene-I (RIG-I) has been shown to suppress HBV replication.[37,81] These data suggest that strategies to boost the innate immunity are a rational therapeutic approach.

Vesatolimod (GS-9620), a toll-like receptor (TLR) 7 agonist, activates intrahepatic dendritic cells, triggering the production of type I and II interferons and activating intrahepatic natural killer (NK) and mucosal-associated invariant T (MAIT) cells. In proof-of-principle studies, vesatolimod was shown to reduce HBV DNA and HBsAg levels in chimpanzees and woodchucks but not in humans.[82–84] Vesatolimod was tested in a phase II, double-blind, randomized, placebo-controlled study in 162 patients stratified by HBsAg levels and serum HBeAg status. Patients received once-weekly oral vesatolimod (1-mg, 2-mg, or 4-mg doses) or placebo for 4, 8, or 12 weeks. No significant decline in HBsAg level was observed at the primary (week 24) or secondary (weeks 4, 8,12, and 48) end points.[85] Differences in response observed in animal and human studies may relate to activity of TLR-7 and doses used in animal and human studies.

GS-9688, a TLR-8 agonist, activates intrahepatic dendritic cells and other myeloid cells leading to production of IL-12/IL-18, activation of NK and MAIT cells, and eventually decline in serum woodchuck hepatitis virus (WHV) DNA and clearance of woodchuck hepatitis surface antigen. GS-9688 is currently under investigation.[86]

Inarigivir (SB9200), an oral dinucleotide RIG-I agonist, has shown antiviral activity against HBV via a combination of activation of innate immunity and as a direct-acting antiviral effect as a nonnucleotide reverse transcriptase inhibitor.[87] The ACHIEVE trial randomized 80 HBeAg-positive and HBeAg-negative patients to receive one of 4 doses of inarigivir (25, 50, 100, and 200 mg) daily or placebo in a 4:1 ratio for 12 weeks, after which all patients were switched to tenofovir for 12 weeks. HBV DNA reduction was achieved in a dose-dependent fashion for both HBeAg-positive and HBeAg-negative patients, with a maximal reduction of 3.26 $\log_{10}$ in the 200-mg dose. HBV RNA levels paralleled reductions in HBV DNA levels but HBsAg decline was not dose dependent, indicating the potential importance of the host response to inarigivir. The medication was well tolerated. Alanine aminotransferase (ALT) flares were observed in 6 treated patients (10%) and 4 placebo patients (25%), and 1 patient required dose discontinuation for ALT level greater than 400 IU. Further development of this compound has been discontinued due to serious adverse events including the death of one patient.[88]

An agonist of the mouse stimulator of IFN genes (STING), 5,6-dimethylxanthenone-4-acetic acid (DMXAA), was found to induce a robust cytokine response in macrophages that efficiently suppressed HBV replication in mouse hepatocytes by reducing the amount of cytoplasmic viral nucleocapsids.[89]

An alternate strategy to augment the intrahepatic innate immune response is to selectively deliver cytokines to HBV-infected hepatocytes using T-cell receptor (TCR)–like antibodies conjugated with cytokines such as IFN-α.[90] These TCR-like antibodies bind to the human leukocyte antigens that present HBV peptides at the surface of the infected hepatocytes and they deliver the cytokines into the microenvironment of the infected cells. Studies in animal models or humans with TCR-like antibodies have not yet been conducted.

In addition, IFN-γ and TNF-α are known to control HBV in a noncytolytic fashion. In Lymphotoxin-b–mediated activation of APOBEC or activation of RIG-I has been shown to suppress HBV replication. Lymphotoxin-a (LTa), lymphotoxin-b (LTb), and cluster of differentiation (CD) 258 are the natural ligands of lymphotoxin-b receptor (LTbR). However, the potential for severe side effects with these cytokines limits their therapeutic use. Superagonistic tetravalent bispecific antibody (BS1) and a bivalent anti-LTbR monoclonal antibody (CBE11) are LTbR agonists. BS1 and CBE11 have been tested in in vitro experiments using HBV-infected differentiated HepaRG (dHepaRG) cells and have been shown to decrease levels of cccDNA, intracellular HBV DNA, pgRNA, and secreted HBeAg by ~90% without toxicity.[37]

ADAPTIVE IMMUNITY CENTRAL TO CONTROL OF HEPATITIS B VIRUS

Control and resolution of acute HBV infection depend on the generation of a complex repertoire of viral-specific B and T cells. HBV-specific CD8 T cells secrete cytokines such as IFN-γ that induce noncytolytic HBV clearance as well as recruitment of other inflammatory immune cells that are critical for clearance of HBV. This process is regulated by HBV-specific CD4 T cells.[91] In chronic HBV infection, there are quantitative and functional defects of the HBV-specific T-cell response that contribute to viral persistence. T-cell exhaustion is a well-characterized phenomenon in chronic HBV infection, and the underlying mechanisms are thought to be the persistent exposure of T cells to HBV antigens[92] and the increased expression of multiple coinhibitory molecules on HBV-specific T cells, programmed cell death protein 1 (PD-1), cytotoxic T lymphocyte–associated antigen 4 (CLTA4), lymphocyte activation gene-3 (LAG-3), CD160, T-cell immunoglobulin domain and mucin 3 (TIM-3), and 2B4.[93,94] The TRAIL-death receptor, TRAIL-2, is upregulated by the exhausted T cells, making them susceptible to TRAIL-dependent NK cell lysis.[95] Several other mechanisms within the liver contribute to diminished T-cell function. The release of enzymes from damaged hepatocytes depletes essential amino acids for T-cell function, such as arginine and tryptophan.[96] Myeloid suppressor cells can also produce arginase, which also depletes arginine.[97] In addition, regulatory T-cells, B cells, and stellate cells can secrete cytokines, such as IL-10 and transforming growth factor-β, that suppress T-cell function.[98,99] Restoration of an adaptive immune responses is crucial for the successful control of HBV.

NONSPECIFIC APPROACHES TO STIMULATE ADAPTIVE IMMUNITY

Nonspecific inhibition of PD-1, programmed death-ligand 1 (PD-L1), T-cell inhibitory receptor Tim-3, and CTLA-4 could restore vigorous immune responses, and this approach has been used in treatment of malignancies. However, a concern with this approach is that nonspecific activation of the immune system may lead to autoimmunity and/or flares of hepatitis.

Given the upregulation of PD-1 in patients with chronic hepatitis B, anti–PD-1 was evaluated to restore exhausted HBV-specific T-cell function.[100,101] The administration of a combination of entecavir with an anti–PD-1 ligand monoclonal antibody together with a WHV DNA vaccine to woodchucks with chronic WHV infection was associated with restoration of WHV-specific T-cell responses and clearance of woodchuck hepatitis surface antigen (WHsAg). No significant increase in serum markers of hepatic injury was observed in treated compared with untreated control animals.[102] Data on safety of nivolumab, a PD-1 inhibitor, in patients with chronic hepatitis B is available from patients with HBV-related HCC. In 1 study, among 51 patients with HBV-related HCC treated with nivolumab, all of whom were receiving nucleos(t)ide analogues with HBV DNA level less than 100 IU/mL, none had reactivation of HBV and no patient experienced anti-HBs seroconversion.[103] A single dose of nivolumab with or without GS-4774 (a therapeutic T-cell vaccine) was evaluated in HBeAg-negative, noncirrhotic patients without HCC in a phase 1 study. The regimen showed a good safety profile and modest decreases of HBsAg levels were observed.[104] The safety of checkpoint inhibitors with prolonged use and whether these medications can be safely administered to patients with cirrhosis, those with underlying autoimmune disease, or who are listed for liver transplant are important issues that need to be addressed.

SPECIFIC APPROACHES TO STIMULATE ADAPTIVE IMMUNITY

Restoring an adequate HBV-specific T-cell response in patients with chronic HBV infection is likely to be challenging because of their low frequency and exhausted phenotype. A possible solution may be the adoptive transfer of newly engineered HBV-specific T cells.[77] Evidence from patients with leukemia and chronic HBV infection who received bone marrow transplants from donors who developed HBV-specific T-cell responses, either from vaccination or prior exposure to HBV with spontaneous recovery, showing clearance of HBsAg and development of anti-HBs, suggests that the approach of adoptive transfer of HBV-specific T cells may be feasible.[105,106] Genetic reprogramming to create functional T cells to eliminate HBV-infected hepatocytes could be achieved through TCR gene transfer or use of chimeric antigen receptor (CAR) T cells. The main difference between the two approaches is the type of antigen receptors used for reprogramming. In the case of TCR gene transfer, it is the native alpha beta chains of the TCR, whereas, in the case of CAR, it is the extracellular domain of virus-specific antibody. HBV-specific T cells with CAR or classic TCRs tested in vitro and in HBV transgenic mice showed selective elimination of HBV-infected cell lines and control of HBV replication with only transient liver damage, respectively.[107,108]

Proof of principle of using adoptive transfer of reprogrammed HBV-specific T cells was shown in a patient with metastatic HCC targeting the malignant cells expressing HBV antigens. Tumor cells were recognized in vivo by lymphocytes engineered to express an HBV-specific TCR. The genetically modified T cells survived, expanded, and mediated a reduction in HBsAg levels without exacerbation of liver inflammation or other toxicity, but clinical efficacy was not observed in this patient.[109]

THERAPEUTIC VACCINATION

Although HBsAg-based vaccines have shown good efficacy at inducing anti-HBs production and protective immunity in vaccinees, the use of vaccines as a therapeutic modality has been generally disappointing. Vaccination has been used therapeutically to break T-cell tolerance to HBV proteins and stimulate HBV-specific T-cell responses with the goal of achieving sustained suppression of HBV replication and ultimately HBsAg loss in patients with chronic HBV infection. However, studies of current protein, DNA, and T-cell vaccines in patients with chronic hepatitis B have been unsuccessful, perhaps because they only targeted HBsAg.[110]

The development of newer DNA vaccines, heterologous prime-boost approaches, vaccines against multiple HBV proteins, and novel adjuvants has renewed interest in vaccines as a therapeutic modality for chronic hepatitis B.[111] DNA vaccines, such as INO-1800 or JNJ-64300535, are in phase 1 trials. INO-1800 is a mixture of recombinant DNA vaccines that encode the HBsAg and the consensus sequence of the hepatitis B core/capsid protein antigen (HBcAg). However, DNA vaccination alone is not very immunogenic. INO-1800, alone or in combination with IL-12 as an immune activator, is currently being tested in adults with chronic hepatitis B. Preliminary results have shown it is safe, well tolerated, and generated virus-specific T cells, including CD8+ killer T cells.[112] JNJ-64300535 is being studied in combination with nucleos(t)ide analogues and results are awaited.[111,113]

A DNA prime-adenovirus boost approach was tested in WHV-transgenic mice and was shown to elicit a potent and functional woodchuck hepatitis core antigen –specific CD8+ T-cell response that resulted in the reduction of the WHV load below the detection limit in more than 70% of animals. In addition, the combination of entecavir and DNA prime-adenovirus boost immunization in chronic WHV carriers resulted in WHsAg-specific and woodchuck hepatitis core antigen–specific CD4+ and CD8+ T-cell responses, which were not detectable in controls animals that received entecavir alone.[114] Woodchucks receiving the combination therapy showed a prolonged suppression of WHV replication and lower WHsAg levels compared with entecavir-treated controls.[114] Moreover, 2 of 4 immunized carriers remained WHV negative after the end of entecavir treatment and developed anti–woodchuck hepatitis surface protein antibodies. A clinical trial using a DNA prime-adenovirus boost approach is planned.

Vaccines using multiple HBV proteins produced by different vectors in combination with adjuvants have shown some efficacy in vitro and in animal models.[77,114,115] GS-4774 (a yeast-based, heat-inactivated, T-cell vaccine containing HBV core, surface, and X protein) and TG-1050 (a nonreplicative adenovirus serotype 5 encoding a unique large fusion protein composed of a truncated HBV core, a modified HBV polymerase, and 2 HBV envelope domains) have been shown to induce immunogenicity in mice and healthy individuals.[116,117] However, results of clinical trials were disappointing.[118–120] GS-4774 at 3 doses (2, 10, and 40 yeast units every 4 weeks for 24 weeks) was compared with tenofovir among HBeAg-positive and HBeAg-negative viremic patients without cirrhosis. The primary end point was HBsAg loss. No HBsAg loss was observed in any of the treatment arms and no significant differences in decline of HBsAg levels were observed between the GS-4774 dosing groups and the tenofovir group. HB-110 (a vaccine composed of 3 plasmids that encode for the HBV envelope proteins S and L, core protein, polymerase, and human IL-12) was evaluated in combination with adefovir and compared with adefovir alone.[121] HBV-specific T-cell responses were induced in a portion of patients and a single patient who received a high dose of HB-110 experienced HBeAg seroconversion.[121] HepTcell (FP-02.2), another candidate vaccine, composed of 9 synthetic peptides derived from the most conserved domains of HBV, is currently in phase I trials.[111] NASVAC (ABX203), a vaccine based on recombinant HBsAg and HBV core proteins, did not prevent viral relapse after discontinuing nucleos(t)ide analogues in HBeAg-negative patients.[122] Further results of therapeutic vaccine trials are awaited but, based on preliminary results, it is unlikely that therapeutic vaccine alone would be effective and a combination approach will be required.

COMBINATION THERAPY

Based on current management of other chronic viral infections, it is likely that a cocktail of antivirals targeting multiple steps in the viral life cycle or a combined antiviral/immunomodulatory approach will be needed to achieve functional cure. Which specific agents will be required and in what sequence in a therapeutic regimen are currently unknown because most of the drugs in the pipeline are in early-phase

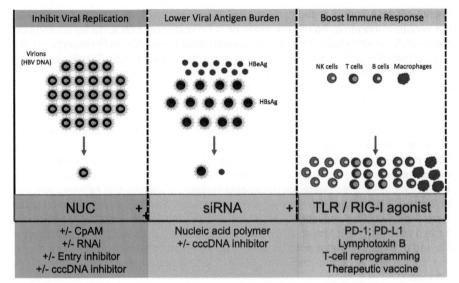

Inhibit Viral Replication	Lower Viral Antigen Burden	Boost Immune Response

Fig. 2. Possible future combination regimens to achieve functional cure. CAR-T, chimeric antigen receptor T cells; NUC, nucleos(t)ide analogue; RNAi, RNA inhibitor.

development. Safety with monotherapy and then in combination therapy will need to be shown before longer-duration studies can be conducted. One therapeutic approach would be to use multiple direct-acting antiviral agents with different mechanisms of action to achieve complete inhibition of intrahepatic HBV replication. A possible regimen might consist of a nucleos(t)ide analogue as a backbone plus 1 or 2 other agents, such as a CpAM, siRNA, entry inhibitor, or cccDNA inhibitor (**Fig. 2**). A second approach might be to combine agents that inhibit viral replication with ones that specifically reduce viral antigen load (see **Fig. 2**). Such a strategy is based on the rationale that a high viral antigen burden may be a contributor to the exhausted immune phenotype characteristic of chronic hepatitis B. Potential regimens might include an siRNA, an NAP, or a cccDNA inhibitor in combination with a direct-acting antiviral. The sequence of administration of agents in such a regimen is unknown. Whether both agents would have to be used in combination initially or as an add-on approach will require future study. Another approach might be to use a combination antiviral/inhibitor of viral antigen burden with an immunomodulator to either boost innate immune immunity (eg, TLR-RIG-I agonist) or to restore the HBV-specific T-cell response, such as a TCR gene transfer or chimeric antigen receptor T (CAR-T) cells or therapeutic vaccines (see **Fig. 2**).

It is also likely that treatment may need to be tailored for different patient populations, such as those who are HBeAg positive or negative, treatment naive versus treatment experienced, those with high or low/suppressed viral replication, those with or without cirrhosis, high versus low viral antigen burden, and perhaps also based on genotype. These are issues that will need to be addressed in future trial designs.

SUMMARY

Although this is an exciting time for drug development in chronic hepatitis B, it is important to remember that, if to have an impact on the global burden of HBV disease, any future treatment regimen will have to be not only efficacious and safe but also tolerable, easy to administer, scalable, and above all affordable. Current antiviral therapy satisfies most of these criteria but must be administered long term and is associated with very low rates of functional cure. There are safety concerns related to some of the therapeutic approaches in development, such as the risk of hepatitis flares, hepatic decompensation, autoimmunity, and drug toxicity, which will need to be addressed. These issues are particularly relevant for resource-limited areas of the world, where most chronic carriers reside and where the infrastructure and cost of additional monitoring may be too burdensome. Although newer therapies that can lead to functional cure are awaited, it is important to not forget some essential steps in the efforts to eliminate HBV: better vaccination coverage, reduce vertical transmission, and improve population-wide testing and linkage to care of patients who require treatment.

AUTHORS' CONTRIBUTIONS

Drafting: E. Spyrou, C.I. Smith, M.G. Ghany. Critical revision: E. Spyrou, C.I. Smith, M.G. Ghany. Final draft: M.G. Ghany.

DISCLOSURE

The authors have no financial discloses. This article has not been submitted to another journal and has not been published in whole novel therapy is or in part elsewhere previously.

REFERENCES

1. Available at: www.who.int/mediacentre/factsheets/fs164/en/. Last Accessed September 30, 2019.
2. Nassal M. HBV cccDNA: viral persistence reservoir and key obstacle for a cure of chronic hepatitis B. Gut 2015;64(12):1972–84.
3. Liang TJ, Block TM, McMahon BJ, et al. Present and future therapies of hepatitis B: from discovery to cure. Hepatology 2015;62(6):1893–908.
4. Wooddell CI, Yuen MF, Chan HL, et al. RNAi-based treatment of chronically infected patients and chimpanzees reveals that integrated hepatitis B virus DNA is a source of HBsAg. Sci Transl Med 2017;9(409) [pii:eaan0241].
5. Yip TC, Wong GL, Chan HL, et al. HBsAg seroclearance further reduces hepatocellular carcinoma risk after complete viral suppression with nucleos(t)ide analogues. J Hepatol 2019;70(3):361–70.
6. Ni Y, Lempp FA, Mehrle S, et al. Hepatitis B and D viruses exploit sodium taurocholate co-transporting polypeptide for species-specific entry into hepatocytes. Gastroenterology 2014;146(4):1070–83.
7. Verrier ER, Colpitts CC, Bach C, et al. A targeted functional RNA interference screen uncovers glypican 5 as an entry factor for hepatitis B and D viruses. Hepatology 2016;63(1):35–48.
8. Yan H, Zhong G, Xu G, et al. Sodium taurocholate cotransporting polypeptide is a functional receptor for human hepatitis B and D virus. Elife 2012;1:e00049.
9. Ko C, Michler T, Protzer U. Novel viral and host targets to cure hepatitis B. Curr Opin Virol 2017;24:38–45.
10. Schulze A, Gripon P, Urban S. Hepatitis B virus infection initiates with a large surface protein-dependent binding to heparan sulfate proteoglycans. Hepatology 2007;46(6):1759–68.

11. Zhong G, Yan H, Wang H, et al. Sodium taurocholate cotransporting polypeptide mediates woolly monkey hepatitis B virus infection of Tupaia hepatocytes. J Virol 2013;87(12):7176–84.

12. Lempp FA, Wiedtke E, Qu B, et al. Sodium taurocholate cotransporting polypeptide is the limiting host factor of hepatitis B virus infection in macaque and pig hepatocytes. Hepatology 2017;66(3):703–16.

13. Sankhyan A, Sharma C, Dutta D, et al. Inhibition of preS1-hepatocyte interaction by an array of recombinant human antibodies from naturally recovered individuals. Sci Rep 2016;6:21240.

14. Ying C, Van Pelt JF, Van Lommel A, et al. Sulphated and sulphonated polymers inhibit the initial interaction of hepatitis B virus with hepatocytes. Antivir Chem Chemother 2002;13(3):157–64.

15. Lucifora J, Esser K, Protzer U. Ezetimibe blocks hepatitis B virus infection after virus uptake into hepatocytes. Antiviral Res 2013;97(2):195–7.

16. Volz T, Allweiss L, Ben MM, et al. The entry inhibitor Myrcludex-B efficiently blocks intrahepatic virus spreading in humanized mice previously infected with hepatitis B virus. J Hepatol 2013;58(5):861–7.

17. Di Stefano G, Colonna FP, Bongini A, et al. Ribavirin conjugated with lactosaminated poly-L-lysine: selective delivery to the liver and increased antiviral activity in mice with viral hepatitis. Biochem Pharmacol 1997;54(3):357–63.

18. Krepstakies M, Lucifora J, Nagel CH, et al. A new class of synthetic peptide inhibitors blocks attachment and entry of human pathogenic viruses. J Infect Dis 2012;205(11):1654–64.

19. Petcu DJ, Aldrich CE, Coates L, et al. Suramin inhibits in vitro infection by duck hepatitis B virus, Rous sarcoma virus, and hepatitis delta virus. Virology 1988; 167(2):385–92.

20. Nkongolo S, Ni Y, Lempp FA, et al. Cyclosporin A inhibits hepatitis B and hepatitis D virus entry by cyclophilin-independent interference with the NTCP receptor. J Hepatol 2014;60(4):723–31.

21. Watashi K, Sluder A, Daito T, et al. Cyclosporin A and its analogs inhibit hepatitis B virus entry into cultured hepatocytes through targeting a membrane transporter, sodium taurocholate cotransporting polypeptide (NTCP). Hepatology 2014;59(5):1726–37.

22. Galun E, Eren R, Safadi R, et al. Clinical evaluation (phase I) of a combination of two human monoclonal antibodies to HBV: safety and antiviral properties. Hepatology 2002;35(3):673–9.

23. Heermann KH, Goldmann U, Schwartz W, et al. Large surface proteins of hepatitis B virus containing the pre-s sequence. J Virol 1984;52(2):396–402.

24. Hong HJ, Ryu CJ, Hur H, et al. In vivo neutralization of hepatitis B virus infection by an anti-preS1 humanized antibody in chimpanzees. Virology 2004;318(1): 134–41.

25. Samuel D, Muller R, Alexander G, et al. Liver transplantation in European patients with the hepatitis B surface antigen. N Engl J Med 1993;329(25):1842–7.

26. Urban S, Bartenschlager R, Kubitz R, et al. Strategies to inhibit entry of HBV and HDV into hepatocytes. Gastroenterology 2014;147(1):48–64.

27. Bogomolov P, VN, Allweiss L, Dandri M, et al. A proof-of-concept Phase 2a clinical trial with HBV/HDV entry inhibitor Myrcludex B. Hepatology 2014;60: 1267A–90A.

28. Wedemeyer H, Schöneweis K, Bogomolov PO, et al. GS-13-Final results of a multicenter, open-label phase 2 clinical trial (MYR203) to assess safety and

efficacy of myrcludex B in cwith PEG-interferon Alpha 2a in patients with chronic HBV/HDV co-infection. J Hepatol 2019;70(1):e81.

29. Zimmerman KA, Fischer KP, Joyce MA, et al. Zinc finger proteins designed to specifically target duck hepatitis B virus covalently closed circular DNA inhibit viral transcription in tissue culture. J Virol 2008;82(16):8013–21.

30. Moyo B, Bloom K, Scott T, et al. Advances with using CRISPR/Cas-mediated gene editing to treat infections with hepatitis B virus and hepatitis C virus. Virus Res 2018;244:311–20.

31. Makarova KS, Haft DH, Barrangou R, et al. Evolution and classification of the CRISPR-Cas systems. Nat Rev Microbiol 2011;9(6):467–77.

32. Lin SR, Yang HC, Kuo YT, et al. The CRISPR/Cas9 system facilitates clearance of the intrahepatic HBV templates in vivo. Mol Ther Nucleic Acids 2014;3:e186.

33. Ely A, Moyo B, Arbuthnot P. Progress with developing use of gene editing to cure chronic infection with hepatitis B virus. Mol Ther 2016;24(4):671–7.

34. Cradick TJ, Keck K, Bradshaw S, et al. Zinc-finger nucleases as a novel therapeutic strategy for targeting hepatitis B virus DNAs. Mol Ther 2010;18(5): 947–54.

35. Chen J, Zhang W, Lin J, et al. An efficient antiviral strategy for targeting hepatitis B virus genome using transcription activator-like effector nucleases. Mol Ther 2014;22(2):303–11.

36. Bloom K, Ely A, Mussolino C, et al. Inactivation of hepatitis B virus replication in cultured cells and in vivo with engineered transcription activator-like effector nucleases. Mol Ther 2013;21(10):1889–97.

37. Lucifora J, Xia Y, Reisinger F, et al. Specific and nonhepatotoxic degradation of nuclear hepatitis B virus cccDNA. Science 2014;343(6176):1221–8.

38. Isorce N, Testoni B, Locatelli M, et al. Antiviral activity of various interferons and pro-inflammatory cytokines in non-transformed cultured hepatocytes infected with hepatitis B virus. Antiviral Res 2016;130:36–45.

39. Xia Y, Stadler D, Lucifora J, et al. Interferon-gamma and tumor necrosis factor-alpha produced by T cells reduce the HBV persistence form, cccDNA, without cytolysis. Gastroenterology 2016;150(1):194–205.

40. Tropberger P, Mercier A, Robinson M, et al. Mapping of histone modifications in episomal HBV cccDNA uncovers an unusual chromatin organization amenable to epigenetic manipulation. Proc Natl Acad Sci U S A 2015;112(42):E5715–24.

41. Belloni L, Allweiss L, Guerrieri F, et al. IFN-alpha inhibits HBV transcription and replication in cell culture and in humanized mice by targeting the epigenetic regulation of the nuclear cccDNA minichromosome. J Clin Invest 2012;122(2): 529–37.

42. Xu Z, Yen TS, Wu L, et al. Enhancement of hepatitis B virus replication by its X protein in transgenic mice. J Virol 2002;76(5):2579–84.

43. Decorsiere A, Mueller H, van Breugel PC, et al. Hepatitis B virus X protein identifies the Smc5/6 complex as a host restriction factor. Nature 2016;531(7594): 386–9.

44. Sekiba K, Otsuka M, Ohno M, et al. Pevonedistat, a neuronal precursor cell-expressed developmentally down-regulated protein 8-activating enzyme inhibitor, is a potent inhibitor of hepatitis B virus. Hepatology 2019;69(5):1903–15.

45. Lee SH, Cha EJ, Lim JE, et al. Structural characterization of an intrinsically unfolded mini-HBX protein from hepatitis B virus. Mol Cells 2012;34(2):165–9.

46. Lucifora J, Arzberger S, Durantel D, et al. Hepatitis B virus X protein is essential to initiate and maintain virus replication after infection. J Hepatol 2011;55(5): 996–1003.

47. Streinu-Cercel A, Gane E, Cheng W, et al. A phase 2a study evaluating the multi-dose activity of ARB-1467 in HBeAg positive and negative virally suppressed subjects with hepatitis B. J Hepatol 2017;66(1):S688–9.
48. Thi EP, Dhillon AP, Ardzinski A, et al. ARB-1740, a RNA interference therapeutic for chronic hepatitis B infection. ACS Infect Dis 2019;5(5):725–37.
49. Mao T, Kao S-C, Cock T-A, et al. BB-HB-331, a DNA-directed RNA interference (ddRNAi) agent targeting hepatitis B virus (HBV), can effectively suppress HBV in vitro and in vivo. Oligonucleotide Therapeutics 2016;24(Supplement 1):S103.
50. Alnylam. Press release: Alnylam and Vir form strategic alliance to advance RNAi therapeutics for infectious diseases. 2017.
51. Yuen M, Chan H, Liu K, et al. Differential reductions in viral antigens expressed from cccDNAVS integrated DNA in treatment naive HBeAg positive and negative patients with chronic HBV after RNA interference therapy with ARC-520. 2016;64(suppl. 2):S390–1.
52. Han K, Cremer J, Elston R, et al. A randomized, double-blind, placebo-controlled, first-time-in-human study to assess the safety, tolerability, and pharmacokinetics of single and multiple ascending doses of GSK3389404 in healthy subjects. Clin Pharmacol Drug Dev 2019;8(6):790–801.
53. Soriano V, Barreiro P, Benitez L, et al. New antivirals for the treatment of chronic hepatitis B. Expert Opin Investig Drugs 2017;26(7):843–51.
54. Mueller H, Wildum S, Luangsay S, et al. A novel orally available small molecule that inhibits hepatitis B virus expression. J Hepatol 2018;68(3):412–20.
55. Diab A, Foca A, Zoulim F, et al. The diverse functions of the hepatitis B core/capsid protein (HBc) in the viral life cycle: implications for the development of HBc-targeting antivirals. Antiviral Res 2018;149:211–20.
56. Ghany MG, Block TM. Disease pathways and mechanisms of potential drug targets. Clin Liver Dis (Hoboken) 2018;12(1):12–8.
57. Zlotnick A, Venkatakrishnan B, Tan Z, et al. Core protein: a pleiotropic keystone in the HBV lifecycle. Antiviral Res 2015;121:82–93.
58. Wang XY, Wei ZM, Wu GY, et al. In vitro inhibition of HBV replication by a novel compound, GLS4, and its efficacy against adefovir-dipivoxil-resistant HBV mutations. Antivir Ther 2012;17(5):793–803.
59. Delaney WET, Edwards R, Colledge D, et al. Phenylpropenamide derivatives AT-61 and AT-130 inhibit replication of wild-type and lamivudine-resistant strains of hepatitis B virus in vitro. Antimicrob Agents Chemother 2002;46(9):3057–60.
60. Billioud G, Pichoud C, Puerstinger G, et al. The main hepatitis B virus (HBV) mutants resistant to nucleoside analogs are susceptible in vitro to non-nucleoside inhibitors of HBV replication. Antiviral Res 2011;92(2):271–6.
61. Berke JM, Tan Y, Verbinnen T, et al. Antiviral profiling of the capsid assembly modulator BAY41-4109 on full-length HBV genotype A-H clinical isolates and core site-directed mutants in vitro. Antiviral Res 2017;144:205–15.
62. Yuen MF, Gane EJ, Kim DJ, et al. Antiviral activity, safety, and pharmacokinetics of capsid assembly modulator NVR 3-778 in patients with chronic HBV infection. Gastroenterology 2019;156(5):1392–403.e7.
63. Zoulim F, Yogaratnam JZ, Vandenbossche JJ, et al. Safety, pharmakokinetics and antiviral activity of novel capsid assembly modulator (CAM) JNJ-56136379 (JNJ-6379) in treatmentnaive chronic hepatitis B (CHB) patients without cirrhosis. J Hepatol 2018;68:S102.
64. Gane E, Liu A, Yuen MF, et al. RO7049389, a core protein allosteric modulator, demonstrates robust anti-HBV activity in chronic hepatitis B patients and is safe and well tolerated. J Hepatol 2018;68:S101.

65. Corporation AB. Arbutus Announces Preliminary Phase 1a/1b Clinical Trial Results for AB-506, an Oral Capsid Inhibitor in Development for People with Chronic Hepatitis B. Company website announcement. 2019.
66. Ma JL, Lalezari J, Nguyen T, et al. Interim safety and efficacy results of the ABI-H0731 phase 2a program exploring the combination of ABI-H0731 with Nuc therapy in treatment-naive and treatment-suppressed chronic hepatitis B patients. J Hepatol 2019;70(1, Supplement):e130.
67. Lanier ER, Ptak RG, Lampert BM, et al. Development of hexadecyloxypropyl tenofovir (CMX157) for treatment of infection caused by wild-type and nucleoside/nucleotide-resistant HIV. Antimicrob Agents Chemother 2010;54(7):2901–9.
68. Ahn SH, Kim W, Jung YK, et al. Efficacy and safety of besifovir dipivoxil maleate compared with tenofovir disoproxil fumarate in treatment of chronic hepatitis B virus infection. Clin Gastroenterol Hepatol 2019;17(9):1850–9.e4.
69. Yuen MF, Kim J, Kim CR, et al. A randomized placebo-controlled, dose-finding study of oral LB80380 in HBeAg-positive patients with chronic hepatitis B. Antivir Ther 2006;11(8):977–83.
70. Yuen MF, Han KH, Um SH, et al. Antiviral activity and safety of LB80380 in hepatitis B e antigen-positive chronic hepatitis B patients with lamivudine-resistant disease. Hepatology 2010;51(3):767–76.
71. Lai CL, Ahn SH, Lee KS, et al. Phase IIb multicentred randomised trial of besifovir (LB80380) versus entecavir in Asian patients with chronic hepatitis B. Gut 2014;63(6):996–1004.
72. Al-Mahtab M, Bazinet M, Vaillant A. Safety and efficacy of nucleic acid polymers in monotherapy and combined with immunotherapy in treatment-naive Bangladeshi patients with HBeAg+ Chronic Hepatitis B infection. PLoS One 2016; 11(6):e0156667.
73. Noordeen F, Scougall CA, Grosse A, et al. Therapeutic antiviral effect of the nucleic acid polymer REP 2055 against Persistent Duck Hepatitis B Virus infection. PLoS One 2015;10(11):e0140909.
74. Quinet J, Jamard C, Burtin M, et al. Nucleic acid polymer REP 2139 and nucleos(T)ide analogues act synergistically against chronic hepadnaviral infection in vivo in Pekin ducks. Hepatology 2018;67(6):2127–40.
75. Jansen L, Vaillant A, Stelma F, et al. O114 : serum HBV-RNA levels decline significantly in chronic hepatitis B patients dosed with the nucleic-acid polymer REP2139-CA. J Hepatol 2015;62:S250.
76. Bazinet M, Pantea V, Placinta G, et al. Preliminary safety and efficacy of REP 2139-Mg or REP 2165-Mg used in combination with tenofovir disoproxil fumarate and pegylated interferon alpha 2a in treatment naïve Caucasian patients with chronic HBeAg negative HBV infection. Paper presented at: Hepatology. 2016;64(s1):1122A. Abstract LB-7.
77. Bertoletti A, Le Bert N. Immunotherapy for chronic hepatitis B virus infection. Gut Liver 2018;12(5):497–507.
78. Cheng X, Xia Y, Serti E, et al. Hepatitis B virus evades innate immunity of hepatocytes but activates cytokine production by macrophages. Hepatology 2017; 66(6):1779–93.
79. Maini MK, Gehring AJ. The role of innate immunity in the immunopathology and treatment of HBV infection. J Hepatol 2016;64(1 Suppl):S60–70.
80. McClary H, Koch R, Chisari FV, et al. Relative sensitivity of hepatitis B virus and other hepatotropic viruses to the antiviral effects of cytokines. J Virol 2000;74(5): 2255–64.

81. Sato S, Li K, Kameyama T, et al. The RNA sensor RIG-I dually functions as an innate sensor and direct antiviral factor for hepatitis B virus. Immunity 2015; 42(1):123–32.

82. Lanford RE, Guerra B, Chavez D, et al. GS-9620, an oral agonist of Toll-like receptor-7, induces prolonged suppression of hepatitis B virus in chronically infected chimpanzees. Gastroenterology 2013;144(7):1508–17, 1517.e1-10.

83. Menne S, Tumas DB, Liu KH, et al. Sustained efficacy and seroconversion with the Toll-like receptor 7 agonist GS-9620 in the Woodchuck model of chronic hepatitis B. J Hepatol 2015;62(6):1237–45.

84. Gane EJ, Lim YS, Gordon SC, et al. The oral toll-like receptor-7 agonist GS-9620 in patients with chronic hepatitis B virus infection. J Hepatol 2015;63(2):320–8.

85. Janssen HLA, Brunetto MR, Kim YJ, et al. Safety, efficacy and pharmacodynamics of vesatolimod (GS-9620) in virally suppressed patients with chronic hepatitis B. J Hepatol 2018;68(3):431–40.

86. Daffis S, Chamberlain J, Zheng J, et al. Sustained efficacy and surface antigen seroconversion in the woodchuck model of chronic hepatitis B with the selective toll-like receptor 8 agonist GS-9688. J Hepatol 2017;66(1):S692–3.

87. Walsh R, Hammond R, Jackson K, et al. Effects of SB9200 (Inarigivir) therapy on immune responses in patients with chronic hepatitis B. J Hepatol 2018;68:S89.

88. Yuen MC, CY, Liu CJ, et al. Ascending dose cohort study of inarigivir - A novel RIG I agonist in chronic HBV patients: final results of the ACHIEVE trial. J Hepatol 2019;70(1, Supplement):e45–79.

89. Guo F, Han Y, Zhao X, et al. STING agonists induce an innate antiviral immune response against hepatitis B virus. Antimicrob Agents Chemother 2015;59(2): 1273–81.

90. Ji C, Sastry KS, Tiefenthaler G, et al. Targeted delivery of interferon-alpha to hepatitis B virus-infected cells using T-cell receptor-like antibodies. Hepatology 2012;56(6):2027–38.

91. Bertoletti A, Ferrari C. Adaptive immunity in HBV infection. J Hepatol 2016;64(1 Suppl):S71–83.

92. Wherry EJ, Ha SJ, Kaech SM, et al. Molecular signature of CD8+ T cell exhaustion during chronic viral infection. Immunity 2007;27(4):670–84.

93. Bengsch B, Martin B, Thimme R. Restoration of HBV-specific CD8+ T cell function by PD-1 blockade in inactive carrier patients is linked to T cell differentiation. J Hepatol 2014;61(6):1212–9.

94. Schurich A, Khanna P, Lopes AR, et al. Role of the coinhibitory receptor cytotoxic T lymphocyte antigen-4 on apoptosis-Prone CD8 T cells in persistent hepatitis B virus infection. Hepatology 2011;53(5):1494–503.

95. Peppa D, Gill US, Reynolds G, et al. Up-regulation of a death receptor renders antiviral T cells susceptible to NK cell-mediated deletion. J Exp Med 2013; 210(1):99–114.

96. Bronte V, Zanovello P. Regulation of immune responses by L-arginine metabolism. Nat Rev Immunol 2005;5(8):641–54.

97. Pallett LJ, Gill US, Quaglia A, et al. Metabolic regulation of hepatitis B immunopathology by myeloid-derived suppressor cells. Nat Med 2015;21(6):591–600.

98. Das A, Ellis G, Pallant C, et al. IL-10-producing regulatory B cells in the pathogenesis of chronic hepatitis B virus infection. J Immunol 2012;189(8):3925–35.

99. Mann DA, Marra F. Fibrogenic signalling in hepatic stellate cells. J Hepatol 2010; 52(6):949–50.

100. Fisicaro P, Valdatta C, Massari M, et al. Antiviral intrahepatic T-cell responses can be restored by blocking programmed death-1 pathway in chronic hepatitis B. Gastroenterology 2010;138(2):682–93, 693.e1-4.
101. Liu J, Zhang E, Ma Z, et al. Enhancing virus-specific immunity in vivo by combining therapeutic vaccination and PD-L1 blockade in chronic hepadnaviral infection. PLoS Pathog 2014;10(1):e1003856.
102. Balsitis S, Gali V, Mason PJ, et al. Safety and efficacy of anti-PD-L1 therapy in the woodchuck model of HBV infection. PLoS One 2018;13(2):e0190058.
103. El-Khoueiry AB, Sangro B, Yau T, et al. Nivolumab in patients with advanced hepatocellular carcinoma (CheckMate 040): an open-label, non-comparative, phase 1/2 dose escalation and expansion trial. Lancet 2017;389(10088): 2492–502.
104. Gane E, Gaggar A, Nguyen AH, et al. A phase1 study evaluating anti-PD-1 treatment with or without GS-4774 in HBeAg negative chronic hepatitis B patients. J Hepatol 2017;66(1):S26–7.
105. Ilan Y, Nagler A, Adler R, et al. Adoptive transfer of immunity to hepatitis B virus after T cell-depleted allogeneic bone marrow transplantation. Hepatology 1993; 18(2):246–52.
106. Lau GK, Lok AS, Liang RH, et al. Clearance of hepatitis B surface antigen after bone marrow transplantation: role of adoptive immunity transfer. Hepatology 1997;25(6):1497–501.
107. Gehring AJ, Xue SA, Ho ZZ, et al. Engineering virus-specific T cells that target HBV infected hepatocytes and hepatocellular carcinoma cell lines. J Hepatol 2011;55(1):103–10.
108. Krebs K, Bottinger N, Huang LR, et al. T cells expressing a chimeric antigen receptor that binds hepatitis B virus envelope proteins control virus replication in mice. Gastroenterology 2013;145(2):456–65.
109. Qasim W, Brunetto M, Gehring AJ, et al. Immunotherapy of HCC metastases with autologous T cell receptor redirected T cells, targeting HBsAg in a liver transplant patient. J Hepatol 2015;62(2):486–91.
110. Lok AS, Zoulim F, Dusheiko G, et al. Hepatitis B cure: from discovery to regulatory approval. Hepatology 2017;66(4):1296–313.
111. Gehring AJ, Protzer U. Targeting innate and adaptive immune responses to cure chronic HBV infection. Gastroenterology 2019;156(2):325–37.
112. Phase I Study of INO-1800 with or Without INO-9112 + EP in Chronic Hepatitis B Subjects. 2015. Available at: ClinicalTrials.gov; https://clinicaltrials.gov/ct2/show/NCT02431312?term=ino-1800&draw=1&rank=1. Accessed September 15, 2019.
113. A First-In-Human Study to Evaluate Safety, Tolerability, Reactogenicity, and Immunogenicity of JNJ-64300535, a DNA Vaccine, Administered by Electroporation-Mediated Intramuscular Injection, in Participants With Chronic Hepatitis B Who Are on Stable Nucleos(t)Ide Therapy and Virologically Suppressed. 2018. Available at: ClinicalTrials.gov; https://clinicaltrials.gov/ct2/show/NCT03463369?term=JNJ-64300535&rank=1. Accessed September 15, 2019.
114. Kosinska AD, Zhang E, Johrden L, et al. Combination of DNA prime–adenovirus boost immunization with entecavir elicits sustained control of chronic hepatitis B in the woodchuck model. PLoS Pathog 2013;9(6):e1003391.
115. Liu J, Kosinska A, Lu M, et al. New therapeutic vaccination strategies for the treatment of chronic hepatitis B. Virol Sin 2014;29(1):10–6.

116. Martin P, Dubois C, Jacquier E, et al. TG1050, an immunotherapeutic to treat chronic hepatitis B, induces robust T cells and exerts an antiviral effect in HBV-persistent mice. Gut 2015;64(12):1961–71.

117. Gaggar A, Coeshott C, Apelian D, et al. Safety, tolerability and immunogenicity of GS-4774, a hepatitis B virus-specific therapeutic vaccine, in healthy subjects: a randomized study. Vaccine 2014;32(39):4925–31.

118. Vandepapeliere P, Lau GK, Leroux-Roels G, et al. Therapeutic vaccination of chronic hepatitis B patients with virus suppression by antiviral therapy: a randomized, controlled study of co-administration of HBsAg/AS02 candidate vaccine and lamivudine. Vaccine 2007;25(51):8585–97.

119. Mancini-Bourgine M, Fontaine H, Scott-Algara D, et al. Induction or expansion of T-cell responses by a hepatitis B DNA vaccine administered to chronic HBV carriers. Hepatology 2004;40(4):874–82.

120. Lok AS, Pan CQ, Han SH, et al. Randomized phase II study of GS-4774 as a therapeutic vaccine in virally suppressed patients with chronic hepatitis B. J Hepatol 2016;65(3):509–16.

121. Yoon SK, Seo YB, Im SJ, et al. Safety and immunogenicity of therapeutic DNA vaccine with antiviral drug in chronic HBV patients and its immunogenicity in mice. Liver Int 2015;35(3):805–15.

122. Wedemeyer H, Hui AJ, Sukeepaisarnjaroen W, et al. Therapeutic vaccination of chronic hepatitis B patients with ABX203 (NASVAC) to prevent relapse after stopping NUCs: contrasting timing rebound between tenofovir and entecavir. J Hepatol 2017;66(1):S101.

Hepatitis Delta
Prevalence, Natural History, and Treatment Options

Julian Hercun, MD*, Christopher Koh, MD, MHSc, Theo Heller, MD

KEYWORDS

• Hepatitis D • Hepatitis B • Chronic liver disease • Investigational treatments

KEY POINTS

• Hepatitis delta is associated with a severe hepatitis and an increased risk of liver-related morbidity.
• Worldwide distribution with global impact caused by immigration from endemic regions.
• Current treatment options have limited efficacy; however, emerging options are promising.

INTRODUCTION

Hepatitis delta virus (HDV) was first described in Italy by Rizzetto and colleagues[1] in a cohort of patients with hepatitis B virus (HBV) with chronic hepatitis in the mid-1970s. At the time of discovery, the delta antibody system was thought to be a new HBV antigen. It was only subsequently concluded that HDV was a separate viral entity from HBV with its own RNA.[2] Since its identification, HDV has represented a diagnostic as well as therapeutic challenge to clinicians worldwide.

Virology

HDV is a spherical particle that is ~36 nm in diameter and contains HDV RNA and small and large HDV antigen (HDAg) proteins (**Fig. 1**). The two antigen isoforms are differentiated by a sequence of 19 amino acids at the carboxyl terminus. The small HDAg is required for RNA synthesis, whereas the large HDAg is required for virion formation and packaging but also acts as an inhibitor of replication.[3] Similar to plant viruses, HDV is able to autocleave its circular RNA into a linear molecule.[4] During viral replication, which occurs in the hepatocyte nuclei,[5] HDV RNA is used for synthesis of both small HDAg and antigenomic RNA via rolling-circle replication.[5] The antigenomic RNA is edited by the host RNA-dependent adenosine deaminase ADAR1, which converts adenosine to inosine, extending the reading frame to produce the large HDAg.[5] The large

Liver Diseases Branch, National Institute of Diabetes and Digestive and Kidney Diseases, National Institutes of Health, 10 Center Drive, Room 4-5722, Bethesda, MD 20892, USA
* Corresponding author.
E-mail address: julian.hercun@nih.gov

Gastroenterol Clin N Am 49 (2020) 239–252
https://doi.org/10.1016/j.gtc.2020.01.004
0889-8553/20/Published by Elsevier Inc.

gastro.theclinics.com

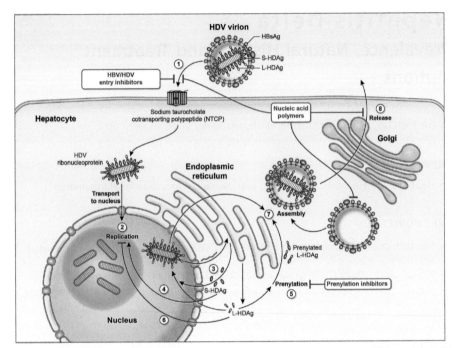

Fig. 1. Replication cycle of HDV and sites of investigative drug targets. (1) HDV attaches to hepatocyte HBV surface proteins and sodium taurocholate cotransporting peptide (NTCP). (2) HDV genome replication in the nucleus via rolling-circle mechanism. (3) HDV antigenome transported out of nucleus and translated into small HDAg and large HDAg. (4) Small HDAg promotes HDV replication in nucleus. (5) Large HDAg prenylated before assembly. (6) Large HDAg inhibits HDV replication. (7) Virus assembly. (8) Virus release from hepatocyte. HBsAg, hepatitis B surface antigen; L-HDAg, large HDAg; S-HDAg, small HDAg.

antigen undergoes isoprenylation (more precisely farnesylation) of the last 4 amino acids near the carboxyl terminus, a crucial step that enables packaging with hepatitis B surface antigen (HBsAg) and therefore virion assembly and export.[6]

The presence of an established HBV infection is a requirement for HDV infection, because HDV uses HBV envelope proteins for virion formation and infectivity. In addition, HDV relies on the same proteins as HBV to enter hepatocytes, including the pre-S1 sequence of the large protein (a target in investigational therapies).[7] To date, 8 distinct genotypes have been described, with HDV1 the most prevalent and widespread[8] (**Fig. 2**).

EPIDEMIOLOGY

Based on earlier prevalence estimates of 5% of patients with HBV being co-infected with HDV, 15 to 20 million people were thought to have HDV.[9] However, a recent meta-analysis has increased this estimate to 10.6% of HBsAg-positive patients.[10] Demographically, twice as many men are affected than women.[11,12] With time, a higher proportion of older patients has been noted; in Italy, 80% are more than 50 years old, whereas 3% are younger than 30 years old.[12] Nonetheless, a younger age at diagnosis has been described in eastern Europe and South Asia.[11] There continues to be great variability in HDV global prevalence, as detailed in **Table 1**.

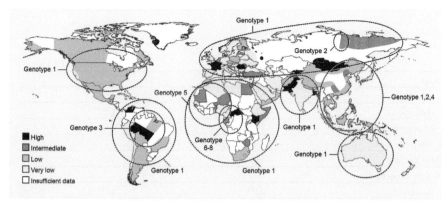

Fig. 2. World map with the estimated HDV infection prevalence and genotype distribution.

With greater awareness of sexually transmitted diseases and the institution of preventive measures, decreases in HDV prevalence have occurred in multiple regions. In Taiwan, prevalence decreased from 24% to 4% between 1983 and 1995,[16] whereas in Italy prevalence decreased from 23% in 1987 to 14% in 1992 to 8% in 1997.[27] Reduced incidence has been reported in Italy, mostly in young adults, mirroring a decrease in incidence of acute HBV.[28]

However, diminished prevalence has not been replicated everywhere. In Germany, a decline from 19% to 7% was noted from 1992 to 1997 but the prevalence has since remained between 8% and 14%,[24] whereas an increase in prevalence was noted in France in the early 2000s.[23] This trend has been attributed to immigration from high-risk endemic regions.[24,25,30]

High-Risk Populations

High-risk groups have been identified, with the human immunodeficiency virus (HIV)–positive intravenous drug user (IVDU) group emerging as an important reservoir for HDV infection,[10] with a prevalence of 42% in the EuroSIDA cohort[35] and 75% in Taiwan.[36] In IVDUs, prevalence ranges from 21% in mainland China[13] to 36% in the United States[34] and 39-69% in Taiwan.[13,36,37] In patients with high-risk sexual behaviors, prevalence was 11% in Taiwan[36] and 3% in men who have sex with men in Europe.[35] Prevalence has decreased from a peak of 85-91% in IVDU in Taiwan in the 1980s,[37] with a similar decrease noted in patients with high-risk sexual behaviors.[16]

Coinfection with other viruses besides HBV is also reported frequently in HDV. In HBV/HIV coinfected cohorts in Europe, HDV prevalence is 14-15%[35,38] and 9% in Taiwan.[39] However, it reaches 61% in an Italian cohort.[26] A high proportion (87-100%) of patients are reported to be viremic[35,39] and with higher rates of active hepatitis.[39] Furthermore, hepatitis C virus coinfection can reach 59%.[32]

Fewer studies have evaluated other high-risk groups; in HBV-positive hemophiliacs, a 19% HDV prevalence was reported,[40] and HDV prevalence ranges from 1.7% in dialysis and kidney transplant patients, to 44.5% in hemodialysis patients in Iran.[41]

DIAGNOSIS

Clinical practice guidelines suggest screening for HDV in all patients with HBV at presentation[42] or high-risk populations with HBV.[43] In practice, patients with a recent diagnosis of HBV are more likely to be screened[29]; however, this only occurs in a minority of high-risk patients with HBV.[32] A biochemical profile that should warrant HDV testing is

Table 1
Global prevalence of hepatitis delta virus

	Prevalence in HBV Carriers (%)	Prevalence in General Population (%)
Asia		
China	0.9[13]	—
Mongolia	61[14]	8[10]
Pakistan	17[15]	—
Taiwan	4[16]	—
Middle East	15[17]	—
South America		
Brazil	42[18]	14[18]
Africa		
Central Africa	38[19]	26[19]
West Africa	10[19]	7[19]
East and South Africa	—	0.05[19]
Gabon	16[20,a]	—
Gambia	2.5[21]	—
Mauritania	33[22]	—
Europe		
France	2[23]	—
Germany	8–14[24]	—
Greece	4[25]	—
Italy	6,[26] 8,[27] 12[28]	—
London	4,[29] 8[30]	—
Switzerland	—	0.06[31,a]
United States	3[32,b]	0.02,[33] 1[34]

[a] Population of pregnant women.
[b] Population of veterans.

abnormal transaminase levels with low or undetectable HBV DNA titers, resulting in an odds ratio of 3.2 for HDV.[32] Inhibition of HBV replication by HDV viremia has been observed, with most patients presenting with low/undetectable HBV DNA.[11,44]

Although serum HDAg determination by immunoblot is the most specific test (92%),[45] other available serologic tests have adequate concordance with HDAg. Anti-HDV immunoglobulin M (IgM) is the most sensitive test (87%); however, it is also the least specific (42%),[45] with a delay in the increase of antibody levels after initial infection.[46] The hot-start reverse transcription polymerase chain reaction (PCR) method for HDV RNA detects viremia in 93% of patients with chronic hepatitis, with high sensitivity in acute hepatitis.[46,47] However, discrepancies in PCR assays worldwide result in underestimation of viral loads, even with the establishment of a World Health Organization standard.[8] A new serologic test has recently been developed by using a quantitative microarray antibody capture assay, with different suggested cutoffs for antibody and viremia detection.[14,21,34]

Transmission

HDV infection occurs in 2 distinct pathways: simultaneously with HBV infection (coinfection) or in patients with established chronic HBV (superinfection) (**Fig. 3**). After an

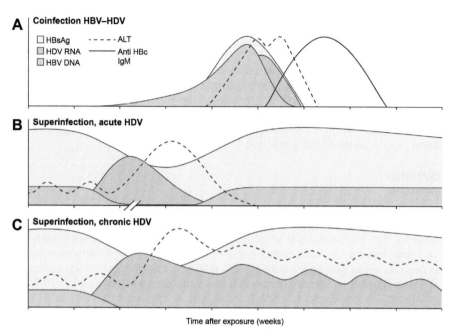

Fig. 3. Patterns of HDV RNA, HBV DNA, ALT during acute coinfection (*A*), acute HDV super-infection leading to HDV clearance (*B*), and chronic HDV infection (*C*). Anti-HBc, antibody to hepatitis B core antigen.

incubation time of 4 to 8 weeks, the presentation is similar in both instances, ranging from asymptomatic to nonspecific symptoms (nausea, asthenia) followed by an icteric phase. In coinfection, anti-HBc IgM (a marker of acute HBV infection) can be found.[48] Fulminant hepatitis is seen more often in coinfection (39% of cases) than with HBV infection alone.[49] The infection is self-limiting in coinfection, with chronicity occurring in less than 5% of cases.[48] This finding contrasts with superinfection, which is often associated with a more severe histologic hepatitis[50] that leads to chronic hepatitis in 80% of cases.[48] HDV RNA and HDAg can be found in both situations, as can anti-HDV IgM, which is not specific for acute infection and can be a marker of chronicity.[48]

NATURAL HISTORY
Cirrhosis

HDV is often associated with severe disease at presentation[25] as well as a fast progression to cirrhosis, which has been estimated to occur in up to 80% of patients and at a rate 15 years earlier than in HBV.[51,52] In longitudinal cohorts, 25% to 40% of patients develop cirrhosis over a mean follow-up of 3 to 28 years.[52–54] Decompensation occurs in half of cirrhotics over a period of 8 years.[55] Patients in South America develop more liver-related events (30.4% of patients),[11] as do patients with genotype I.[44] HDV viremia is associated with a greater likelihood of progression to cirrhosis.[56] In cirrhotics with HDV viremia, liver failure and all-cause mortality are increased,[32,44,53] and mortality in cirrhosis is twice as high as in HBV cirrhosis.[51] In an Italian cohort, transplant-free survival was 49% at 5 years.[57] In contrast, a subset of patients with chronic hepatitis develop a more benign clinical course[27,57] and avoid decompensation for 10 years even after developing cirrhosis.[57]

Hepatocellular Carcinoma

Hepatocellular carcinoma (HCC) caused by HDV develops at an annual rate of 2.8%[53] and a 5-year 13% risk been described in cohorts of cirrhotic patients.[51] HDV leads to a 3-fold increased risk for HCC[32,51] and is an independent risk factor for HCC.[32,38] However, once HCC has developed, tumor progression and survival are comparable to patients with HBV.[58] Persistent HBV replication has been associated with HCC,[55,56] as has lack of interferon treatment.[55] However, HCC was not linked to HDV in a Taiwanese population with high prevalence of HBV[59] and occurs at a similar age as HBV-related HCC in cases of superinfection.[60]

TREATMENT
Interferon

Although no therapy for HDV infection is currently approved by the US Food and Drug Administration (FDA), interferon (IFN) alfa is the only therapy endorsed by expert guidelines.[42,43] High-dose IFN-a2 (9 million international units 3 times weekly) for 1 year has shown a survival benefit in persons infected with HDV.[61] Better compliance has been achieved with pegylated IFN (PEG-IFN) alfa (1.5 μg/kg or 180 μg subcutaneously weekly), with similar side effects of flulike symptoms and leukopenia.[62,63] Treatment results in undetectable HDV RNA at end of treatment in 19% to 57% of patients,[62–66] with sustained response in 17% to 43% at 6 months of follow-up. However, sustained viral clearance persists in 28% of patients at 1 year,[66] and only a minority of patients remain HDV RNA negative years after treatment response.[67] Loss of HBsAg is the best indicator of remaining HDV RNA negative,[67,68] which is achieved in around 10% of patients.[67] Patients with higher HBV DNA loads seem to respond significantly faster to PEG-IFN than patients with HDV viremia only.[69] Tolerance and outcomes are not improved with the addition of ribavirin, adefovir, or entecavir.[63,66,70]

Patients with cirrhosis have a lower rate of response to treatment and have more adverse clinical liver-related events.[63,71] Maintaining HDV clearance results in a lower likelihood of liver-related morbidity or mortality,[71] and response to treatment leads to stabilization and improvement of fibrosis.[61,72] Clinical events occur at an annual rate of 2.5% (4.9% in cirrhosis),[67] significantly less frequently than in patients treated exclusively with nucleos(t)ide analogs or untreated patients.[54]

Length of treatment has been debated, with 2 years of PEG-IFN treatment resulting in 33% HDV clearance (with a nonsignificant difference in combination with tenofovir), and most patients achieving viral clearance during the first year of treatment.[72] Extension of treatment to 5 years results in a virological response in 30% to 50% of cases.[68,71]

Nucleos(t)ide Inhibitors

The use of nucleos(t)ide inhibitors for the treatment of HDV results in inhibition of HBV replication with minimal effects on HDV replication.[73] Adefovir,[66,74,75] lamivudine,[73] and tenofovir[75] do not affect HDV viremia significantly. Furthermore, liver-related outcomes and mortality are higher in patients with HDV than in cirrhotic patients monoinfected with HBV on treatment.[75]

Investigational Therapies

Because of the less than desirable results with IFN-alfa–based therapies, new approaches for the treatment of HDV have been studied. Although remaining investigational, these drugs that stimulate host functions or target the HDV replication cycle (see **Fig. 1**) have yielded encouraging results.

Interferon lambda

Although initially shown to induce interferon-stimulated genes resulting in antiviral and immunomodulatory activities in HBV and HCV, IFN-lambda therapy has been shown to reduce HDV RNA in vivo.[76] In an initial trial, a 24-week regimen of IFN-lambda achieved similar virologic response at 24 weeks after treatment (36%), with reduced side effects compared with IFN-alfa.[77] At present, a clinical trial (NCT03600714) is evaluating IFN-lambda in combination with lonafarnib and ritonavir (discussed later).

Hepatitis B virus/hepatitis delta virus entry inhibitors

The identification of specific receptors for virus binding has led to the development of molecules preventing the entry of HBV and HDV into hepatocytes. The myristoylated N-terminal pre-S1 domain of the large HBV surface protein binds to hepatocytes[7] at a site identified as the sodium taurocholate cotransporting polypeptide (NTCP).[78] Myrcludex B (bulevirtide), a myristoylated lipopeptide containing amino acids of the pre-S1 domain, showed tolerability and inhibition of HBV and HDV replication in vitro in a phase I study.[79] During a phase II study, a daily 2-mg subcutaneous injection of bulevirtide for 24 weeks alone or in combination with PEG-IFN-a2a significantly decreased HDV RNA in all participants, with 5 of 7 (71%) patients achieving HDV RNA clearance in the combination group and 2 out of 8 (25%) in the bulevirtide group.[80] A subsequent phase II study evaluated bulevirtide in doses of 2, 5, or 10 mg daily in combination with tenofovir for 24 weeks. Although resulting in a dose-dependent decline in HDV RNA, relapses occurred in up to 80% of patients after 12 weeks of follow-up.[81] At present, a phase II study evaluating the combination of bulevirtide (2 or 5 mg daily) alone or in combination with PEG-IFN-a2a for 48 weeks (NCT02888106) is recruiting in Russia. A European phase IIb study evaluating bulevirtide (2 or 10 mg daily) with or without PEG-IFN-a2a for 48 weeks (NCT03852433) and a phase III study evaluating bulevirtide (2 or 10 mg daily) for a total duration of 96 to 144 weeks (NCT03852719) are currently recruiting.

Prenylation inhibitors

As previously described, prenylation of the C terminus of the large HDAg is required in order to enable binding with the HBsAg and therefore formation of HDV virions.[6] First tested in mice, prenylation inhibitors, specifically farnesyltransferase inhibitors, FTI-277 and FTI-2153, contributed in HDV RNA clearance.[82] A proof-of-concept phase IIa study with oral lonafarnib treatment for 28 days revealed a significant dose-dependent reduction in HDV RNA compared with placebo.[83] Dose-dependent gastrointestinal side effects were noted, including nausea, diarrhea, and weight loss. Although HDV RNA decrease correlated with higher lonafarnib serum concentrations, side effects decreased its tolerability. With the addition of ritonavir, an inhibitor of cytochrome P450 3A4, the use of lower doses of lonafarnib has resulted in similar if not higher serum concentrations with improved gastrointestinal tolerability.[84] A follow-up phase II study has evaluated various dosing regimens of oral lonafarnib and ritonavir with the addition of PEG-IFN-a2a for a total of 12 to 24 weeks. A low dose of oral lonafarnib (25–50 mg twice daily) resulted in a reduction of viral load with reduced gastrointestinal side effects, with an even greater HDV RNA reduction with the addition of PEG-IFN-a2a.[85] Although a greater than 2 log decrease in HDV RNA was noted in 64% of patients, subgroup analysis revealed a higher response rate in patients with a baseline viral load less than 4 log.[86] Additional studies have focused on dose titration, with the description of superior viral load reduction with 50 mg of lonafarnib once daily compared with higher doses,[87] whereas a subsequent study showed that dose escalation up to 100 mg twice daily is feasible.[88]

Studies currently enrolling include a phase III study evaluating the combination of lonafarnib and ritonavir with or without PEG-INF-a2a (NCT03719313), and a phase II study evaluating the combination of investigational agents: PEG-IFN-lambda, lonafarnib, and ritonavir (NCT03600714).

Nucleic acid polymers

The antiviral effects of nucleic acid polymers include blocking the release of HBsAg, clearing circulating HBsAg, and assisting in control of viral infection. REP 2139 (at doses of 500 mg intravenously weekly for 15 weeks followed by 250 mg intravenously weekly for an additional 15 weeks) has been evaluated in combination with PEG-IFN-a2a, resulting in loss of HBsAg in 41% and negative HDV RNA in 58% of patients 1 year after completion of treatment,[89] all of whom remain HDV RNA negative at 18 months.[90] Although adverse effects caused by PEG-IFN were noted, no serious adverse effects caused by REP 2139 or previously reported symptoms caused by heavy metal intoxication during treatment were recorded. A follow-up study, NCT02876419, is evaluating response at 3 years.

TRANSPLANT

In the absence of successful therapies or nonclinical investigational therapies for HDV, the remaining available therapy is liver transplant. Indications for transplant include decompensated cirrhosis as well as HCC. An 88% 5-year posttransplant survival has been reported,[91] with some investigators describing a survival advantage as opposed to HBV monoinfection.[92]

Effective posttransplant HBV prophylaxis is crucial to prevent reinfection of the graft, with high morbidity and mortality before its introduction, and spontaneous clearance of HBV/HDV in only 18% of cases.[93] However, the use of hepatitis B immune globulin (HBIg) has reduced the reappearance of HBV/HDV to 13.2% of cases,[91] and the addition of nucleos(t)ide analogs to HBIg further reduces recurrence to 5.8% of cases.[94] A longer duration of HBIg has been recommended as a shorter use was associated with HDV recurrence[94] and because intrahepatic HDAg can remain detectable once HDV serum markers are negative.[95] Although isolated HDV viremia has been described in a few reports, possibly dependent on the capacity of PCR to detect low levels of HBV,[91] HBV reactivation is required for clinically apparent liver disease.[91,93]

SUMMARY

HDV remains a global health problem in the twenty-first century. Although improvements in public health have limited the spread of HBV, awareness needs to be raised to the clinical outcomes associated with coinfection with HDV. Although there remains a dire need for better treatments, recent advances yield encouraging results and give hope for better control of HDV.

DISCLOSURE

The authors report no conflicts of interest and have no financial support to disclose.

REFERENCES

1. Rizzetto M, Canese MG, Arico S, et al. Immunofluorescence detection of new antigen-antibody system (delta/anti-delta) associated to hepatitis B virus in liver and in serum of HBsAg carriers. Gut 1977;18(12):997–1003.

2. Rizzetto M, Canese MG, Gerin JL, et al. Transmission of the hepatitis B virus-associated delta antigen to chimpanzees. J Infect Dis 1980;141(5):590–602.
3. Chao M, Hsieh SY, Taylor J. Role of two forms of hepatitis delta virus antigen: evidence for a mechanism of self-limiting genome replication. J Virol 1990; 64(10):5066–9.
4. Sharmeen L, Kuo MY, Dinter-Gottlieb G, et al. Antigenomic RNA of human hepatitis delta virus can undergo self-cleavage. J Virol 1988;62(8):2674–9.
5. Casey JL. Control of ADAR1 editing of hepatitis delta virus RNAs. Curr Top Microbiol Immunol 2012;353:123–43.
6. Glenn JS, Watson JA, Havel CM, et al. Identification of a prenylation site in delta virus large antigen. Science 1992;256(5061):1331–3.
7. Engelke M, Mills K, Seitz S, et al. Characterization of a hepatitis B and hepatitis delta virus receptor binding site. Hepatology 2006;43(4):750–60.
8. Le Gal F, Brichler S, Sahli R, et al. First international external quality assessment for hepatitis delta virus RNA quantification in plasma. Hepatology 2016;64(5): 1483–94.
9. Sureau C, Negro F. The hepatitis delta virus: Replication and pathogenesis. J Hepatol 2016;64(1 Suppl):S102–16.
10. Chen HY, Shen DT, Ji DZ. Prevalence and burden of hepatitis D virus infection in the global population: a systematic review and meta-analysis. Gut 2019;68(3): 512–21.
11. Wranke A, Pinheiro Borzacov LM, Parana R, et al. Clinical and virological heterogeneity of hepatitis delta in different regions world-wide: The Hepatitis Delta International Network (HDIN). Liver Int 2018;38(5):842–50.
12. Stroffolini T, Sagnelli E, Sagnelli C, et al. Hepatitis delta infection in Italian patients: towards the end of the story? Infection 2017;45(3):277–81.
13. Chen F, Zhang J, Guo F, et al. Hepatitis B, C, and D virus infection showing distinct patterns between injection drug users and the general population. J Gastroenterol Hepatol 2017;32(2):515–20.
14. Chen X, Oidovsambuu O, Liu P, et al. A novel quantitative microarray antibody capture assay identifies an extremely high hepatitis delta virus prevalence among hepatitis B virus-infected mongolians. Hepatology 2017;66(6):1739–49.
15. Mumtaz K, Hamid SS, Adil S, et al. Epidemiology and clinical pattern of hepatitis delta virus infection in Pakistan. J Gastroenterol Hepatol 2005;20(10):1503–7.
16. Huo TI, Wu JC, Lin RY, et al. Decreasing hepatitis D virus infection in Taiwan: an analysis of contributory factors. J Gastroenterol Hepatol 1997;12(11):747–51.
17. Amini N, Alavian SM, Kabir A, et al. Prevalence of hepatitis d in the eastern mediterranean region: systematic review and meta analysis. Hepat Mon 2013;13(1): e8210.
18. Braga WS, Castilho Mda C, Borges FG, et al. Hepatitis D virus infection in the Western Brazilian Amazon - far from a vanishing disease. Rev Soc Bras Med Trop 2012;45(6):691–5.
19. Stockdale AJ, Chaponda M, Beloukas A, et al. Prevalence of hepatitis D virus infection in sub-Saharan Africa: a systematic review and meta-analysis. Lancet Glob Health 2017;5(10):e992–1003.
20. Makuwa M, Caron M, Souquiere S, et al. Prevalence and genetic diversity of hepatitis B and delta viruses in pregnant women in Gabon: molecular evidence that hepatitis delta virus clade 8 originates from and is endemic in central Africa. J Clin Microbiol 2008;46(2):754–6.
21. Mahale P, Aka P, Chen X, et al. Hepatitis D virus infection, cirrhosis and hepatocellular carcinoma in The Gambia. J Viral Hepat 2019;26(6):738–49.

22. Lunel-Fabiani F, Mansour W, Amar AO, et al. Impact of hepatitis B and delta virus co-infection on liver disease in Mauritania: a cross sectional study. J Infect 2013; 67(5):448–57.

23. Servant-Delmas A, Le Gal F, Gallian P, et al. Increasing prevalence of HDV/HBV infection over 15 years in France. J Clin Virol 2014;59(2):126–8.

24. Wedemeyer H, Heidrich B, Manns MP. Hepatitis D virus infection–not a vanishing disease in Europe! Hepatology 2007;45(5):1331–2 [author reply: 1332–3].

25. Manesis EK, Vourli G, Dalekos G, et al. Prevalence and clinical course of hepatitis delta infection in Greece: a 13-year prospective study. J Hepatol 2013;59(5): 949–56.

26. Nicolini LA, Taramasso L, Schiavetti I, et al. Epidemiological and clinical features of hepatitis delta in HBsAg-positive patients by HIV status. Antivir Ther 2015; 20(2):193–7.

27. Gaeta GB, Stroffolini T, Chiaramonte M, et al. Chronic hepatitis D: a vanishing Dis-ease? An Italian multicenter study. Hepatology 2000;32(4 Pt 1):824–7.

28. Mele A, Mariano A, Tosti ME, et al. Acute hepatitis delta virus infection in Italy: incidence and risk factors after the introduction of the universal anti-hepatitis B vaccination campaign. Clin Infect Dis 2007;44(3):e17–24.

29. El Bouzidi K, Elamin W, Kranzer K, et al. Hepatitis delta virus testing, epidemi-ology and management: a multicentre cross-sectional study of patients in London. J Clin Virol 2015;66:33–7.

30. Cross TJ, Rizzi P, Horner M, et al. The increasing prevalence of hepatitis delta vi-rus (HDV) infection in South London. J Med Virol 2008;80(2):277–82.

31. Bart PA, Jacquier P, Zuber PLF, et al. Seroprevalence of HBV (anti-HBc, HBsAg and anti-HBs) and HDV infections among 9006 women at delivery. Liver 1996;16: 110–6.

32. Kushner T, Serper M, Kaplan DE. Delta hepatitis within the Veterans Affairs med-ical system in the United States: Prevalence, risk factors, and outcomes. J Hepatol 2015;63(3):586–92.

33. Njei B, Do A, Lim JK. Prevalence of Hepatitis Delta Infection in the United States: national health and nutrition examination survey, 1999-2012. Hepatology 2016; 64(2):680–1.

34. Mahale P, Aka PV, Chen X, et al. Hepatitis D Viremia among injection drug users in San Francisco. J Infect Dis 2018;217(12):1902–6.

35. Soriano V, Grint D, d'Arminio Monforte A, et al. Hepatitis delta in HIV-infected in-dividuals in Europe. AIDS 2011;25(16):1987–92.

36. Lin HH, Lee SS, Yu ML, et al. Changing hepatitis D virus epidemiology in a hep-atitis B virus endemic area with a national vaccination program. Hepatology 2015; 61(6):1870–9.

37. Kao JH, Chen PJ, Lai MY, et al. Hepatitis D virus genotypes in intravenous drug users in taiwan: decreasing prevalence and lack of correlation with hepatitis B vi-rus genotypes. J Clin Microbiol 2002;40(8):3047–9.

38. Beguelin C, Moradpour D, Sahli R, et al. Hepatitis delta-associated mortality in HIV/HBV-coinfected patients. J Hepatol 2017;66(2):297–303.

39. Lee CY, Tsai HC, Lee SS, et al. Higher rate of hepatitis events in patients with hu-man immunodeficiency virus, hepatitis B, and hepatitis D genotype II infection: a cohort study in a medical center in southern Taiwan. J Microbiol Immunol Infect 2015;48(1):20–7.

40. Troisi CL, Hollinger FB, Hoots WK, et al. A multicenter study of viral hepatitis in a United States hemophilic population. Blood 1993;81(2):412–8.

41. Pierre A, Feldner A, Carvalho Filho RJ, et al. Prevalence of hepatitis delta virus among hemodialysis and renal transplant patients. Int J Artif Organs 2018; 41(3):171–4.
42. European Association for the Study of the Liver. EASL 2017 clinical practice guidelines on the management of hepatitis B virus infection. J Hepatol 2017; 67(2):370–98.
43. Terrault NA, Lok ASF, McMahon BJ, et al. Update on prevention, diagnosis, and treatment of chronic hepatitis B: AASLD 2018 hepatitis B guidance. Hepatology 2018;67(4):1560–99.
44. Su CW, Huang YH, Huo TI, et al. Genotypes and viremia of hepatitis B and D viruses are associated with outcomes of chronic hepatitis D patients. Gastroenterology 2006;130(6):1625–35.
45. Jardi R, Buti M, Rodriguez F, et al. Comparative analysis of serological markers of chronic delta infection: HDV-RNA, serum HDAg and anti-HD IgM. J Virol Methods 1994;50(1–3):59–66.
46. Simpson LH, Battegay M, Hoofnagle JH, et al. Hepatitis delta virus RNA in serum of patients with chronic delta hepatitis. Dig Dis Sci 1994;39(12):2650–5.
47. Zignego AL, Dubois F, Samuel D, et al. Serum hepatitis delta virus RNA in patients with delta hepatitis and in liver graft recipients. J Hepatol 1990;11(1): 102–10.
48. Negro F. Hepatitis D virus coinfection and superinfection. Cold Spring Harb Perspect Med 2014;4(11):a021550.
49. Pasetti G, Calzetti C, Degli Antoni A, et al. Clinical features of hepatitis delta virus infection in a northern Italian area. Infection 1988;16(6):345–8.
50. Dienes HP, Purcell RH, Popper H, et al. The significance of infections with two types of viral hepatitis demonstrated by histologic features in chimpanzees. J Hepatol 1990;10(1):77–84.
51. Fattovich G, Giustina G, Christensen E, et al. Influence of hepatitis delta virus infection on morbidity and mortality in compensated cirrhosis type B. The European Concerted Action on Viral Hepatitis (Eurohep). Gut 2000;46(3):420–6.
52. Fattovich G, Boscaro S, Noventa F, et al. Influence of hepatitis delta virus infection on progression to cirrhosis in chronic hepatitis type B. J Infect Dis 1987;155(5): 931–5.
53. Romeo R, Del Ninno E, Rumi M, et al. A 28-year study of the course of hepatitis Delta infection: a risk factor for cirrhosis and hepatocellular carcinoma. Gastroenterology 2009;136(5):1629–38.
54. Wranke A, Serrano BC, Heidrich B, et al. Antiviral treatment and liver-related complications in hepatitis delta. Hepatology 2017;65(2):414–25.
55. Niro GA, Smedile A, Ippolito AM, et al. Outcome of chronic delta hepatitis in Italy: a long-term cohort study. J Hepatol 2010;53(5):834–40.
56. Romeo R, Foglieni B, Casazza G, et al. High serum levels of HDV RNA are predictors of cirrhosis and liver cancer in patients with chronic hepatitis delta. PLoS One 2014;9(3):e92062.
57. Rosina F, Conoscitore P, Cuppone R, et al. Changing pattern of chronic hepatitis D in Southern Europe. Gastroenterology 1999;117(1):161–6.
58. Huo TI, Wu JC, Lai CR, et al. Comparison of clinico-pathological features in hepatitis B virus-associated hepatocellular carcinoma with or without hepatitis D virus superinfection. J Hepatol 1996;25(4):439–44.
59. Chen DS, Lai MY, Sung JL. Delta agent infection in patients with chronic liver diseases and hepatocellular carcinoma–an infrequent finding in Taiwan. Hepatology 1984;4(3):502–3.

60. Wu JC, Chen TZ, Huang YS, et al. Natural history of hepatitis D viral superinfection: significance of viremia detected by polymerase chain reaction. Gastroenterology 1995;108(3):796–802.

61. Farci P, Roskams T, Chessa L, et al. Long-term benefit of interferon alpha therapy of chronic hepatitis D: regression of advanced hepatic fibrosis. Gastroenterology 2004;126(7):1740–9.

62. Castelnau C, Le Gal F, Ripault MP, et al. Efficacy of peginterferon alpha-2b in chronic hepatitis delta: relevance of quantitative RT-PCR for follow-up. Hepatology 2006;44(3):728–35.

63. Niro GA, Ciancio A, Gaeta GB, et al. Pegylated interferon alpha-2b as monotherapy or in combination with ribavirin in chronic hepatitis delta. Hepatology 2006;44(3):713–20.

64. Farci P, Mandas A, Coiana A, et al. Treatment of chronic hepatitis D with interferon alfa-2a. N Engl J Med 1994;330(2):88–94.

65. Yurdaydin C, Bozkaya H, Karaaslan H, et al. A pilot study of 2 years of interferon treatment in patients with chronic delta hepatitis. J Viral Hepat 2007;14(11):812–6.

66. Wedemeyer H, Yurdaydin C, Dalekos GN, et al. Peginterferon plus adefovir versus either drug alone for hepatitis delta. N Engl J Med 2011;364(4):322–31.

67. Heidrich B, Yurdaydin C, Kabacam G, et al. Late HDV RNA relapse after peginterferon alpha-based therapy of chronic hepatitis delta. Hepatology 2014;60(1):87–97.

68. Heller T, Rotman Y, Koh C, et al. Long-term therapy of chronic delta hepatitis with peginterferon alfa. Aliment Pharmacol Ther 2014;40(1):93–104.

69. Lutterkort GL, Wranke A, Hengst J, et al. Viral dominance patterns in chronic hepatitis delta determine early response to interferon alpha therapy. J Viral Hepat 2018;25(11):1384–94.

70. Gunsar F, Akarca US, Ersoz G, et al. Two-year interferon therapy with or without ribavirin in chronic delta hepatitis. Antivir Ther 2005;10(6):721–6.

71. Yurdaydin C, Keskin O, Kalkan C, et al. Interferon treatment duration in patients with chronic delta hepatitis and its effect on the natural course of the disease. J Infect Dis 2018;217(8):1184–92.

72. Wedemeyer H, Yurdaydin C, Hardtke S, et al. Peginterferon alfa-2a plus tenofovir disoproxil fumarate for hepatitis D (HIDIT-II): a randomised, placebo controlled, phase 2 trial. Lancet Infect Dis 2019;19(3):275–86.

73. Niro GA, Ciancio A, Tillman HL, et al. Lamivudine therapy in chronic delta hepatitis: a multicentre randomized-controlled pilot study. Aliment Pharmacol Ther 2005;22(3):227–32.

74. Grattagliano I, Palmieri VO, Portincasa P, et al. Adefovir dipivoxyl for the treatment of delta-related liver cirrhosis. Ann Pharmacother 2006;40(9):1681–4.

75. Brancaccio G, Fasano M, Grossi A, et al. Clinical outcomes in patients with hepatitis D, cirrhosis and persistent hepatitis B virus replication, and receiving long-term tenofovir or entecavir. Aliment Pharmacol Ther 2019;49(8):1071–6.

76. Giersch K, Homs M, Volz T, et al. Both interferon alpha and lambda can reduce all intrahepatic HDV infection markers in HBV/HDV infected humanized mice. Sci Rep 2017;7(1):3757.

77. Etzion O, Hamid SS, Lurie Y, et al. End of study results from LIMT HDV study: 36% durable virologic response at 24 weeks post-treatment with pegylated interferon

lambda monotherapy in patients with chronic hepatitis delta virus infection. J Hepatol 2019;70(1):e32.

78. Yan H, Zhong G, Xu G, et al. Sodium taurocholate cotransporting polypeptide is a functional receptor for human hepatitis B and D virus. Elife 2012; 1:e00049.

79. Blank A, Markert C, Hohmann N, et al. First-in-human application of the novel hepatitis B and hepatitis D virus entry inhibitor myrcludex B. J Hepatol 2016; 65(3):483–9.

80. Bogomolov P, Alexandrov A, Voronkova N, et al. Treatment of chronic hepatitis D with the entry inhibitor myrcludex B: First results of a phase Ib/IIa study. J Hepatol 2016;65(3):490–8.

81. Wedemeyer H, Bogomolov P, Blank A, et al. Final results of a multicenter, open-label phase 2b clinical trial to assess safety and efficacy of Myrcludex B in combination with Tenofovir in patients with chronic HBV/HDV co-infection. J Hepatol 2018;68:s3.

82. Bordier BB, Ohkanda J, Liu P, et al. In vivo antiviral efficacy of prenylation inhibitors against hepatitis delta virus. J Clin Invest 2003;112(3):407–14.

83. Koh C, Canini L, Dahari H, et al. Oral prenylation inhibition with lonafarnib in chronic hepatitis D infection: a proof-of-concept randomised, double-blind, placebo-controlled phase 2A trial. Lancet Infect Dis 2015;15(10):1167–74.

84. Yurdaydin C, Keskin O, Kalkan C, et al. Optimizing lonafarnib treatment for the management of chronic delta hepatitis: The LOWR HDV-1 study. Hepatology 2018;67(4):1224–36.

85. Yurdaydin C, Idilman R, Keskin O, et al. A phase 2 dose-optimization study of lonafarnib with ritonavir for the treatment of chronic delta hepatitis—end of treatment results from the LOWR HDV-2 study. J Hepatol 2017;66(1):S33–4.

86. Yurdaydin C, Kalkan C, Karakaya F, et al. Subanalysis of the LOWR HDV-2 study reveals high response rates to Lonafarnib in patients with low viral loads. J Hepatol 2018;68:S89.

87. Koh C, Surana P, Han T, et al. A phase 2 study exploring once daily dosing of ritonavir boosted lonafarnib for the treatment of chronic delta hepatitis – end of study results from the LOWR HDV-3 study. J Hepatol 2017;66(1):S101–2.

88. Wedemeyer H, Port K, Deterding K, et al. A phase 2 dose-escalation study of lonafarnib plus ritonavir in patients with chronic hepatitis D: final results from the Lonafarnib with ritonavir in HDV-4 (LOWR HDV-4) study. J Hepatol 2017;66(1).

89. Bazinet M, Pantea V, Cebotarescu V, et al. Safety and efficacy of REP 2139 and pegylated interferon alfa-2a for treatment-naive patients with chronic hepatitis B virus and hepatitis D virus co-infection (REP 301 and REP 301-LTF): a non-randomised, open-label, phase 2 trial. Lancet Gastroenterol Hepatol 2017; 2(12):877–89.

90. Bazinet M, Pantea V, Cebotarescu V, et al. Establishment of persistent functional remission of HBV and HDV infection following REP 2139 and pegylated interferon alpha 2a therapy in patients with chronic HBV/HDV co-infection: 18 month follow-up results from the REP 301-LTF study. J Hepatol 2018;68:S509.

91. Samuel D, Zignego AL, Reynes M, et al. Long-term clinical and virological outcome after liver transplantation for cirrhosis caused by chronic delta hepatitis. Hepatology 1995;21(2):333–9.

92. Rifai K, Wedemeyer H, Rosenau J, et al. Longer survival of liver transplant recipients with hepatitis virus coinfections. Clin Transpl 2007;21(2):258–64.

93. Ottobrelli A, Marzano A, Smedile A, et al. Patterns of hepatitis delta virus rein-
    fection and disease in liver transplantation. Gastroenterology 1991;101(6):
    1649–55.
94. Cholongitas E, Goulis I, Antoniadis N, et al. Nucleos(t)ide analog(s) prophylaxis
    after hepatitis B immunoglobulin withdrawal against hepatitis B and D recurrence
    after liver transplantation. Transpl Infect Dis 2016;18(5):667–73.
95. Mederacke I, Filmann N, Yurdaydin C, et al. Rapid early HDV RNA decline in the
    peripheral blood but prolonged intrahepatic hepatitis delta antigen persistence
    after liver transplantation. J Hepatol 2012;56(1):115–22.

Progress Toward Hepatitis C Virus Elimination

Therapy and Implementation

Marianne Martinello, MBBS, FRACP, PhD*, Sahar Bajis, BPharm, MPH, PhD,
Gregory J. Dore, BSc, MBBS, MPH, FRACP, PhD

KEYWORDS

- Hepatitis C • Treatment • Direct-acting antivirals • Elimination • Global health
- People who inject drugs • Sustainable development goals
- Universal health coverage

KEY POINTS

- The adoption of the World Health Organization (WHO) hepatitis C virus (HCV) elimination 2030 targets has galvanized considerable global and national responses.
- The introduction of direct-acting antiviral (DAA) therapy has generated the impetus for global HCV elimination, but primary prevention strategies, including high harm-reduction coverage for people who inject drugs remain essential.
- Twelve countries are considered on track to achieve HCV elimination targets by 2030, including both high-income and low- to middle-income countries.
- Novel strategies to enhance HCV screening and linkage to care are crucial.
- Innovative financing mechanisms, low-cost HCV diagnostics, and low-cost DAA therapy are pivotal in achieving global HCV elimination.

INTRODUCTION

In 2015, 71 million people were estimated to be living with chronic hepatitis C virus (HCV) infection worldwide.[1] With ongoing transmission related largely to injecting drug use and unsafe health care injection practices, approximately 2 million people are newly infected each year.[2] Mortality from HCV-related cirrhosis and its complications, including hepatocellular carcinoma, is estimated at 475,000 deaths per year.[3] In light of the global disease burden attributed to hepatitis B virus (HBV) and HCV infection, the World Health Organization (WHO) adopted the first global hepatitis strategy in 2016 and proposed the "elimination of viral hepatitis as a public health threat" by 2030 (**Table 1**).[4]

Viral Hepatitis Clinical Research Program, The Kirby Institute, UNSW Sydney, Sydney, Australia
* Corresponding author. The Kirby Institute, UNSW Sydney, Wallace Wurth Building, Sydney, New South Wales 2052, Australia.
E-mail address: mmartinello@kirby.unsw.edu.au

Table 1
World Health Organization hepatitis C virus elimination targets[4]

	2015 Baseline	2020 Target	2030 Target
Impact Targets			
Incidence	-	30% reduction	80% reduction
New cases of HCV infection, n	1 750 000	1 230 000	<350,000
Mortality	-	10% reduction	65% reduction
HCV-related deaths,[a] n	399,000	359,100	139,650
Service Delivery Targets			
Diagnosis Proportion diagnosed with HCV	20%	30%	90%
Treatment Uptake Proportion with HCV diagnosed and initiated on treatment	7%	Not specified (3 million[b])	80% (cumulative)
Blood Safety Donations screened with quality assurance	97%	95%	100%
Injection Safety Proportion of unsafe injections	5%	0%	0%
Harm Reduction Number of sterile needles and syringes distributed per PWID per year	27	200	300

[a] Death predominantly caused by hepatocellular carcinoma and cirrhosis.
[b] Total cumulative HCV treatment uptake target by 2020.

The development and availability of highly effective direct-acting antiviral (DAA) therapy has revolutionized the management of HCV infection, providing the therapeutic tools required for elimination.[5] Despite major advances in HCV therapy, globally, the proportion of people living with HCV who have been diagnosed and treated is inadequate.[6] In 2016, the number of new HCV infections continued to exceed DAA-based cure.[7] In the absence of a vaccine, HCV elimination will require a combination of enhanced prevention and broad scale-up of DAA therapy (treatment-as-prevention).

This article summarizes current management of HCV infection; defines the epidemiologic concepts of control, elimination, and eradication; and discusses strategies required to achieve global HCV elimination. Examples of successful national HCV strategies are presented, highlighting the facilitators and barriers to implementation of HCV elimination strategies.

DIRECT-ACTING ANTIVIRAL THERAPY FOR CHRONIC HEPATITIS C VIRUS INFECTION: THE CURRENT STATE OF PLAY

The goal of treatment is cure of HCV infection (with achievement of a sustained virological response [SVR], defined as undetectable HCV RNA in blood 12 or 24 weeks after treatment) in order to prevent HCV-related hepatic and extrahepatic complications, prevent onward transmission, and improve quality of life.[8] SVR is associated with improvements in liver fibrosis stage, quality of life and survival, and reduction in HCV-related morbidity.[9,10]

The treatment paradigm for individuals with chronic HCV infection has evolved rapidly in the last decade (**Fig. 1**). The first-generation HCV protease inhibitors,

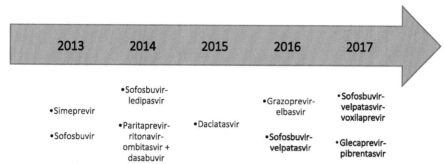

2013	2014	2015	2016	2017
•Simeprevir	•Sofosbuvir-ledipasvir	•Daclatasvir	•Grazoprevir-elbasvir	•Sofosbuvir-velpatasvir-voxilaprevir
•Sofosbuvir	•Paritaprevir-ritonavir-ombitasvir + dasabuvir		•Sofosbuvir-velpatasvir	•Glecaprevir-pibrentasvir

Fig. 1. Milestones in HCV direct-acting antiviral development. Between 2013 and 2017, 5 NS3/4a protease inhibitors (simeprevir, ritonavir-boosted paritaprevir, grazoprevir, voxilaprevir, glecaprevir), 6 NS5A inhibitors (ledipasvir, ombitasvir, daclatasvir, elbasvir, velpatasvir, pibrentasvir), and 2 NS5B polymerase inhibitors (nucleotide: sofosbuvir; non-nucleotide: dasabuvir) were approved by the US Food and Drug Administration for treatment of chronic HCV infection in adults. Combinations of 2 or 3 DAAs from different classes for 8 to 24 weeks achieve cure (sustained virological response) in more than 90% of people treated. Pan-genotypic DAA regimens are highlighted in **bold**.

telaprevir and boceprevir, were approved for use in combination with pegylated-interferon and ribavirin in 2011[11]; however, these agents were rapidly rendered obsolete given inferior efficacy and poor tolerability. In 2014, the first interferon-free regimens, sofosbuvir-ledipasvir and sofosbuvir plus simeprevir, were approved for the treatment of genotype 1 HCV infection, followed by the first pan-genotypic regimen, sofosbuvir-velpatasvir, in 2016.

Major milestones in DAA development include

Very high cure rates (SVR ≥95%) in both treatment-naïve and experienced individuals across all genotypes
Short duration of treatment for 8 to 12 weeks for first-line therapy (with 8 weeks of glecaprevir/pibrentasvir for treatment-naïve individuals with no cirrhosis)
Oral administration of once-a-day pan-genotypic regimens (without ribavirin) with few to no adverse effects
Extremely low rates of HCV resistance

Currently, 3 pan-genotypic fixed-dose combination DAA regimens are available: sofosbuvir-velpatasvir, glecaprevir-pibrentasvir, and sofosbuvir-velpatasvir-voxilaprevir (**Table 2**). Sofosbuvir-velpatasvir-voxilaprevir was specifically developed as a second-line or salvage regimen for people with virological failure following previous DAA therapy.

Direct-Acting Antiviral Therapy for People Who Inject Drugs

Importantly, DAA therapy is safe and effective among priority populations, including people who inject drugs (PWID) and people living with HIV.[12,13] Of the 71 million people living with chronic HCV infection, 6.1 million people have recently injected drugs.[14] Despite improvements in HCV therapy, HCV treatment uptake among PWID remains suboptimal. Barriers to treatment uptake include physician reluctance to provide HCV therapy to PWID[15] and payer restrictions in some countries and jurisdictions based on ongoing drug use or receiving OST.[16,17] This arises from historic concerns about interferon-based treatment adherence, poorer outcomes compared with the general population, and the risk of HCV reinfection.[15,18]

Table 2
US Food and Drug Administration-approved hepatitis C virus NS3/4A protease inhibitors, NS5B polymerase inhibitors, and NS5A inhibitors: administration and dosage in adults

Drug Name	Formulation	Routine Adult Dosage		Precautions and Dose Adjustments
Single drug class				
NS5B polymerase inhibitors				
Sofosbuvir	400 mg tablet	400 mg once daily	Impaired renal function	Not recommended for GFR <30 mL/min, hemodialysis
			Impaired hepatic function	No dose adjustment
			Pregnancy and lactating women	Pregnancy category B
Dasabuvir	250 mg tablet	250 mg twice daily	Impaired renal function	No dose adjustment
			Impaired hepatic function	Contraindicated in moderate and severe hepatic impairment
			Pregnancy and lactating women	Pregnancy category B
NS5A inhibitor				
Daclatasvir	30 mg tablet	60 mg once daily	Impaired renal function	No dose adjustment
	60 mg tablet		Impaired hepatic function	No dose adjustment
			Pregnancy and lactating women	Contraindicated
Multiple drug classes in fixed-dose combination				
NS3/4A protease inhibitor + NS5A inhibitor				
Ombitasvir + paritaprevir + ritonavir	12.5 mg/75 mg/50 mg tablet	25 mg/150 mg/100 mg daily (2 tablets once daily)	Impaired renal function	No dose adjustment
			Impaired hepatic function	Contraindicated in moderate and severe hepatic impairment
			Pregnancy and lactating women	Pregnancy category B
Grazoprevir + elbasvir	100 mg/50 mg tablet	100 mg/50 mg daily (1 tablet once daily)	Impaired renal function	No dose adjustment
			Impaired hepatic function	Contraindicated in moderate and severe hepatic impairment
			Pregnancy and lactating women	No data

Drug	Tablet	Daily dose	Condition	Recommendation
Glecaprevir + pibrentasvir	100 mg/40 mg tablet	300 mg/120 mg daily (3 tablets once daily)	Impaired renal function	No dose adjustment
			Impaired hepatic function	Not recommended in moderate hepatic impairment; Contraindicated in severe hepatic impairment
			Pregnancy and lactating women	Pregnancy category B
NS5B polymerase inhibitor + NS5A inhibitor				
Sofosbuvir + ledipasvir	400 mg/90 mg tablet	400 mg/90 mg daily (1 tablet once daily)	Impaired renal function	Not recommended for GFR <30 mL/min, haemodialysis sis
			Impaired hepatic function	No dose adjustment
			Pregnancy and lactating women	Pregnancy category B
Sofosbuvir + velpatasvir	400 mg/100 mg tablet	400 mg/100 mg daily (1 tablet once daily)	Impaired renal function	Not recommended for GFR <30 mL/min, hemodialysis
			Impaired hepatic function	Administer with ribavirin in moderate-to-severe impairment
			Pregnancy and lactating women	No data
NS5B polymerase inhibitor + NS5A inhibitor + NS3/4A protease inhibitor				
Sofosbuvir + velpatasvir + voxilaprevir	400 mg/100 mg/ 100 mg tablet	400 mg/100 mg/ 100 mg daily (1 tablet once daily)	Impaired renal function	No dose adjustment in mild-moderate renal impairment; No data in severe renal impairment
			Impaired hepatic function	Not recommended in moderate-severe hepatic impairment
			Pregnancy and lactating women	No data

Degree of hepatic impairment: mild refers to Child Pugh Class A; moderate refers to Child Pugh Class B, and severe refers to Child Pugh Class C.

A recent meta-analysis of clinical trials and observational studies demonstrated favorable DAA treatment outcomes; among people receiving OST, treatment completion was 97%, and SVR by ITT was 91%.[19] In people with recent drug use (injecting and noninjecting), treatment completion and SVR by ITT was 98% and 88%, respectively. Clinical trials (vs observational studies) and older age were associated with higher ITT SVR (94% vs 89%). The lower SVR observed among people who have recently used drugs (both injecting and noninjecting), is likely attributable to post-treatment loss to follow-up (ie, between end-of-treatment and SVR12) and not virological failure. This emphasizes the need to improve retention in post-treatment care through innovative models of care tailored to the unique needs of PWID. Integration of HCV care within drug user health services has been shown to be effective in engaging and retaining people in HCV care.[20,21] Importantly, OST should not be a precondition to receiving HCV treatment, particularly given many people who report recent injecting are not opioid dependent and therefore are not candidates for OST.

Treatment as Prevention

Treatment as prevention incorporates treatment as a tool for limiting spread of an infection in generalized epidemics, by reducing the pool of infection in the community and subsequent risk of transmission.[22] For an HCV treatment-as-prevention strategy to be effective there must be broad coverage of HCV testing and expedient linkage to care and treatment, and targeted interventions in populations with high HCV prevalence and incidence. In populations of PWID, for instance, interventions must also include high coverage of harm-reduction strategies to reduce pretreatment prevalence and prevent reinfection.

DAA treatment uptake must improve if the WHO 2030 elimination targets are to be met. In 2015 and 2016, almost 3 million people initiated DAA treatment.[23] As such, treated HCV infections are only keeping pace with new HCV infections.[7] Most people living with HCV infection remain undiagnosed and untreated. In jurisdictions with unrestricted access to DAAs, encouraging initial reports highlight high DAA uptake among HIV-positive men-who-have-sex-with-men (MSM) with corresponding reductions in HCV viremic prevalence and incidence, providing preliminary empirical evidence in support of HCV treatment as prevention.[24–26] As linkage to care and engagement with health services are generally high among HIV-positive MSM, the short- and long-term success of HCV elimination service implementation in this population should provide important information for use in other settings.

CONTROL, ELIMINATION, AND ERADICATION

The WHO viral hepatitis elimination targets need to be viewed in the context of established epidemiologic definitions. Definitions of control, elimination, and eradication in the field of infectious diseases are presented in **Table 3**.[27] Although the WHO has called for elimination of HCV as a public health threat, the targets set are in keeping with HCV epidemiologic control. The use of the term elimination may relate to the aspirational element associated with the former term, and ensures consistency with global efforts in relation to HBV, HIV, malaria, and tuberculosis.

HCV elimination should be biologically feasible. When considering elimination of an infectious disease, 3 fundamental biologic and technical factors underpin feasibility, including the availability of an effective intervention, the availability of practical sensitive and specific diagnostic tools, and the role of people in the life cycle of the pathogen. In relation to HCV, effective therapeutic and prevention interventions are

Table 3
Dahlem workshop on the eradication of infectious diseases[27]

Epidemiologic Term	Definition	Example(s)
Control	The reduction of disease incidence, prevalence, morbidity, or mortality to a locally acceptable level as a result of deliberate efforts; continued intervention measures are required to maintain the reduction	Diarrheal diseases Schistosomiasis
Elimination of disease	Reduction to zero of the incidence of a specified disease in a defined geographic area as a result of deliberate efforts; continued intervention measures are required	Neonatal tetanus
Elimination of infection	Reduction to zero of the incidence of infection caused by a specific agent in a defined geographic area as a result of deliberate efforts; continued measures to prevent re-establishment of transmission are required	Measles Poliomyelitis
Eradication	Permanent reduction to zero of the worldwide incidence of infection caused by a specific agent as a result of deliberate efforts; intervention measures are no longer needed	Smallpox
Extinction	The specific infectious agent no longer exists in nature or in the laboratory	None

available to curb HCV transmission; HCV diagnostics are evolving to allow broader access and implementation, and infected people are the exclusive reservoir of HCV.

When discussing the WHO HCV elimination targets, it is also important to remember that inherent to the definitions of control and elimination is the need for continued intervention measures to prevent re-emergence and re-establishment of transmission. The need for continued interventions after reaching control or elimination targets can pose a public health challenge. Misunderstanding, inadequate surveillance, insufficient financial resources, and lack of political will can lead to neglect or cessation of intervention activities and resultant re-emergence of the target disease. Global progress in combating infectious diseases has been uneven, with many millions (predominantly in low- and middle-income countries [LMICs]) unable to access appropriate treatment and prevention. Historically, the fight against infectious diseases has been impeded by social, legal, and economic barriers, with significant funding gaps. These issues are paramount in designing national and global HCV elimination strategies, to ensure equitable access to HCV care and treatment.

Hepatitis C Virus Microelimination

Microelimination refers to targeted and tailored treatment and prevention interventions, which allow for the effective implementation and evaluation in specific populations or geographic regions in accordance with local epidemiology and resources.[28] Given the enormous task of HCV elimination, the approach of microelimination in specified populations has been proposed in both countries with comprehensive national HCV elimination strategies (eg, Australia, Iceland, and Scotland), and in countries (particularly LMICs) struggling to mobilize domestic and international resources and infrastructure to implement nation-wide strategy.[28] The microelimination approach permits the setting of smaller targets for subpopulations, with achievable targets geared toward national elimination. Features of a successful microelimination strategy include multistakeholder involvement and the development of a well-resourced plan that overcomes individual, structural, and organizational barriers to care experienced by the target population.[28] A monitoring and evaluation plan must be implemented with achievable targets based on mathematical modeling data, where appropriate.

Selection of a population for microelimination should be based on local epidemiology, national priorities, and health system resources, and as such varies in countries. Mathematical modeling suggests that substantial reductions in HCV incidence and prevalence could be achieved by targeted HCV treatment scale-up among those at highest risk of ongoing transmission, including PWID and HIV-positive MSM, across a wide range of settings.[29–32] For instance, regardless of prevalence, modeling studies show that treating less than 100 cases per 1000 PWID per year results in considerable HCV prevalence and incidence reductions.[32] Currently, microelimination efforts are underway in the Tayside region of Scotland to eliminate HCV among high-risk groups, with focus on PWID.[33] Interventions in various settings include nurse-led models of care, pharmacist-led treatment of OST clients in community pharmacies, and treatment in prisons and addiction treatment centers. The aim is to increase the number treated required to reduce prevalence to below 10% and incidence to below 1% over 3 years. A microelimination initiative in an Australian prison demonstrated a reduction in HCV viremia from 12% to less than 1% over a 22-month period with rapid DAA scale-up.[34] Notably, 5 reinfection cases were observed, highlighting ongoing HCV exposure risks and pertinence of the implementation of harm reduction strategies.

WHAT IS NEEDED TO ACHIEVE GLOBAL HEPATITIS C VIRUS ELIMINATION?

Biological and technical feasibility alone is insufficient; a successful elimination strategy must also consider health system capabilities and political and socioeconomic factors.[27,35] HCV elimination challenges include

Limited reliable epidemiologic data
Inadequate HCV testing and diagnosis
Limited access to treatment and harm reduction for PWID
Inadequate HCV education and training for health care providers
Continued iatrogenic transmission in LMICs
Stigma and discrimination against people living with HCV and people at high-risk of HCV (including PWID and MSM)
Variable leadership from governments and policy makers
Financial constraints

Although HCV control and elimination are conceptually simple, with unequivocal outcome, global operational challenges make implementation difficult.

The launch of the WHO HCV elimination targets has galvanized global efforts. Many countries have developed HCV or viral hepatitis national strategies, a fundamental step toward elimination. Recent modeling indicates that global HCV elimination targets are achievable, but will require implementation of a comprehensive package of interventions to enhance engagement of populations along the HCV care cascade. Importantly, several countries are pivotal to HCV elimination because of their large burden of infection, including China, India, Pakistan, and Egypt.

Increase Hepatitis C Virus Testing, Diagnosis, and Linkage to Care

High levels of HCV diagnosis and linkage to care are a prerequisite to a successful HCV elimination strategy. Modeling studies have demonstrated the limited impact of DAA therapy on HCV epidemics in settings of low HCV diagnosis and treatment up-take.[36,37] In 2015, of the 71 million people living with HCV infection, only 20% (14 million) were diagnosed, with marked disparities between high-income countries (43% diagnosed) and LMICs (8% diagnosed).[23] In China, Pakistan, Egypt, India, and Russia, the 5 countries with the largest number of individuals living with HCV infection,[38] less than 25% of those infected were diagnosed.[39]

Several strategies have demonstrated effectiveness in increasing HCV diagnosis and linkage to care.[40,41] In primary care and hospital-based settings, automated HCV testing reminders and screening based on risk assessment or birth cohort have increased HCV testing and diagnosis.[40] In drug and alcohol services, utilizing comprehensive multidisciplinary programs, including counseling, education, and peer-support, can achieve high HCV testing and assessment.[41] Other strategies that have facilitated linkage to HCV care and treatment include noninvasive liver disease screening using transient elastography[42] and patient navigation programs.[43,44] Simplified HCV diagnostic procedures, including point-of-care and dried blood spot testing, have also been effective in increasing HCV testing, diagnosis, and linkage to care.[41,45,46]

Develop Low-Cost and Simplified Hepatitis C Virus Diagnostics

Strategies to scale-up testing and diagnosis must address the complex high-cost diagnostic paradigm and be tailored to local epidemiology and budgetary considerations. The current HCV testing algorithm is a 2-step process, with anti-HCV antibody testing followed by HCV RNA to confirm current infection. Several studies from high-income countries have shown that between 46% to 73% of people testing HCV antibody positive received confirmatory HCV RNA testing.[47] Barriers to testing include the requirement of multiple visits to diagnose, difficulty in accessing phlebotomy services, lack of decentralized laboratories, and limited knowledge among primary care providers and limited financial resources.[47] Although education[48–50] and innovative laboratory testing algorithms (involving reflex HCV RNA testing) may improve HCV diagnosis, further diagnostic simplification is required to achieve HCV elimination.

In recognition of the need for large-scale testing uptake, cheaper (less than US$5–10), and less sensitive (lower limit of detection 1000 IU/mL) diagnostic HCV RNA tests have recently been recommended by peak bodies.[8] There has also been renewed interest in HCV core antigen as a stable, affordable (US$25- US$50) alternative to HCV RNA testing, particularly in LMICs.[51] In addition, the availability of pan-genotypic DAA therapy should markedly simplify diagnostic and monitoring requirements and reduce cost, by removing the need for HCV genotyping, quantitative HCV RNA assessment, and on-treatment HCV RNA monitoring. Further, there is discussion regarding the absolute requirement for SVR12 test given the high efficacy of current DAA regimens and global DAA scale-up needs.

Point-of-care tests for HCV infection, particularly for HCV RNA, have the potential to simplify testing algorithms and increase diagnoses and linkage to care and treatment.[52,53] Point-of-care HCV testing can include oral fluid rapid diagnostic testing,[54] finger-stick whole-blood rapid diagnostic testing,[54,55] on-site venepuncture-based testing,[56] and finger-stick capillary whole-blood testing.[56,57] The Xpert HCV VL Finger-stick utilizes a finger-stick whole-blood sample and delivers a result in less than an hour.[57] Simplified point-of-care diagnostic algorithms can potentially be integrated in a variety of settings including, community health centers, drug treatment clinics, prisons, remote and rural regions, and homelessness settings. Countries could reduce costs by using existing infrastructure and equipment available for other infectious diseases, including HIV[58,59] and tuberculosis.[58,60]

Optimize Hepatitis C Virus Screening Strategies

Different screening strategies for HCV infection have been recommended based on regional epidemiology, and include screening of at-risk populations, birth cohorts, and general populations in areas with intermediate- (2%-5%) to-high prevalence (>5%).[61,62] For instance, in the United States, the US Centers for Disease Control and Prevention and the Preventive Services Task Force currently recommend 1-time anti-HCV antibody testing for all people born between 1945 and 1965 (birth cohort screening) and targeted testing for people at high risk of HCV acquisition (risk-based screening).[62] However, if HCV prevalence is high or elimination is the ultimate goal, cost-effectiveness analysis supports 1-time screening of all adults (≥18 years) in addition to risk-based screening.[63]

Populations at high risk of HCV infection require targeted screening interventions. PWID should be screened for HCV with anti-HCV antibody, and in the context of ongoing injecting drug use, 6 to 12 monthly screenings with anti-HCV antibody should be performed to assess for incident infection.[8] In some high-income settings with high chronic HCV prevalence among PWID, qualitative HCV RNA testing could be justified for screening. In Australia, a modeling study indicated that replacing anti-HCV antibody testing with point-of-care HCV RNA testing for screening PWID would save AUS$62 million, and gain 11,000 quality-adjusted life years.[64] All newly diagnosed HIV-positive individuals should be screened for HCV antibody.[8] HIV-positive MSM at risk of HCV acquisition should be reviewed for 6 to 12 months with assessments for ALT levels and anti-HCV antibody.[8,65] Screening protocols for HCV infection in specific high-risk populations, including young PWID, PWID in incarceration, and HIV-positive GBM, should be considered, potentially utilizing point-of-care diagnostics to enhance HCV diagnosis, prevention, and surveillance as part of a microelimination strategy.

Lower Direct-Acting Antiviral Pricing and Access for All

Because of the high DAA pricing and potential impact on national health budgets, governments and insurers in many countries initially restricted access to DAA therapy based on liver disease stage, drug and alcohol use, and prescriber type.[16,17] However, this is inconsistent with recent international recommendations from peak bodies, which support treatment for all people living with HCV,[8] nor is it a sensible public health approach, based on mathematical modeling.[66,67]

Substantial reductions in DAA pricing have occurred in most countries, primarily in LMICs because of the introduction of generic DAAs.[23] Even in high-income countries, discounting of greater than 50% is common, with some countries including Australia negotiating large discounts.[68] Depending on the setting, DAA treatment prices have also been reduced through price negotiation with pharmaceutical companies, increased competition among pharmaceutical companies and generic producers, acquisition of voluntary licenses, and occasional compulsory licenses. In order to scale-up DAA treatment, most countries will require further price discounting and innovative financing models to ensure unrestricted access (eg, through a risk-sharing arrangement as in Australia or volume taxation as in France). In some settings, however, there is no facility for government-based health care plans (for example, Medicaid in the United States) to negotiate with pharmaceutical companies. Legislative changes may be required in order to improve access to DAA therapy, as has occurred in Canada and the United States.[69,70]

The completion of DAA development pathways by the major pharmaceutical companies should not be an impediment to further innovation. Further therapeutic strategy development, including evaluation of shorter-duration (4–6 weeks) DAA therapy and exploration of technologies for delivery of long-acting antiviral therapy isessential. Investment partnerships between governments, industry, and private organizations are required to propel innovation.

Prevent Hepatitis C Virus Infection and Reinfection

Interventions to prevent HCV infection are available and cost-effective and must be included in a national elimination strategy, tailored to the epidemiology.

Harm reduction services

DAA therapy will play a key elimination role in relation to its treatment-as-prevention benefits; however, high harm reduction coverage is crucial. OST is associated with a 50% reduction in HCV acquisition risk, while OST and high-coverage NSP (defined as adequate sterile needles/syringes to cover all injections) are associated with a 74% reduction in HCV acquisition risk.[71] Despite the evidence base, harm reduction remains appallingly inadequate globally. Less than 1% of PWID reside in countries with high coverage of both NSP and OST.[72] Further, only 9 countries have high NSP coverage (ie, distributed more than 200 needles/syringe per PWID annually), and 20 countries provide high coverage OST.[72] Lack of political will, stigma, discrimination, and criminalization of injection drug use have limited accessibility and coverage in many jurisdictions.

Integrated models of care

HCV treatment for PWID should be integrated into existing services, concurrently managing substance dependency, mental health, and other medical comorbidities. Lower HCV reinfection risk has been observed among recent PWID receiving OST and mental health counseling services.[73] The provision of HCV services within existing services (eg, drug treatment clinics, NSPs, prisons, and homelessness services) compared with referral to traditional tertiary hospital clinics may more effectively facilitate the ongoing health care needs of PWID and reduce the risk of (re)infection. Acknowledgment of the individual circumstances of PWID as opposed to rigid criteria will aid in the success of long-term HCV management strategies and drug user health overall.

Patient education and counseling

Education and counseling can reduce risky injecting behaviors among people with HCV infection.[74,75] Injecting risk behaviors do not increase following the initiation of HCV therapy. It is important, however, for health care providers, peer-support workers, and community drug user organizations to design and deliver education and counseling to PWID commencing DAA about the potential risks of HCV reinfection.

Post-treatment surveillance and treatment of reinfection

People at risk for HCV reinfection should have at least annual monitoring of HCV RNA and ALT.[8] Monitoring for reinfection following HCV treatment is not standardized and may be infrequent. In a Scottish cohort, only 61% of PWID were screened at least once in 4.5 years after SVR follow-up.[76] Although the optimal testing interval for detection of reinfection is unknown, more frequent testing may identify a greater number of reinfections, providing the potential for earlier retreatment.

One of the barriers to testing for reinfection may be jurisdictional limitations on DAA access, driven largely by the current high prices of treatment.[17] DAA retreatment should be made available to all people with reinfection, without stigma or discrimination. Key health care bodies and medical societies should consider implicit recommendations regarding retreatment of reinfection to help facilitate reimbursement by payers.

Prevent health care-associated hepatitis C virus transmission

Unsafe health care practices account for a substantial proportion of incident HCV infections in LMICs.[77] In 2010, an estimated 5% of all health care injections were given with unsterilized or reused equipment, resulting in an estimated 315,000 new HCV infections, most of which were in the Eastern Mediterranean and Southeast Asia regions.[77]

Enhanced investment in context-specific training of health care providers and awareness campaigns for the general population, effective screening and HCV diagnostics, disposable materials (with reuse-prevention devices) and effective sterilization procedures will be required to reduce health care-associated HCV transmission and meet the WHO HCV elimination targets regarding blood product and injection safety.

Monitoring and Evaluation

Surveillance data are needed to set national health priorities, policy decision-making, and health service implementation. Evaluation of HCV elimination will require monitoring of DAA uptake and effectiveness, particularly among populations at risk of transmission, monitoring of HCV viremic prevalence and incidence, and monitoring of the population-level impact of DAA therapy on HCV-related morbidity and mortality. Many countries will need to implement new or improve upon existing surveillance networks to gain reliable epidemiologic data, identify and respond to new epidemics, and accurately analyze the change in burden of HCV infection in response to public health interventions.

Financing for Hepatitis C Virus Infection

A massive barrier to the comprehensive scale-up of interventions in countries is insufficient funding for HCV. According to a recent WHO analysis, an additional US$6 billion per year will be needed in LMIC until 2030, as part of universal health coverage, in order to achieve viral hepatitis targets.[78] With universal health coverage high on the agenda for sustainable development goals, mobilization of domestic funding by creating fiscal space (including taxation on tobacco) is an important strategy.[79] Access to DAAs is particularly problematic for upper middle-income and high-income countries where generics cannot be introduced. Innovative financing mechanisms for HCV (DAAs and diagnostics) that also limit out-of-pocket expenditure are urgently needed. Unlike dedicated international pooled funding for HIV and vaccines, significant support for HCV from the Global Fund or other foundations does not exist. Suggested methods to mobilize funding include

More efficient and effective allocation of health resources

Harness global coalition of stakeholders with the involvement of civil society in advocacy

Case demonstration of the financial impact HCV has on the national gross domestic product (GDP) as has been demonstrated in Egypt

Pooling of public-private funding for LMIC (governments and private foundation) (UNITAID shows some promise for this financing mechanism)[79]

Social and Political Will

Political and civil society support

The success of HCV elimination hinges on high levels of sustained political and civil society engagement. As of March 2017, of 194 WHO member states, only 43 (22%)

had formulated national viral hepatitis elimination plans, and an additional 36 (19%) reported that they were in development.[80] National viral hepatitis strategies are critical to define national priorities, outline public health interventions, enable the effective and efficient use of resources, allocate roles and responsibilities to stakeholders, and enable measurement of progress. Political support and advocacy are being generated in many settings, and organizations such as UNITE-Parliamentarians Network to End HIV/AIDS, Viral Hepatitis and Tuberculosis are providing critical advocacy and leadership.

Integration in health systems
Given limited resources in many countries, HCV elimination strategies should be integrated in existing health systems, as opposed to establishing a new disease-specific program. Elimination efforts can support primary health care by providing basic services and improving surveillance, training personnel, and expanding immunization programs. To increase access and reduce health inequities, delivery of hepatitis and harm reduction services can be tailored to different populations and settings through integration, decentralization, and task shifting.

Deliver hepatitis C virus education and training to health care providers
Education needs to be delivered to health care providers regarding best practice in the diagnosis, management, and prevention of HCV infection. Poor knowledge and limited competence among health care providers regarding the natural history and testing algorithm for HCV infection may impede diagnosis.[48–50] For example, providers may fail to order confirmatory HCV RNA testing following a positive anti-HCV antibody test to accurately determine HCV viremic status (and subsequent requirement for treatment).[50] Lack of confirmatory testing risks inappropriately labeling people with prior exposure to HCV as hepatitis C positive, or risks failing to diagnose, educate, and treat people with active HCV infection. Education should be culturally appropriate and specific to the epidemiologic setting, involve both health care providers and the effected community, and address issues of stigma and discrimination.

Remove stigma and discrimination and decriminalize drug use
Access to health services, implementation and expansion of evidence-based harm reduction programs, and drug policy reform are necessary in efforts to eliminate HCV infection.[81] Despite the evidence base, political resistance to harm reduction service in many countries, stigma, discrimination, and criminalization of drug use have reduced accessibility and limited coverage. Fear of arrest and prosecution may reduce uptake of prevention services, resulting in decreased needle-syringe distribution and increased needle-syringe sharing.[82] Incarceration of PWID places them in an environment with high HCV prevalence and incidence, and limited HCV treatment or harm reduction services.[83] Consulting and involving community drug user organizations in the design and implementation of HCV prevention strategies will be essential, ensuring public health efforts meet the needs of the target population. Drug reform policies must be considered, including decriminalization of drug use or alternatives to imprisonment, development of policies and laws that decriminalize use of needles and syringes (to permit NSP service provision), and legalizing OST for those who are opioid dependent.

PROGRESS TOWARD HEPATITIS C VIRUS ELIMINATION

The total number of people treated for HCV infection increased from 1.8 million to 2.1 million between 2016 and 2017. Encouragingly, this increase mostly occurred in middle-income countries (with the majority in Egypt and Pakistan); however, the number treated in many high-income countries has either stagnated or declined. As those already diagnosed are treated, the big task ahead toward achieving elimination is rapid scale-up of screening and linkage to care.

Around 80% of high-income countries are not on track to meet HCV elimination targets by 2030.[84] At the end of 2017, 12 countries were considered on track to achieve WHO HCV elimination 2030 targets, including several high-income countries (Australia, France, Iceland, Italy, Japan, South Korea, Spain, Switzerland, and the United Kingdom) and 3 LMICs (Egypt, Georgia, and Mongolia) (**Fig. 2**).[39,84] In general, those countries on track to achieve the 2030 HCV elimination targets have demonstrated a strong coordinated multisectoral response, with national HCV treatment strategies, allocation of funding and resources, integration into broader health systems, active pursuit of measures to improve DAA access and lower DAA pricing, and political support (**Tables 4** and **5**).[7,85–88] Accumulated success in individual countries or regions should generate the momentum required for ongoing international support.

Australia

In March 2016, government-subsidized DAA regimens were made available to all Australians (≥18 years of age) living with chronic HCV infection, with no liver disease stage, drug and alcohol, or prescriber restrictions, and at no or minimal cost to the individual (AUS$0 - AUS$39.50/mo). By the end of 2018, approximately 70,000 people (30% of chronic HCV cases in Australia) had received treatment.

Australia is considered an international leader in its public health response to HCV. Strong political leadership and national strategic development since 2000, combined with well-established partnerships between government, clinical, academic and

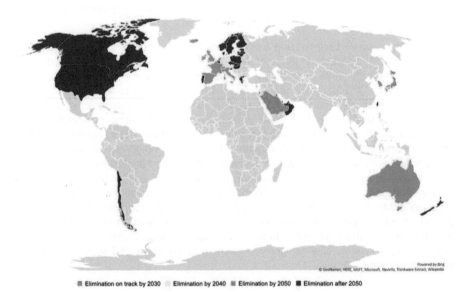

■ Elimination on track by 2030   Elimination by 2040   ■ Elimination by 2050   ■ Elimination after 2050

Fig. 2. Timing of HCV elimination in 45 high-income countries and territories. (*Reprinted from Razavi et al. Global timing of hepatitis C virus elimination: estimating the year countries will achieve the World Health Organization elimination targets. JOURNAL OF HEPATOLOGY; 2019: ELSEVIER SCIENCE.*)

Table 4
Examples of countries on track to achieve the World Health Organization 2030 hepatitis C virus elimination targets

Countries on Track to Achieve WHO 2030 Elimination Targets	High-Income Countries					Low-Middle Income Countries	
	Australia	France	Iceland	Spain	Switzerland	Georgia	Mongolia
HCV-infected population, n							
2014	230,000	220,000	1100	400,000	43,000	175,000	200,000
2016	200,000	200,000	750	350,000	40,000	150,000	190,000
Diagnosed, %	80%	70%	75%	33%	70%	33%	26%
Treated, %	16%	8%	40%	8%	5%	12%	4%
New HCV infections, n	6000	5100	50	2200	700	6000	3200
HCV-related deaths, n	800	800	2	1450	230	210	1300
National HCV strategy	✔	✔	✔	✔	✗	✔	✔
National clinical guidelines	✔	✔	✔	✔	✔	✔	✔
National expert advisory group	✔	✔	✔	✔	✔	✔	✔
Main population group/s affected							
PWID	✔	✔	✔	✔	✔	✔	
HIV-positive GBM	✔	✔			✔		
Prisoners	✔		✔				
Blood product recipients						✔	✔
Government subsidized DAA therapy	✔	✔	✔	✔	Health insurance	Gilead funded	✔
Unrestricted DAA therapy (year)	✔ (2016)	✔ (2017)	✔ (2016)	✔ (2017)	✔ (2017)	✔ (2016)	✔ (2016)
DAA prescriber type							
Specialist	✔	✔	✔	✔	✔	✔	✔
GP primary care	✔	✗	✗	✗	✗	✗	✗
Harm reduction programs for PWID							
NSP	✔	✔	✔ (limited)	✔	✔	✔	✔
OST	✔	✔	✔	✔	✔	✔	✗

Abbreviations: GBM, gay and bisexual men; GP, general practitioner; NSP, needle and syringe program; OST, opiate substitution therapy.

community stakeholders have been pivotal to Australia's success. Centralized national independent assessment of new therapies for government subsidization together with rigorous price negotiations between the Australian government and the pharmaceutical industry were instrumental in the development of what has been labeled the Netflix model, a risk-sharing agreement to spend AUS$1 billion over 5 years (ie, 2016–2020 inclusive) on DAA drugs in exchange for an unlimited supply.[85]

Table 5 Key components required for national hepatitis C virus elimination strategy	
Screening	General population-based screening • Birth cohort • All adults (≥18 y), especially in intermediate (2%-5%) and high prevalence settings (>5%) Risk-based screening, with regular testing of high-risk populations • People who inject drugs • People who are incarcerated • HIV-positive gay and bisexual men
Diagnosis	Low cost, simple, accurate HCV diagnostics Efficient linkage to care Education of health care providers
Treatment	DAA therapy • Cost-effective; access for all • Expansion of treatment services and capacity building • Specialist and nonspecialist prescribers • Education of health care providers and affected community • Targeted strategies among high prevalence and incidence populations • Retreatment of reinfection
Prevention	Harm reduction • Needle and syringe program, opioid substitution therapy • Behavioral interventions Education • Counseling • Peer support Integrated care • Mental health assessment Blood and injection safety
Epidemiology, modeling, and surveillance	Baseline epidemiology (including number of people living with HCV, HCV-related morbidity and mortality, transmission risks) Modeling to plan beneficial, cost-effective strategies (including screening programs) Regular (at least annual) reporting Monitoring of DAA uptake and effectiveness, HCV viremic prevalence and incidence (primary and reinfection), HCV-related morbidity and mortality
Social and political will	Sustainable funding Expert advisory panel Decentralization of programs with establishment of local HCV networks Education and public awareness campaign • Specific to epidemiologic setting • Involving community and health care providers Adequate infrastructure with dedicated personnel

High harm reduction coverage and high diagnosis rate (>80% of chronic HCV population) are also important features. The high initial DAA uptake, including among marginalized PWID populations,[89] is testament to the importance of this foundation.

Extremely high DAA treatment uptake in the initial months of the DAA program was followed by an anticipated decline in the number treated per month as the large clinic-based warehouses of patients were treated (**Fig. 3**).[85] Recent modeling indicates that a treatment level of 13,000 to 14,000 cases per year in Australia will be required to achieve HCV elimination targets.[90] To maintain DAA treatment uptake, enhanced

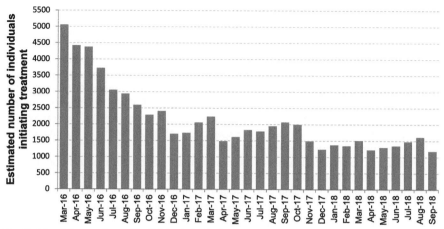

Fig. 3. Monthly number of individuals initiating DAA treatment in Australia.

case finding outside of traditional tertiary clinics will be required; encouragingly, the proportion of DAA initiations by general practitioners has increased, and the age of people treated has declined, suggesting broader community access. Between 2015 and 2018, HCV RNA prevalence among PWID attending needle and syringe programs and completing the Australian Needle and Syringe Program Survey has declined from 51% to 20%.[91] The key to HCV elimination in Australia will be sustained DAA treatment scale-up among high-risk populations, in particular harder-to-reach groups such as people who are homeless or incarcerated. DAA treatment in the prison setting continues to expand; with evidence in New South Wales by the end of 2018, 1 in 4 people initiated on DAA therapy were incarcerated.

Egypt

In efforts to rapidly scale-up treatment in Egypt, the Ministry of Health in 2016 removed liver disease stage restrictions for DAA treatment and began large-scale targeted screening programs of university students, prisoners, hospital inpatients, blood donors, and general screening of people living in rural areas. With these public health initiatives, 4.5 million Egyptians were screened for HCV, and over 400,000 people newly diagnosed with chronic HCV infection.[39] Of the 6 million people estimated to be living with chronic HCV in Egypt, more than 2 million people have been treated since 2015.[39] This demonstrates what can be achieved in a high HCV prevalence lower-middle income country with strong political leadership, low generic drug cost and domestic production, development of an effective infrastructure for broad screening, and nation-wide treatment facilities.

An enormous task lies ahead as treatment numbers in Egypt have dropped, highlighting the need to further scale-up screening and diagnosis. In October 2018, the Ministry of Health launched a nationwide mass screening and treatment campaign called "100 Million Health." By September 2019, the plan was to screen all adults at least 18 years of age, equating to an estimated 52 million individuals. The campaign incorporates anti-HCV antibody testing and assessment of hypertension, diabetes, and obesity, and involves more than 5000 test sites including rural clinics. Screening in rural remote areas will be performed using a finger-stick anti-HCV antibody rapid test (SD Bioline - US$0.60/test), and identifying viremic cases, costing US$15 per test. Primary prevention through enhanced infection control in health care is essential to the success of this massive initiative.

France

France incorporated HCV and hepatitis B virus (HBV) in a national action plan and provided universal unrestricted access to DAA therapy in 2016. Strong political support in collaboration with civil society manifested in a public communication strategy, including television and radio awareness campaigns with prevention a priority message for the general population. The French government invested €750 million in treating 15,000 patients per year. To counter the impact of public health expenditure, the government established a volume taxation mechanism called 'W,' which fixes a cap on pharmaceutical profit (ie, if the expenditure on HCV regimens surpasses the budget, the surplus would be taxed at 100%).[92]

France also implemented targeted interventions to reach marginalized populations of PWID including integrated HCV care in harm reduction programs (needle and syringe programs and OST clinics), and free anonymous testing. HCV education for primary health care physicians and workers was made a priority. France has also recently allowed nonspecialists to prescribe DAAs, which removes a barrier to broadening treatment in the community.

Georgia

In 2016, an estimated 150,000 people were living with chronic HCV in Georgia (anti-HCV antibody prevalence 5%), most of whom were PWID.[39] In 2015, Georgia launched its national HCV elimination strategy in partnership with several organizations including the US Centers for Disease Control and Prevention, Gilead Sciences, and The Global Fund on the background of strong political and social support.[88] The national program incorporates unrestricted access to DAA treatment, HCV screening, national surveillance and monitoring, and public awareness campaigns.[93] DAA treatment has been provided free of charge, and in June 2016, liver disease restrictions were lifted. Between 2015 and March 2018, approximately 45,000 people initiated treatment (30% of HCV infected population), and 29,000 were cured.[94]

Unfortunately, the proportion diagnosed with HCV prior to the launch of the national strategy was low (10%–15%). A steady decline in the number of people commencing treatment was seen in the last 3 months of 2016, similar to the warehouse effect observed in other countries. In response, efforts to scale-up HCV screening and treatment have commenced, with provision of outreach services for at-risk populations, including PWID. Subsequently, the proportion of people living with HCV who are diagnosed has risen to over 33%.[39]

Iceland

In Iceland, a national HCV treatment as prevention project is underway (TraPHepC; clinicaltrials.gov registry identifier: NCT02647879).[87] Most of the estimated 800 to 1300 people living with HCV in Iceland are PWID, of whom 80% are diagnosed.[87] By increasing DAA uptake to 188 per 1000 PWID per year (equivalent to 75 of the estimated 400 PWID in Iceland per year), an 80% reduction in incidence will be achieved by 2020.[95] Between 2016 and 2018, 632 people initiated DAA treatment, representing 80% of the estimated total HCV population.[96] The prevalence of HCV viraemia among current PWID admitted for treatment of substance misuse or dependency has dropped from approximately 48% in 2015% to 16% in 2017.[96] Screening and harm reduction will need to increase in concert with DAA scale-up. The small population size and high proportion diagnosed are strong foundations on which to build a national HCV elimination program.

Mongolia

Mongolia, with a high burden of HCV infection (HCV viremic prevalence >10%) and hepatocellular carcinoma among the general population, has demonstrated the impact of societal and political will in establishing an HCV elimination strategy in a lower-middle income country, with approximately 20,000 people having received DAA treatment (of an estimated 200,000 total population). With the publication of the Hepatitis Prevention, Control and Elimination Program 2016 to 2020, the Mongolian government allocated 232 billion Mongolian tögrög (approximately US$96 million) in funding, added HBV and HCV therapy to the national health insurance scheme (which covers most of the population), and petitioned for significant discounting in the cost of DAA therapy (generic sofosbuvir-ledipasvir, US$65).

SUMMARY

Although considerable progress has been made in the global HCV elimination response, further political and societal support and financial domestic and international investment are needed to rapidly increase the number of countries on track for HCV elimination. Delayed diagnosis of HCV and presentation with HCV-related complications remain commonplace, thereby hindering global efforts to reduce morbidity and mortality. Many countries have not yet seized the opportunity to initiate government-subsidized HCV treatment services, while HCV testing coverage and diagnosis remains extremely low in most regions. Models of care simplifying HCV testing and treatment are required to achieve viral hepatitis elimination as a major public health threat by 2030. Countries must push to achieve DAA access for all, and in the process, overcome barriers imposed by high drug pricing, liver disease stage and drug use restrictions, and stigma. Countries that have made considerable headway are those with a strong government response, national elimination and treatment strategies, and policies to improve HCV testing and DAA access. Ultimately, to maximize the population-level impact of DAA therapy and achieve the WHO elimination targets, HCV screening, diagnosis, and treatment must dramatically improve.

A concerted coordinated international public health response will be required between governments, researchers, health care providers, policy makers, community members, advocates, and industry partners. Optimism and aspiration fuel human effort. Although the WHO has moved the epidemiologic goalposts, striving for HCV elimination is a worthy endeavor.

ACKNOWLEDGMENTS

The Kirby Institute is funded by the Australian Government Department of Health and Aging. The views expressed in this publication do not necessarily represent the position of the Australian Government. The content is solely the responsibility of the authors. M. Martinello and G.J. Dore are supported through National Health and Medical Research Council Fellowships (M. Martinello: Early Career Fellowship; G.J. Dore: Practitioner Fellowship).

COMPETING INTERESTS

No conflicts (M. Martinello, S. Bajis). G.J. Dore is an advisory board member and has received honoraria from Abbvie, Gilead, and Merck; has received research grant funding from Abbvie, Gilead, and Merck; and travel sponsorship from Gilead, Abbvie, and Merck.

REFERENCES

1. The Polaris Observatory HCV Collaborators. Global prevalence and genotype distribution of hepatitis C virus infection in 2015: a modelling study. Lancet Gastroenterol Hepatol 2017;2(3):161–76.
2. Martinello M, Hajarizadeh B, Grebely J, et al. Management of acute HCV infection in the era of direct-acting antiviral therapy. Nat Rev Gastroenterol Hepatol 2018; 15(7):412–24.
3. Stanaway JD, Flaxman AD, Naghavi M, et al. The global burden of viral hepatitis from 1990 to 2013: findings from the Global Burden of Disease Study 2013. Lancet 2016;388(10049):1081–8.
4. World Health Organization. Global health sector strategy on viral hepatitis 2016-2021. Towards ending viral hepatitis. Geneva, Switzerland: World Health Organization; 2016.
5. Gotte M, Feld JJ. Direct-acting antiviral agents for hepatitis C: structural and mechanistic insights. Nat Rev Gastroenterol Hepatol 2016;13(6):338–51.
6. World Health Organization. WHO global hepatitis report 2017. WHO. 2017. Available at: http://www.who.int/hepatitis/publications/global-hepatitis-report2017/en/. Accessed April 23, 2017.
7. Hill AM, Nath S, Simmons B. The road to elimination of hepatitis C: analysis of cures versus new infections in 91 countries. J Virus Erad 2017;3(3):117–23.
8. Pawlotsky J-M, Negro F, Aghemo A, et al. EASL recommendations on treatment of Hepatitis C 2018. J Hepatol 2018;69(2):461–511.
9. Cacoub P, Desbois AC, Comarmond C, et al. Impact of sustained virological response on the extrahepatic manifestations of chronic hepatitis C: a meta-analysis. Gut 2018;67(11):2025–34.
10. Smith-Palmer J, Cerri K, Valentine W. Achieving sustained virologic response in hepatitis C: a systematic review of the clinical, economic and quality of life benefits. BMC Infect Dis 2015;15:19.
11. Moradpour D, Grakoui A, Manns MP. Future landscape of hepatitis C research - Basic, translational and clinical perspectives. J Hepatol 2016;65(1):S143–55.
12. Grebely J, Hajarizadeh B, Dore GJ. Direct-acting antiviral agents for HCV infection affecting people who inject drugs. Nat Rev Gastroenterol Hepatol 2017; 14(11):641–51.
13. Martinello M, Hajarizadeh B, Grebely J, et al. HCV cure and reinfection among people with HIV/HCV coinfection and people who inject drugs. Curr HIV/AIDS Rep 2017;14(3):110–21.
14. Grebely LS, Larney S, Peacock A, et al. Global, regional, and country-level estimates of hepatitis C infection among people who have recently injected drugs. Addiction 2018;114(1):150–66.
15. Asher AK, Portillo CJ, Cooper BA, et al. Clinicians' views of Hepatitis C virus treatment candidacy with direct-acting antiviral regimens for people who inject drugs. Subst Use Misuse 2016;51(9):1218–23.
16. Marshall AD, Cunningham EB, Nielsen S, et al. Restrictions for reimbursement of interferon-free direct-acting antiviral drugs for HCV infection in Europe. Lancet Gastroenterol Hepatol 2018;3(2):125–33.
17. Barua S, Greenwald R, Grebely J, et al. Restrictions for Medicaid reimbursement of sofosbuvir for the treatment of hepatitis C virus infection in the United States. Ann Intern Med 2015;163(3):215–23.
18. Grebely J, Oser M, Taylor LE, et al. Breaking down the barriers to Hepatitis C Virus (HCV) treatment among individuals with HCV/HIV coinfection: action required

at the system, provider, and patient levels. J Infect Dis 2013;207(suppl_1): S19–25.

19. Hajarizadeh B, Cunningham EB, Reid H, et al. Direct-acting antiviral treatment for hepatitis C among people who use or inject drugs: a systematic review and meta-analysis. Lancet Gastroenterol Hepatol 2018;3(11):754–67.

20. Nouch S, Gallagher L, Erickson M, et al. Factors associated with lost to follow-up after hepatitis C treatment delivered by primary care teams in an inner-city multi-site program, Vancouver, Canada. Int J Drug Policy 2018;59:76–84.

21. Christensen S, Buggisch P, Mauss S, et al. Direct-acting antiviral treatment of chronic HCV-infected patients on opioid substitution therapy: Still a concern in clinical practice? Addiction 2018;113(5):868–82.

22. The HIV Modelling Consortium Treatment as Prevention Editorial Writing Group. HIV treatment as prevention: models, data, and questions-towards evidence-based decision-making. PLoS Med 2012;9(7):e1001259.

23. WHO. Progress report on access to hepatitis C treatment: focus on overcoming barriers in low- and middle-income countries, March, 2018. Geneva (Switzerland): World Health Organization; 2018. WHO/CDS/HIV/18.4.

24. Boerekamps A, Van den Berk GE, Fanny LN, et al. Declining HCV incidence in Dutch HIV positive men who have sex with men after unrestricted access to HCV therapy. Clin Infect Dis 2018;66(9):1360–5.

25. Pradat P, Huleux T, Raffi F, et al. Incidence of new hepatitis C virus infection is still increasing in French MSM living with HIV. AIDS 2018;32(8):1077–82.

26. Martinello M, Bartlett S, Dore G, et al. Universal access to DAA therapy paves the way for HCV control and elimination among people living with HIV in Australia. J Hepatol 2018;68(Suppl 1):S312 [Abstract].

27. Dowdle WR. The principles of disease elimination and eradication. Bull World Health Organ 1998;76(Suppl 2):22–5.

28. Lazarus JV, Wiktor S, Colombo M, et al. Micro-elimination - a path to global elimination of hepatitis C. J Hepatol 2017;67(4):665–6.

29. Martin NK, Thornton A, Hickman M, et al. Can hepatitis C virus (HCV) direct-acting antiviral treatment as prevention reverse the HCV epidemic among men who have sex with men in the United Kingdom? Epidemiological and modeling insights. Clin Infect Dis 2016;62(9):1072–80.

30. Zelenev A, Li J, Mazhnaya A, et al. Hepatitis C virus treatment as prevention in an extended network of people who inject drugs in the USA: a modelling study. Lancet Infect Dis 2018;18(2):215–24.

31. Fraser H, Martin NK, Brummer-Korvenkontio H, et al. Model projections on the impact of HCV treatment in the prevention of HCV transmission among people who inject drugs in Europe. J Hepatol 2018;68(3):402–11.

32. Ward Z, Platt L, Sweeney S, et al. Impact of Current and Scaled-Up Levels of Hepatitis C Prevention and Treatment Interventions for People Who Inject Drugs in Three UK Settings-What Is Required to Achieve the WHO's HCV Elimination Targets? Addiction 2018;113(9):1727–38.

33. Iliceto A, Bagert B. Successful treatment of HTLV-1 associated myelopathy with chronic immunosuppression. Neurology 2017;88(16).

34. Bartlett SR, Fox P, Cabatingan H, et al. Demonstration of near-elimination of hepatitis C virus among a prison population: the lotus glen correctional centre Hepatitis C treatment project. Clin Infect Dis 2018;67(3):460–3.

35. Aylward B, Hennessey KA, Zagaria N, et al. When is a disease eradicable? 100 years of lessons learned. Am J Public Health 2000;90(10):1515–20.

36. Wedemeyer H, Duberg AS, Buti M, et al. Strategies to manage hepatitis C virus (HCV) disease burden. J Viral Hepat 2014;21:60–89.

37. Durham DP, Skrip LA, Bruce RD, et al. The impact of enhanced screening and treatment on Hepatitis C in the United States. Clin Infect Dis 2016;62(3):298–304.

38. Gower E, Estes C, Blach S, et al. Global epidemiology and genotype distribution of the hepatitis C virus infection. J Hepatol 2014;61(1):S45–57.

39. Centre for Disease Analysis. Polaris observatory. 2018. Available at: http://cdafound.org/polaris-hepc-dashboard/. Accessed May 1, 2018.

40. Zhou K, Fitzpatrick T, Walsh N, et al. Interventions to optimise the care continuum for chronic viral hepatitis: a systematic review and meta-analyses. Lancet Infect Dis 2016;16(12):1409–22.

41. Bajis S, Dore GJ, Hajarizadeh B, et al. Interventions to enhance testing, linkage to care and treatment uptake for hepatitis C virus infection among people who inject drugs: a systematic review. Int J Drug Policy 2017;47:34–46.

42. Foucher J, Reiller B, Jullien V, et al. FibroScan used in street-based outreach for drug users is useful for hepatitis C virus screening and management: a prospective study. J Viral Hepat 2009;16(2):121–31.

43. Trooskin SB, Poceta J, Towey CM, et al. Results from a geographically focused, community-based HCV screening, linkage-to-care and patient navigation program. J Gen Intern Med 2015;30(7):950–7.

44. Falade-Nwulia O, Mehta SH, Lasola J, et al. Public health clinic-based hepatitis C testing and linkage to care in Baltimore. J Viral Hepat 2016;23(5):366–74.

45. Bottero J, Boyd A, Gozlan J, et al. Simultaneous human immunodeficiency virus-hepatitis B-hepatitis C point-of-care tests improve outcomes in linkage-to-care: results of a randomized control trial in persons without healthcare coverage. Open Forum Infect Dis 2015;2(4):ofv162.

46. Meyer JP, Moghimi Y, Marcus R, et al. Evidence-based interventions to enhance assessment, treatment, and adherence in the chronic Hepatitis C care continuum. Int J Drug Pol 2015;26(10):922–35.

47. Grebely J, Applegate TL, Cunningham P, et al. Hepatitis C point-of-care diagnostics: in search of a single visit diagnosis. Expert Rev Mol Diagn 2017;17(12): 1109–15.

48. Cox J, Graves L, Marks E, et al. Knowledge, attitudes and behaviours associated with the provision of hepatitis C care by Canadian family physicians. J Viral Hepat 2011;18(7):e332–40.

49. Gupta L, Shah S, Ward JE. Educational and health service needs of Australian general practitioners in managing hepatitis C. J Gastroenterol Hepatol 2006; 21(4):694–9.

50. Shehab TM, Sonnad SS, Lok AS. Management of hepatitis C patients by primary care physicians in the USA: results of a national survey. J Viral Hepat 2001;8(5): 377–83.

51. Freiman JM, Tran TM, Schumacher SG, et al. Hepatitis C core antigen testing for diagnosis of hepatitis C virus infection: a systematic review and meta-analysis. Ann Intern Med 2016;165(5):345–55.

52. Schito M, Peter TF, Cavanaugh S, et al. Opportunities and challenges for cost-efficient implementation of new point-of-care diagnostics for HIV and tuberculosis. The J Infect Dis 2012;205(Suppl 2):S169–80.

53. Medecins Sans Frontieres. Putting HIV and HCV to the test: a product guide for point-of-care CD4 tests and laboratory-based point-of-care HIV and HCV Viral Load Tests 2017. Geneva (Switzerland).

54. Shivkumar S, Peeling R, Jafari Y, et al. Accuracy of rapid and point-of-care screening tests for hepatitis C: a systematic review and meta-analysis. Ann Intern Med 2012;157(8):558–66.

55. Poiteau L, Soulier A, Rosa I, et al. Performance of rapid diagnostic tests for the detection of antibodies to hepatitis C virus in whole blood collected on dried blood spots. J viral Hepat 2016;23(5):399–401.

56. Grebely, Lamoury FMJ, Hajarizadeh B, et al. Evaluation of the Xpert HCV Viral Load point-of-care assay from venepuncture-collected and finger-stick capillary whole-blood samples: a cohort study. Lancet Gastroenterol Hepatol 2017;2(7):514–20.

57. Lamoury FM, Bajis S, Hajarizadeh B, et al. LiveRLife Study Group. Evaluation of the Xpert HCV Viral Load Finger-Stick Point-of-Care Assay. J Infect Dis 2018; 217(12):1889–96.

58. Drain PK, Hyle EP, Noubary F, et al. Diagnostic point-of-care tests in resource-limited settings. Lancet Infect Dis 2014;14(3):239–49.

59. Gliddon HD, Peeling RW, Kamb ML, et al. A systematic review and meta-analysis of studies evaluating the performance and operational characteristics of dual point-of-care tests for HIV and syphilis. Sex Transm Infect 2017;93(S4):S3–15.

60. Drobniewski F, Cooke M, Jordan J, et al. Systematic review, meta-analysis and economic modelling of molecular diagnostic tests for antibiotic resistance in tuberculosis. Health Technol Assess 2015;19(34):1–188, vii-viii.

61. WHO. WHO guidelines on hepatitis B and C testing. Geneva (Switzerland): World Health Organisation; 2017.

62. AASLD-IDSA. Recommendations for testing, managing, and treating hepatitis C. 2016. Available at: http://www.hcvguidelines.org/. Accessed December 30, 2016.

63. Barocas JA, Tasillo A, Eftekhari Yazdi G, et al. Population level outcomes and cost-effectiveness of expanding the recommendation for age-based hepatitis C testing in the United States. Clin Infect Dis 2018;67(4):549–56.

64. Scott N, Doyle JS, Wilson DP, et al. Reaching hepatitis C virus elimination targets requires health system interventions to enhance the care cascade. Int J Drug Policy 2017;47:107–16.

65. European AIDS Clinical Society. EACS guidelines version 9.0 2017 2017.

66. Martin NK, Vickerman P, Dore GJ, et al. Prioritization of HCV treatment in the direct-acting antiviral era: an economic evaluation. J Hepatol 2016;65(1):17–25.

67. Scott N, McBryde ES, Thompson A, et al. Treatment scale-up to achieve global HCV incidence and mortality elimination targets: a cost-effectiveness model. Gut 2016;66(8):1507–15.

68. Moon S, Erickson E. Universal medicine access through lump-sum remuneration — Australia's approach to Hepatitis C. N Engl J Med 2019;380(7):607–10.

69. Aleccia J. Judge orders Washington Medicaid to provide lifesaving hepatitis C drugs for all. 2016. Available at: http://www.seattletimes.com/seattle-news/health/judge-orders-apple-health-to-cover-hepatitis-c-drugs-for-all/. Accessed September 11, 2017.

70. Jones S. Jones introduces legislation to treat hepatitis C sooner. 2016. Available at: http://sylviajonesmpp.ca/2016/06/08/jones-introduces-legislation-to-treat-hepatitis-c-sooner/. Accessed September 11, 2017.

71. Platt L, Minozzi S, Reed J, et al. Needle and syringe programmes and opioid substitution therapy for preventing HCV transmission among people who inject drugs: findings from a Cochrane Review and meta-analysis. Addiction 2018; 113(3):545–63.

72. Larney S, Peacock A, Leung J, et al. Global, regional, and country-level coverage of interventions to prevent and manage HIV and hepatitis C among people who inject drugs: a systematic review. Lancet Glob Health 2017;5(12):e1208–20.

73. Islam N, Krajden M, Shoveller J, et al. Incidence, risk factors, and prevention of hepatitis C reinfection: a population-based cohort study. Lancet Gastroenterol Hepatol 2017;2(3):200–10.

74. Bruneau J, Zang G, Abrahamowicz M, et al. Sustained drug use changes after hepatitis C screening and counseling among recently infected persons who inject drugs: a longitudinal study. Clin Infect Dis 2014;58(6):755–61.

75. Roux P, Le Gall JM, Debrus M, et al. Innovative community-based educational face-to-face intervention to reduce HIV, hepatitis C virus and other blood-borne infectious risks in difficult-to-reach people who inject drugs: results from the ANRS-AERLI intervention study. Addiction 2016;111(1):94–106.

76. Weir A, McLeod A, Innes H, et al. Hepatitis C reinfection following treatment induced viral clearance among people who have injected drugs. Drug Alcohol Depend 2016;165:53–60.

77. Pepin J, Abou Chakra CN, Pepin E, et al. Evolution of the global burden of viral infections from unsafe medical injections, 2000-2010. PLoS One 2014;9(6): e99677.

78. Tordrup D, Hutin Y, Stenberg K, et al. Additional resource needs for viral hepatitis elimination through universal health coverage: projections in 67 low-income and middle-income countries, 2016–30. Lancet Glob Health 2019;7(9):e1180–8.

79. Cooke GS, Andrieux-Meyer I, Applegate TL, et al. Accelerating the elimination of viral hepatitis: a Lancet Gastroenterology & Hepatology Commission. Lancet Gastroenterol Hepatol 2019;4(2):135–84.

80. World Health Organisation. Global hepatitis report 2017 2017. Geneva (Switzerland). CC BY-NC-SA 3.0 IGO.

81. Grebely J, Dore GJ, Morin S, et al. Elimination of HCV as a public health concern among people who inject drugs by 2030 - what will it take to get there? J Int AIDS Soc 2017;20(1):22146.

82. DeBeck K, Cheng T, Montaner JS, et al. HIV and the criminalisation of drug use among people who inject drugs: a systematic review. Lancet HIV 2017;4(8): e357–74.

83. Larney S, Kopinski H, Beckwith CG, et al. Incidence and prevalence of hepatitis C in prisons and other closed settings: results of a systematic review and meta-analysis. Hepatology 2013;58(4):1215–24.

84. Razavi H, Sanchez Y, Pangerl A, et al. Global timing of hepatitis C virus elimination: estimating the year countries will achieve the World Health Organization elimination targets. Paper presented at: The International Liver Congress, 10-14 April 2019:Vienna, Austria. SAT-620.

85. Dore GJ, Hajarizadeh B. Elimination of Hepatitis C Virus in Australia: laying the foundation. Infect Dis Clin North Am 2018;32(2):269–79.

86. Elsharkawy A, El-Raziky M, El-Akel W, et al. Planning and prioritizing direct-acting antivirals treatment for HCV patients in countries with limited resources: lessons from the Egyptian experience. J Hepatol 2018;68(4):691–8.

87. Olafsson S, Tyrfingsson T, Runarsdottir V, et al. Treatment as Prevention for Hepatitis C (TraP Hep C) - a nationwide elimination programme in Iceland using direct-acting antiviral agents. J Intern Med 2018;283(5):500–7.

88. Nasrullah M, Sergeenko D, Gamkrelidze A, et al. HCV elimination — lessons learned from a small Eurasian country, Georgia. Nat Rev Gastroenterol Hepatol 2017;14:447.

89. Iversen J, Dore GJ, Catlett B, et al. Association between rapid utilisation of direct hepatitis C antivirals and decline in the prevalence of viremia among people who inject drugs in Australia. J Hepatol 2019;70(1):33–9.

90. Kwon JA, Dore GJ, Grebely J, et al. Australia on track to achieve WHO HCV elimination targets following rapid initial DAA treatment uptake: a modelling study. J Viral Hepat 2019;26(1):83–92.

91. Heard S, Iversen J, Geddes L, et al. Australian needle syringe program survey national data report 2014-2018: prevalence of HIV, HCV and injecting and sexual behaviour among NSP attendees. Sydney (Australia): Kirby Institute, UNSW Sydney; 2019.

92. Delile JM. Réduction des risques et des dommages (RdRD) et approche intégrative. In: Audition publique: La réduction des risques et des dommages liés aux conduites addictives. Paris: Fédération Française d'Addictologie. Available at: http://www.asud.org/2016/04/07/audition-publique-2-0-sur-la-reduction-des-risques-et-des-dommages-lies-aux-conduites-addictives/. Accessed September 7, 2019

93. Mitruka K, Tsertsvadze T, Butsashvili M, et al. Launch of a nationwide hepatitis c elimination program — Georgia, april 2015. MMWR Morb Mortal Wkly Rep 2015; 64(28):753–7.

94. Tsertsvadze T, Gamkrelidze A, Chkhartishvili N, et al. Hepatitis C care cascade in the country of Georgia after 2 years of starting national hepatitis C elimination program. J Hepatol 2018;68:S53.

95. Scott N, Ólafsson S, Gottfreðsson M, et al. Modelling the elimination of hepatitis C as a public health threat in Iceland: a goal attainable by 2020. J Hepatol 2018; 68(5):932–9.

96. Gottfredsson M, Tyrfingsson T, Runarsdottir V, et al. Major decrease in prevalence of hepatitis C Viremia in key populations following the second year of treatment as prevention for Hepatitis C (TraP HepC) program in Iceland. Open Forum Infect Dis 2018;5(suppl_1):S30.

Hepatitis C

How Good Are Real-Life Data and Do Generics Work

Ashley N. Tran, MD[a], Joseph K. Lim, MD[a,b],*

KEYWORDS

- Hepatitis C • Drug therapy • Antiviral therapy • Direct-acting antivirals
- Real-world cohorts • Generics

KEY POINTS

- Oral direct-acting antiviral regimens are associated with high rates of sustained virologic response in phase III registration trials of chronic hepatitis C virus infection.
- Sustained virologic response is associated with significant improvement in clinical outcomes, including reduced risk for liver cirrhosis, liver failure, hepatocellular carcinoma, and liver-related and all-cause mortality.
- Observational studies confirm similar safety and efficacy as that reported in clinical trials with contemporary oral direct-acting antiviral regimens across genotypes, geography, and special populations.
- Preliminary data suggest that generic oral direct-acting antiviral formulations seem to have equivalent efficacy as their originator drugs.
- Additional real-world studies are needed to clarify optimal treatment regimens in difficult-to-treat populations, as well as in direct-acting antiviral-experienced patients who fail salvage treatment.

INTRODUCTION

Chronic hepatitis C virus (HCV) infection affects 71 million individuals worldwide and is associated with significant morbidity and mortality owing to complications from cirrhosis, hepatic decompensation, and hepatocellular carcinoma (HCC).[1] The goal of antiviral therapy is to achieve a sustained virologic response (SVR), which has been shown to improve clinical outcomes, including liver-related and all-cause mortality. Over the last 5 years, treatment of HCV has shifted to direct-acting antiviral (DAA)

a Section of Digestive Diseases, Yale Liver Center, Yale University School of Medicine, New Haven, CT, USA; b Yale Viral Hepatitis Program, Yale University School of Medicine, 333 Cedar Street, LMP 1080, New Haven, CT 06520-8019, USA
* Corresponding author. Yale Viral Hepatitis Program, Yale University School of Medicine, 333 Cedar Street, LMP 1080, New Haven, CT 06520-8019.
E-mail address: joseph.lim@yale.edu

Gastroenterol Clin N Am 49 (2020) 279–299
https://doi.org/10.1016/j.gtc.2020.01.006
0889-8553/20/© 2020 Elsevier Inc. All rights reserved.

regimens, which have led to a greater than 90% SVR in clinical trials (**Tables 1** and **2**). These therapies have superior efficacy, tolerability, and safety compared with historical interferon-based regimens. The success of DAA regimens have led to their widespread use across genotypes and in populations traditionally viewed as difficult to treat, including those with HIV coinfection, renal failure, and decompensated cirrhosis. Currently, there are 8 oral DAA regimens approved for HCV treatment by the US Food and Drug Administration and recommended by guidelines of the American Association for the Study of Liver Diseases (AASLD) and Infectious Diseases Society of American (IDSA) (**Table 3**). Although these advances in therapy raise the prospect of HCV eradication, many questions still remain about real-world efficacy and safety.

Data from real-world studies can provide valuable information to patients, clinicians, and policymakers about therapeutic efficacy in clinical practice. Real-world studies offer complementary evidence to randomized controlled trials, which often have limited external validity owing to restrictive inclusion and exclusion criteria.[2] The populations enrolled in clinical trials may not be representative of real-world patients who may have complex medical and psychiatric comorbidities, and are more likely to have advanced liver disease. Data from real-world studies can come from diverse patient cohorts and registries that exist worldwide and can provide a practical and longitudinal assessment of clinical outcomes.[3] In this review, we summarize HCV treatment efficacy and safety of DAAs using data published from real-world studies across genotypes 1 to 4 and special populations, and review available data assessing the effectiveness of generic DAA formulations.

REAL-WORLD EFFICACY BY GENOTYPE
Genotype 1

HCV genotype 1 (GT1) is the most prevalent worldwide affecting 83.4 million persons, accounting for 46.2% of all HCV cases.[4] GT1 has been widely pursued for treatment optimization, and multiple phase III trials have demonstrated a more than 90% SVR with several generations of oral DAA regimens. Similar efficacy has also been observed in clinical practice across various settings (**Table 4**). HCV-TARGET is a prospective, observational, multicenter international cohort study of patients with chronic HCV undergoing antiviral therapy. Terrault and colleagues[5] evaluated 2255 patients, the majority of whom had cirrhosis and were treatment experienced. Patients were treated with sofosbuvir (SOF)/ledipasvir (LDV) with and without ribavirin (RBV) for 8, 12, and 24 weeks, and the SVR was 96% among patients treated with SOF/LDV and 97% in those treated with SOF/LDV + RBV. The addition of RBV was not associated with increased efficacy, and furthermore was associated with a higher incidence of reported adverse events. A subsequent study evaluating a subset of GT1 treatment-naïve, cirrhotic patients also failed to demonstrate an increased SVR with the use of RBV.[6]

The US Veterans Health Administration (VHA) represents the largest provider of care for patients with chronic HCV in the United States, and has provided valuable real-world efficacy data in this population. Ioannou and colleagues[7] reviewed 13,974 patients with GT1 HCV who were treated with SOF/LDV with and without RBV for 8, 12 and 24 weeks. An SVR was achieved in 92.8% and no differences were observed between regimen type, prior treatment status, and presence of cirrhosis. Another study performed by Backus and colleagues[8] reported SVR rates of 91.3% for SOF/LDV and 92.% in SOF/LDV + RBV in a cohort of 4834 treatment-naïve VA patients who were treated for 8 and 12 weeks. This study reported a statistically significant decrease in the SVR among patients treated with shorter course (8 weeks) versus

Table 1
Efficacy of SOF-containing regimens in phase III clinical trials

Author, Year	GT	Regimen	Duration (wk)	Cirrhosis	Treatment History	N	SVR (%)
ION-1 (Afdhal et al,[57] 2014)	1	SOF/LDV	12	With/without	Naïve	214	99.0
		SOF/LDV	24	With/without	Naïve	217	98.0
		SOF/LDV + RBV	12	With/without	Naïve	217	97.0
		SOF/LDV + RBV	24	With/without	Naïve	217	99.0
ION-2 (Afdhal et al,[58] 2014)	1	SOF/LDV	12	With/without	Experienced	109	94.0
		SOF/LDV	24	With/without	Experienced	111	99.0
		SOF/LDV + RBV	12	With/without	Experienced	109	96.0
		SOF/LDV + RBV	24	With/without	Experienced	111	99.0
ION-3 (Kowdley et al,[59] 2014)	1	SOF/LDV	8	Without	Naïve	215	94.0
		SOF/LDV	12	Without	Naïve	216	95.0
		SOF/LDV + RBV	8	Without	Naïve	216	93.0
ASTRAL-1 (Feld et al,[60] 2015)	1a	SOF/VEL	12	With/without	Both	210	98.0
	1b	SOF/VEL	12	With/without	Both	118	99.0
	2	SOF/VEL	12	With/without	Both	104	100.0
	4	SOF/VEL	12	With/without	Both	116	100.0
	5	SOF/VEL	12	With/without	Both	35	97.0
	6	SOF/VEL	12	With/without	Both	41	100.0
ASTRAL-2,3 (Foster et al,[61] 2015)	2	SOF/VEL	99.0%	With/without	Both	134	99.0
	3	SOF/VEL	12	With/without	Both	277	95.0
ASTRAL-4 (Curry et al,[62] 2015)	1a	SOF/VEL	12	With	Both	50	88.0
	1a	SOF/VEL	24	With	Both	55	93.0
	1b	SOF/VEL	12	With	Both	18	89.0
	1b	SOF/VEL	24	With	Both	16	88.0
	2	SOF/VEL	12	With	Both	4	100.0
	2	SOF/VEL	24	With	Both	4	75.0
	3	SOF/VEL	12	With	Both	14	50.0
	3	SOF/VEL	24	With	Both	12	50.0
	4	SOF/VEL	12	With	Both	4	100.0
	4	SOF/VEL	24	With	Both	2	100.0
	6	SOF/VEL	24	With	Both	1	100.0
ALLY-3 (Nelson et al,[18] 2015)	3	SOF/DCV	12 wk	With/without	Naïve	101	90.0
		SOF/DCV	12 wk	With/without	Experienced	51	86.0
ALLY-3+ (Leroy et al,[63] 2016)	3	SOF/DCV + RBV	12 wk	With/without	Both	24	87.5
		SOF/DCV + RBV	16 wk	With/without	Both	26	92.3
POLARIS-1 (Bourliere et al,[64] 2017)	1a	SOF/VEL/VOX	12 wk	With/without	Experienced	101	96.0
	1b	SOF/VEL/VOX	12 wk	With/without	Experienced	45	100.0
	2	SOF/VEL/VOX	12 wk	With/without	Experienced	5	100.0
	3	SOF/VEL/VOX	12 wk	With/without	Experienced	78	95.0
	4	SOF/VEL/VOX	12 wk	With/without	Experienced	22	91.0
	5	SOF/VEL/VOX	12 wk	With/without	Experienced	1	100.0
	6	SOF/VEL/VOX	12 wk	With/without	Experienced	6	100.0

(continued on next page)

Table 1
(continued)

Author, Year	GT	Regimen	Duration (wk)	Cirrhosis	Treatment History	N	SVR (%)
POLARIS-2	1a	SOF/VEL/VOX	8 wk	With/without	Both	169	92.0
(Jacobson	1b	SOF/VEL/VOX	8 wk	With/without	Both	63	97.0
et al,[65] 2017)	2	SOF/VEL/VOX	8 wk	With/without	Both	63	97.0
	3	SOF/VEL/VOX	8 wk	With/without	Both	92	99.0
	4	SOF/VEL/VOX	8 wk	With/without	Both	63	94.0
	5	SOF/VEL/VOX	8 wk	With/without	Both	18	94.0
	6	SOF/VEL/VOX	8 wk	With/without	Both	30	100.0
POLARIS-3	3	SOF/VEL/VOX	8 wk	With/without	Both	110	96.0
(Jacobson							
et al,[65] 2017)							
POLARIS-4	1a	SOF/VEL/VOX	12 wk	With/without	Experienced	54	98.0
(Bourliere	1b	SOF/VEL/VOX	12 wk	With/without	Experienced	24	96.0
et al,[64] 2017)	2	SOF/VEL/VOX	12 wk	With/without	Experienced	31	100.0
	3	SOF/VEL/VOX	12 wk	With/without	Experienced	54	96.0
	4	SOF/VEL/VOX	12 wk	With/without	Experienced	19	100.0

Abbreviations: DCV, daclatasvir; LDV, ledipasvir; RBV, ribavirin; SOF, sofosbuvir; VEL, velpatasvir; VOX, voxilaprevir.

standard course (12 weeks) DAA therapy, although the absolute difference was only 3.4%.

Shorter courses of 8-week DAA therapy is currently recommended for a subset of GT1 treatment-naïve patients without cirrhosis. The TRIO Health network is a prospective, US multicenter that reported SVR results in a cohort of 826 GT1 treatment-naïve patients who were treated with SOF/LDV for 8 or 12 weeks, and revealed no difference between groups (95.2% vs 95.3%; P = NS).[9] Similar findings were also observed in the German Hepatitis C-Registry (DHC-R), who reported no differences in the overall SVR between 8- and 12-week regimens of SOF/LDV (98.3% vs 98.1%; P = NS) among 2404 patients with GT1 treatment-naïve HCV, although a lower SVR was reported with the 8-week regimen among patients with cirrhosis.[10] These findings support current guideline recommendations for the use of 12-week SOF/LDV regimens in patients with cirrhosis.

Similar efficacy has been observed in real-world cohort studies evaluating other novel oral DAA regimens. The French HEPATHER cohort evaluated the use of SOF/daclatasvir (DCV) with and without RBV in 768 GT1 patients, and reported an overall SVR of 95%, without any observed differences in patients with or without RBV and 12- versus 24-week treatment duration among noncirrhotic patients; however, extended duration SOF/DCV was associated with a higher SVR among cirrhotic patients (95% vs 88%).[11] A retrospective study by Kramer and colleagues[12] evaluated the efficacy of elbasvir (EBR)/grazoprevir (GZR) with and without RBV in a cohort of 2324 VA patients, and revealed an overall SVR of 96.2% and more than 95% across subgroups, including those with prior DAA experience, decompensated cirrhosis, or severe renal impairment. Similarly, an analysis of 349 patients treated with EBR/GZR for 12 weeks in the TRIO network demonstrated an overall SVR of 99%.[13] Few data are available, with the most recently approved DAA regimens such as glecaprevir (GLE)/pibrentasvir (PIB) and sofosbuvir (SOF)/velpatasvir (VEL). D'Ambrosio and colleagues[14] reported a 100% SVR in 352 GT1 Italian patients treated with GLE/PIB for 8, 12, or 16 weeks and Berg and colleagues[15] reported a 99.7% SVR in the DHC-R cohort of 286 patients with

Table 2
Efficacy of EBR/GZR and GLE/PIB in phase III clinical trials

Author, Year	GT	Regimen	Duration (wk)	Cirrhosis	Treatment History	N	SVR (%)
C-EDGE (Zeuzem et al,[66] 2015)	1a	EBR/GZR	12	With/without	Naïve	157	92.0
	1b	EBR/GZR	12	With/without	Naïve	131	99.0
	4	EBR/GZR	12	With/without	Naïve	18	100.0
	6	EBR/GZR	12	With/without	Naïve	10	80.0
C-EDGE (Kwo et al,[67] 2017)	1a	EBR/GZR	12	With/without	Experienced	60	91.7
		EBR/ GZR + RBV	12	With/without	Experienced	60	93.3
		EBR/GZR	16	With/without	Experienced	48	93.8
		EBR/ GZR + RBV	16	With/without	Experienced	55	100.0
	1b	EBR/GZR	12	With/without	Experienced	34	100.0
		EBR/ GZR + RBV	12	With/without	Experienced	29	96.6
		EBR/GZR	16	With/without	Experienced	47	97.9
		EBR/ GZR + RBV	16	With/without	Experienced	37	100.0
	4	EBR/GZR	12	With/without	Experienced	8	87.5
		EBR/ GZR + RBV	12	With/without	Experienced	15	93.3
		EBR/GZR	16	With/without	Experienced	5	60.0
		EBR/ GZR + RBV	16	With/without	Experienced	8	100.0
	6	EBR/GZR	16	With/without	Experienced	2	100.0
		EBR/ GZR + RBV	16	With/without	Experienced	2	100.0
		EBR/ GZR + RBV	12	With/without	Experienced	15	93.3
C-CORAL (Wei et al,[68] 2019)	1a	EBR/GZR	12	With/without	Naïve	37	91.9
	1b	EBR/GZR	12	With/without	Naïve	389	98.2
	4	EBR/GZR	12	With/without	Naïve	3	100.0
	6	EBR/GZR	12	With/without	Naïve	51	66.7
EXPEDITION-1 (Forns et al,[69] 2017)	1	GLE/PIB	12	With	Both	90	99.0
	2	GLE/PIB	12	With	Both	31	100.0
	4	GLE/PIB	12	With	Both	16	100.0
	5	GLE/PIB	12	With	Both	2	100.0
	6	GLE/PIB	12	With	Both	7	100.0
ENDURANCE-1 (Zeuzem et al,[70] 2018)	1	GLE/PIB	8	Without	Both	335	99.1
		GLE/PIB	12	Without	Both	332	99.7
ENDURANCE-3 (Zeuzem et al,[70] 2018)	3	GLE/PIB	8	Without	Both	157	95.0
		GLE/PIB	12	Without	Both	233	95.0

(continued on next page)

Table 2
(continued)

Author, Year	GT	Regimen	Duration (wk)	Cirrhosis	Treatment History	N	SVR (%)
SURVEYOR-II, 3 (Wyles et al,[71] 2018)	3	GLE/PIB	12	With	Naïve	40	98.0
		GLE/PIB	12	Without	Experienced	22	91.0
		GLE/PIB	16	Without	Experienced	22	95.0
		GLE/PIB	16	With	Experienced	47	96.0
Asselah et al,[72] 2018	2	GLE/PIB	8	Without	Both	145	98.0
	2	GLE/PIB	12	Without	Both	196	99.0
	4	GLE/PIB	8	Without	Both	46	93.0
	4	GLE/PIB	12	Without	Both	76	99.0
	5	GLE/PIB	8	Without	Both	2	100.0
	5	GLE/PIB	12	Without	Both	26	100.0
	6	GLE/PIB	8	Without	Both	10	90.0
	6	GLE/PIB	12	Without	Both	19	100.0

Abbreviations: EBR, elbasvir; GLE, glecaprevir; GZR, grazoprevir; PIB, pibrentasvir; RBV, ribavirin.

Table 3
AASLD/IDSA and EASL treatment recommendations by genotype

GT with and Without Cirrhosis (Child-Pugh a)	Regimen	RBV	Duration (wk)
1	SOF/VEL	No	12
	SOF/LDV	No	8–12
	GLE/PIB	No	8–12
	EBR/GZR	Yes	12–16
	PrOD	Yes	12
	SIM + SOF	No	12
	SOF/DCV	No	12
2	SOF/VEL	No	12
	GLE/PIB	No	8–12
	SOF/DCV	No	12–24
3	SOF/VEL	No	12
	GLE/PIB	No	8–16
	SOF/DCV	Yes	12–24
	SOF/VEL/VOX	No	12
4	SOF/LDV	No	12
	EBR/GZR	No	12
	SOF/VEL	No	12
	GLE/PIB	No	8–12
	PrOD	Yes	12
5 and 6	SOF/LDV	No	12
	SOF/VEL	No	12
	GLE/PIB	No	8–12

Abbreviations: DCV, daclatasvir; EBR, elbasvir; GLE, glecaprevir; GZR, grazoprevir; LDV, ledipasvir; PIB, pibrentasvir; PrOD, paritaprevir/ritonavir/ombitasvir with dasabuvir; RBV, ribavirin; SOF, sofosbuvir; VEL, velpatasvir; VOX, voxilaprevir.

Data from AASLD-IDSA. Recommendations for testing, managing, and treating hepatitis C. Available from: http://www.hcvguidelines.org. Accessed Jan 16 2020; and European Association for the Study of the Liver. EASL Recommendations on Treatment of Hepatitis C 2018. J Hepatol 2018;69(2):461-511.

Table 4
Real-world efficacy for treatment of chronic HCV infection with GT1

Cohort (Author, Year)	Regimen	n	SVR (%)	Duration (wk)
VA (Ioannou et al,[7] 2016)	SOF/LDV	8140	94.3	8
			95.0	12
			94.6	24
	SOF/LDV + RBV	2692	92.9	12
			95.8	24
VA (Backus et al,[8] 2016)	SOF/LDV	3763	92.1	8
			94.3	12
	SOF/LDV + RBV	602	94.2	12
HCV-TARGET (Terrault et al,[5] 2016)	SOF/LDV	1927	96.0	8
			97.0	12
			95.0	24
	SOF/LDV + RBV	328	97.0	12
			95.0	24
HCV-Target (Lim et al,[6] 2018)	SOF/LDV	459	98.0	12
			94.1	24
	SOF/LDV + RBV	130	97.1	12
			95.0	24
Trio (Tapper et al,[73] 2016)	SOF/LDV	1521	94.1	12
	SOF/LDV + RBV	76	97.4	12
Trio (Curry et al,[9] 2017)	SOF/LDV	826	95.2	8
			95.3	12
German Hepatitis C Registry (Honer zu Siederdissen et al,[74] 2018)	SOF/LDV	2218	93.9	8
			95.2	12
			94.6	24
	SOF/LDV + RBV	429	91.6	12
			92.9	24
German Hepatitis C Registry (Buggisch et al,[10] 2018)	SOF/LDV	2383	98.3	8
			85.5	12
Spanish National Registry (Calleja et al,[75] 2017)	SOF/LDV	869	92.4	8
			96.1	12
			95.6	24
	SOF/LDV + RBV	889	95.7	12
HEPATHER (Pol et al,[11] 2017)	SOF/DCV	599	92.0	12
			95.0	24
	SOF/DCV + RBV	169	94.0	12
			99.0	24
German Hepatitis C Registry (Honer zu Siederdissen et al,[74] 2018)	SOF/DCV	471	96.1	12
			95.0	24
	SOF/DCV + RBV	31	93.5	24
VA (Kramer et al,[12] 2018)	EBR/GZR	1801	97.9	12
			95.7	16
	EBR/GZR + RBV	113	93.7	12
			87.1	16
Trio (Flamm et al,[13] 2018)	EBR/GZR	404	99.0	12
			90.0	16
	EBR/GZR	43	100	12
			92.0	16

(continued on next page)

Table 4
(continued)

Cohort (Author, Year)	Regimen	n	SVR (%)	Duration (wk)
NAVIGATORE-Lombardia (D'Ambrosio et al,[14] 2019)	GLE/PIB	321	95.6	8, 12 and 16
DHC-R (Berg et al,[15] 2019)	GLE/PIB	286	99.7	8 and 12
VA (Belperio et al,[22] 2019)	SOF/VEL/VOX	490	90.7	12

Abbreviations: DCV, daclatasvir; EBR, elbasvir; GZR, grazoprevir; LDV, ledipasvir; PIB, pibrentasvir; RBV, ribavirin; SOF, sofosbuvir; VEL, velpatasvir; VOX, voxilaprevir.

GT1 HCV. Although these early real-world results are very promising, the high reported SVR rates with GLE/PIB have been observed in treatment-naïve noncirrhotic individuals and additional validation in cirrhotic and treatment-experienced patients are needed.

Genotype 2

In patients infected with genotype 2 (GT2), SOF/VEL and GLE/PIB are currently recommended by the AASLD/IDSA as first-line regimens, and SOF/DCV is considered an alternative regimen, although remains commonly used in global settings outside the United States and Europe (**Table 5**). The largest real-world study was performed by Belperio and colleagues,[16] who evaluated 2939 VA patients treated with either SOF/DCV or SOF/VEL, with and without RBV, for 12 or 24 weeks. Overall, an SVR was achieved in 93.9% of patients and rates did not differ between SOF/DCV or SOF/VEL (94.5% vs 94.4%; P = NS), although higher treatment discontinuation was observed with SOF/DCV. Although the addition of RBV was not associated with an increased SVR, treatment extension to 24 weeks was associated with a

Table 5
Real-world efficacy for treatment of chronic HCV infection with GT2

Cohort (Author, Year)	Regimen	N	SVR (%)	Duration (wk)
VA (Belperio et al,[16] 2019)	SOF/DCV	271	96.1	12
			100.0	16
			97.7	24
	SOF/DCV + RBV	44	90.9	12
			80.0	16
			100.0	24
	SOF/VEL	2368	97.9	12
			93.2	16
			100.0	24
	SOF/VEL + RBV	256	93.0	12
			100.0	16
			88.9	24
NAVIGATORE-Lombardia (D'Ambrosio et al,[14] 2019)	GLE/PIB	183	94.5	8, 12 and 16
DHC-R (Berg et al,[15] 2019)	GLE/PIB	36	100	8 and 12
VA (Belperio et al,[22] 2019)	SOF/VEL/VOX	20	90	12

Abbreviations: DCV, daclatasvir; GLE, glecaprevir; PIB, pibrentasvir; RBV, ledipasvir; SOF, sofosbuvir; VEL, velpatasvir; VOX, voxilaprevir.

higher SVR compared with the 12-week regimen among patients with cirrhosis (95.8% vs 82.6%). In addition, both the Italian and DHC-R cohorts reported high SVR rates of greater than 98% in patients treated with GLE/PIB for GT2, although these studies were completed predominantly in treatment-naïve, noncirrhotic individuals.[14,15] Additional reports from cohort studies evaluating treatment-experienced and/or cirrhotic populations with GT2 HCV may further clarify real-world efficacy across subgroups.

Genotype 3

HCV genotype 3 (GT3) infection represents the second most prevalent genotype in the world, has been identified as the most challenging to treat, and is associated with a higher risk for liver-associated outcomes, including HCC. SOF/VEL and GLE/PIB are first-line regimens recommended for the treatment of GT3 HCV per AASLD/IDSA guidelines, although SOF/DCV remains a commonly used regimen in global settings. In contrast with clinical trial results from the ALLY-3 protocol revealing an increase in the SVR with SOF/DCV/RBV versus SOF/DCV, real-world studies have revealed conflicting data regarding an additive role for RBV[17,18] (**Table 6**). In the European Compassionate Use Protocol, a similar SVR was observed between GT3 patients treated with SOF/DCV or SOF/DCV/RBV for 24 weeks (88% vs 89%; P = NS).[17] The French ATU cohort also revealed no difference in the SVR between SOF/DCV with or without RBV for 24 weeks (89% vs 82%; P = NS).[19] In contrast, 2 studies have revealed a signal for improved efficacy for RBV-containing regimens in

Table 6
Real-world efficacy for treatment of chronic HCV infection with GT3

Cohort (Author, Year)	Regimen	n	SVR (%)	Duration (wk)
VA (Belperio et al,[16] 2019)	SOF/DCV	431	93.6	12
			93.8	16
			90.9	24
	SOF/DCV + RBV	514	89.8	12
			89.4	16
			94.6	24
	SOF/VEL	1424	95.3	12
			88.5	16
			80.0	24
	SOF/VEL + RBV	455	90.3	12
			82.1	16
			89.5	24
French ATU (Hézode et al,[19] 2017)	SOF/DCV	262	72.7	12
			88.8	24
	SOF/DCV + RBV	71	60.0	12
			82.0	24
European Compassionate Use Protocol (Welzel et al,[17] 2016)	SOF/DCV	56	88.0	24
	SOF/DCV + RBV	37	89.0	24
DHC-R (Cornberg et al,[20] 2017)	SOF/DCV ± RBV	262	87.8	12 and 24
German GECCO (Wehmeyer et al,[76] 2018)	SOF/DCV	22	81.2	12 and 24
	SOF/DCV + RBV	67	86.6	
NAVIGATORE-Lombardia (D'Ambrosio et al,[14] 2019)	GLE/PIB	53	86.8	8, 12 and 16
DHC-R (Berg et al,[15] 2019)	GLE/PIB	176	98.9	8 and 12
VA (Belperio et al,[22] 2019)	SOF + VEL + VOX	46	91.3	12

GT3 HCV treatment. Belperio and colleagues[16] reported an incremental increase in the SVR by regimen: 84.8% (28/33) in SOF/DCV for 24 weeks, 86.4% (95/110) SOF/DCV/RBV for 12 weeks, and 93.9% (107/114) SOF/DCV/RBV for 24 weeks. The DHC-R cohort also reported a trend toward a higher SVR with SOF/DCV/RBV versus SOF/DCV for GT3 HCV, although statistical significance was not achieved.[20] Differences in the reported effect of RBV on the SVR may reflect important distinctions in studied populations, including varying proportions of patients with cirrhosis and/or hepatic decompensation; therefore, further clarification of optimal regimens is needed through real-world studies.[21]

The efficacy of SOF/VEL for GT3 HCV has been validated in several phase III randomized controlled trials. Real-world studies from the US VHA largely confirm the efficacy of SOF/VEL in this population. Belperio and colleagues[22] reported high SVR rates with SOF/VEL with or without RBV (92% vs 86.4%; P = NS) in a cohort of 1735 US veterans with GT3 HCV. Another VHA study investigated the efficacy of SOF/VEL/voxilaprevir (VOX) in 46 DAA-experienced GT3 patients and reported an overall SVR of 93.3%, with a lower SVR observed only in the subgroup previously treated with SOF/VEL. Finally, a small study evaluating efficacy of GLE/PIB in an Italian cohort of 48 GT3 patients reported an overall SVR of 95.8%.[14]

Genotype 4

Real-world data on treatment efficacy in genotype 4 (GT4)-infected patients are limited (**Table 7**).[23] Crespo and colleagues[24] evaluated 252 GT4-infected patients who were treated with paritaprevir/ritonavir/ombitasvir with dasabuvir or SOF/LDV with or without RBV, and for 12 or 24 weeks. The overall SVR was 96.2% and 95.4% for the paritaprevir/ritonavir/ombitasvir with dasabuvir and SOF/LDV regimens, respectively, with a lower SVR observed in patients with cirrhosis regardless of RBV or treatment duration. In a separate study evaluating a Saudi Arabian GT4 cohort of patients with advanced cirrhosis or decompensated cirrhosis, SOF/LDV was associated with a 92.5% SVR without impact of RBV.[25] Data from the French ATU cohort of 176 GT4 patients with advanced cirrhosis revealed a reported SVR of 90% and 97% with SOF/DCV and SOF/DCV/RBV regimens, respectively.[26] Both EBR/GZR and

Table 7				
Real-world efficacy for treatment of chronic HCV infection with GT4				
Cohort (Author, Year)	**Regimen**	**n**	**SVR (%)**	**Duration (wk)**
VA (Ioannou et al,[7] 2016)	SOF/LDV + RBV	103	97.0	12
Spanish National Registry (Crespo et al,[24] 2017)	PrOD + RBV	122	96.2	12 and 24
	SOF/LDV ± RBV	130	95.4	8, 12 and 24
SOLID registry (Sanai et al,[25] 2018)	SOF/LDV ± RBV	213	90.5	12
			100	24
French ATU (Hézode,[26] 2017)	SOF/DCV	137	90.0	12 and 24
	SOF/DCV + RBV	34	97.0	12 and 24
Trio (Flamm et al,[13] 2018)	EBR/GZR	21	95.0	12
VA (Kramer et al,[12] 2018)	EBR/GZR	50	100	12
NAVIGATORE-Lombardia (D'Ambrosio et al,[14] 2018)	GLE/PIB	79	89.9	8, 12, and 16
DHC-R (Berg et al,[15] 2019)	GLE/PIB	26	100	8 and 12
VA (Belperio et al,[22] 2019)	SOF + VEL + VOX	12	100	12

Abbreviation: PrOD, paritaprevir/ritonavir/ombitasvir with dasabuvir.

GLE/PIB have additionally been associated with high rates of SVR 95% to 100% in the VHA, Trio, DHC-R, and Lombardia networks.[12–15] These collective data confirm overall efficacy of current oral DAA regimens for GT4 HCV in diverse real-world settings, although owing to small sample sizes with limited representation of treatment-experienced patients and special populations, additional studies are warranted to clarify optimal management.

Genotypes 5 and 6

Genotype 5 (GT5) and genotype 6 (GT6) represent the least frequent HCV genotypes globally, and are significantly under-represented in both clinical trials and real-world studies. Whereas HCV GT5 is concentrated in southern and eastern sub-Saharan Africa,[27] HCV GT6 is most commonly seen in East and Southeast Asia, and accounts for 20% to 50% of chronic HCV in Laos, Cambodia, Thailand, Vietnam, and Myanmar.[4,27] Current guidelines of the AASLD/IDSA and EASL recommend GLE/PIB as first-line therapy for the treatment of chronic GT5 and GT6 HCV infection.[28,29] Very limited real-world data are currently available for these genotypes; in a small DHC-R cohort of 13 GT5 or GT6 patients, the overall SVR observed with GLE/PIB was 100%.[15] More studies are needed to verify real-world efficacy of GLE/PIB and other regimens for GT5 and GT6 HCV.

GENERIC DRUGS

Despite major advances in therapy, access to treatment remains a barrier owing to high costs of DAAs. Two pharmaceutical companies, Gilead and Bristol-Myers Squibb, have granted voluntary licenses to generic manufacturers to produce SOF, LDV, VEL (Gilead), and DCV to low- and middle-income countries.[30] Additionally, unlicensed production and the import of generics represent an option in countries where specific DAAs are not patented.[31] Countries have also been able to negotiate prices and issue government use or compulsory licenses, which allow for local companies to manufacture or import generics under conditions stated by national patent laws. Although the increase in competition has led to a downward trend in prices, cost remains a barrier to access in many middle- and high-income countries, and wide disparities exist between the prices of the originator and generic versions among different countries in the same income groups.[30]

Available studies reveal that generic DAAs seem to have similar efficacy with comparable SVR rates as their originator drugs in clinical trials and real-world studies (**Table 8**). Multiple observational studies have demonstrated SVR rates between 90% and 100% in patients infected with GT 1 to 6 who were treated with generic DAAs in low- and middle-income countries worldwide. The largest real-world study was performed by Omar and colleagues,[32] who reported an SVR rate of 95.1% in 18,738 Egyptian patients infected with GT4 and treated with generic SOF/DCV with or without RBV; tolerability and adherence were remarkably high in this cohort, with only 1.45% premature treatment discontinuation. A large observational study of 11,105 GT1 to GT4 patients in India treated with generic SOF/DCV with or without RBV revealed an overall SVR of 93%.[33] Similarly high SVR rates of greater than 95% were observed in real-world studies evaluating generic SOF/VEL in GT1 to GT6 HCV monoinfected patients from Taiwan and Myanmar,[34,35] and in HCV/HIV coinfected patients from Taiwan.[36]

Several international cohorts have also demonstrated high efficacy rates in generic DAAs. Data from the REDEMPTION-1 trial reported an overall SVR of 94.2% in 419 GT1 to GT6 infected patients treated with imported generic SOF, LDV, DCV, and

Table 8
Real-world efficacy of generic oral DAA regimens for chronic HCV infection

Author, Year	Country	Regimen	Population	Study Design	n	SVR12 (%)
Premkumar et al,[33] 2017	India	SOF/DCV/RBV	GT1-4	Observational	11,105	93
Goel et al,[77] 2017	India	SOF/DCV ± RBV	GT3	Observational	100	91.9
Zeng et al,[78] 2017	China	SOF/LDV ± RBV	GT1b	Observational	192	96.9
Freeman et al,[37] 2016	International	SOF/LDV or SOF/DCV	GT1-6	Observational	448	90–100
Hajarizadeh et al,[79] 2017	Iran	SOF/DCV	GT1 and 3 Cirrhosis or after transplantation	Observational	104	98
Hill et al,[38] 2017	International	SOF/LDV or SOF/DCV	GT1-6	Observational	616	99
Liu et al,[36] 2018	Taiwan	SOF/VEL ± RBV	HCV and HCV/HIV	Observational	228	97.1–98.1
Abozeid et al,[80] 2018	Egypt	SOF/DCV, ± RBV, LDV/SOF ± RBV	GT4	Observational	395	98.2
Ahmed et al,[81] 2018	Egypt	SOF/DCV	GT4	Observational	183	96
El-Nahaas et al,[82] 2018	Egypt	SOF/DCV	GT4	Observational	134	100
Gupta et al,[84] 2018	India	SOF/RBV, LDV, DCV	GT1 and 3	Observational	499	95.9
Liu et al,[35] 2018	Taiwan	SOF/RBV, SOF/LDV, SOF/DCV, SOF/VEL	GT1-6	Observational	517	95.4
Omar et al,[32] 2018	Egypt	SOF/DCV ± RBV	GT4	Observational	18,378	95.1
Marciano et al,[83] 2018	Argentina	SOF/DCV, SOF/DCV/RBV, or SOF/RBV	GT1	Observational	321	90
Hlaing et al,[34] 2019	Myanmar	SOF/DCV ± RBV, SOF/VEL ± RBV	GT3 and 6 cirrhosis	Observational	522	95
Lashen et al,[39] 2019	Egypt	SOF/LDV ± RBV, DCV + SOF ± RBV	GT4	Observational	648	97.8

RBV in Russia, Australia, and southeast Asia.[37] One report by Hill and colleagues[38] revealed an overall SVR of 99% in 616 GT1 to GT6 patients who were treated with generic SOF/LDV and SOF/DCV with or without RBV acquired through online buyer's clubs supplied from Bangladesh, China, and Egypt. Finally, real-world studies have demonstrated that generic DAAs are highly effective in special patient populations, such as patients with decompensated cirrhosis, transplant recipients, intravenous drug users, and patients with renal impairment.[31,33]

Although multiple cohorts worldwide have shown the efficacy of generic DAAs that are generally similar to the SVR rates observed with originator drugs in clinical trials and real-world practice, additional studies are needed to evaluate adherence, safety, and long-term clinical outcomes. To date, no placebo-controlled, blinded, randomized, controlled trials have compared generic versus originator DAA regimens for HCV, and existing observational studies have revealed significant variability in sourcing owing to international differences in licensing and drug patent laws.[31] Concerns remain for the potential for the manufacture and distribution of counterfeit DAAs, as well as both logistical and medical monitoring challenges associated with patient-initiated procurement of DAA medications through online buyers' clubs.[38] Further investigation is needed to evaluate a broader range of generic sources and larger representative cohorts that include difficult-to-treat populations. Nevertheless, low-cost generic DAAs have thus far demonstrated similar efficacy and tolerability compared with originator drugs and are very likely represent an essential component to public health efforts to accomplish the World Health Organization targets for HCV elimination by 2030.[38,39]

SPECIAL POPULATIONS
HIV/Hepatitis C Virus Coinfection

HCV is common among those infected with HIV and the global prevalence of HIV/HCV coinfection is estimated at 2.5 to 5.0 million. The rate of coinfection is 10% to 30% in patients with HIV and as high as 90% in those who inject drugs.[40] Compared with monoinfected patients, those with HIV/HCV coinfection experience more rapid progression of liver fibrosis, hepatic decompensation, and HCC. Although the rate of progression is mitigated in virologically controlled patients, the risk of hepatic decompensation in coinfected patients treated with antiretroviral therapy (ART) remains higher than in HCV monoinfected patients.[41] Finally, liver failure is the leading cause of mortality in this population and once hepatic decompensation occurs, HIV coinfected patients experience higher mortality compared with those with HCV alone.[42]

Multiple clinical trials have demonstrated the safety and efficacy of DAAs in coinfected patients with similar SVR rates as those with HCV monoinfection.[40] These findings have been confirmed in a series of real-world observational studies, and importantly have clarified safety and efficacy in patients on a spectrum of ART regimens. Bhattacharya and colleagues[43] demonstrated a 90.9% SVR in a population of 969 HIV/HCV GT1 coinfected veterans treated with SOF/LDV with or without RBV. In a French multicenter observational cohort of HIV/HCV GT1-6 coinfected patients treated with SOF/DCV or SOF/LDV, with and without RBV, 93.5% achieved a SVR.[44] No differences in the SVR were observed between patients receiving protease inhibitor-based, non-nucleoside reverse transcriptase inhibitor-based, and integrase inhibitor-based ART regimens, respectively. Furthermore, data from the German GECCO cohort of GT1 and GT4 coinfected patients (mean CD4 count 601) suggested the possibility of short duration treatment; reported an SVR rate of 96.4% in subset of GT1 and 4 patients who were treated with 8 weeks of SOF/LDV.[45]

Although the AASLD/IDSA and EASL guidelines recommend that HIV/HCV-coinfected patients should be treated similarly to those with HCV monoinfection, it is important to note that HCV reinfection after achieving an SVR may be higher in those coinfected with HIV and have one or more risk factors.[28,29] In the GECCO cohort, 32 of 1960 patients who achieved an SVR with a SOF-based regimen experienced HCV reinfection, 81.2% of whom were coinfected with HIV; injection drug use and men who have sex with men were significant risk factors for reinfection.[46] Overall, treatment of HCV/HIV coinfected patients with oral DAA regimens is associated with excellent efficacy similar, to that observed with HCV monoinfected patients. Careful assessment and management of potential drug–drug interactions with ART therapy is warranted in collaboration with an HIV treating clinician. Patients with additional risk factors for reinfection should be regularly monitored as per AASLD/IDSA guidance.

Renal Impairment

The prevalence of chronic kidney disease (CKD) and end-stage renal disease (ESRD) is higher among patients with HCV compared with the general population. Studies have shown that patients with HCV with CKD have an accelerated rate in the loss of renal function and have an increased risk for progressing to ESRD. Furthermore, there is an increased risk of all-cause mortality in patients with HCV on dialysis, and HCV impairs the survival of renal allografts and transplant recipients.[47] Treatment guidelines for the use of oral DAA regimens in CKD patients with an estimated glomerular filtration rate of greater than 30 mL/min are generally the same as CKD patients without CKD without a dose adjustment; however, the AASLD recommends the use of EBR/GZR or GLE/PIB in those with an estimated glomerular filtration rate of less than 30 mL/min and/or ESRD requiring dialysis.[28] SOF-based DAA regimens are commonly used for HCV therapy, but safety concerns for worsening renal failure exist owing to renal excretion of SOF with significant accumulation of its systemic metabolite GS-331007 in patients with CKD. The HCV-TARGET group studied the efficacy and safety of SOF containing regimens in patients with renal impairment and ESRD. The overall reported SVR was 82%, which did not vary significantly with baseline renal dysfunction, although patients with a glomerular filtration rate of less than 45 mL/min experienced more adverse events, including worsening renal function, anemia, and discontinuation of RBV.[48] Similarly, the VA ERCHIVES study group reported high SVR rates of 89% to 100% in 2281 patients with stage 3 CKD and 257 patients with stage 4 or 5 CKD treated with SOF/LDV with or without RBV, but SOF-based treatment was associated with higher rates of worsening renal function and anemia, independent of RBV.[49]

EBR/GZR is associated with an excellent safety and efficacy profile in real-world studies. Kramer and colleagues[12] reported high SVR rates in US veteran with HCV GT1 to CT4 with CKD, including a 96.7% SVR in 393 patients with stage 3 CKD and a 96.3% SVR in 407 patients with stage 4 or 5 CKD. Similar findings were reported from the TRIO network, which revealed a 99% SVR in 114 patients with HCV with stage 4 or 5 CKD.[13] Limited real-world data examining the safety and efficacy of GLE/PIB are available; preliminary data presented by an Italian cohort study group at the 2019 International Liver Congress meeting revealed a 96.4% SVR in patients with ESRD treated with GLE/PIB without an increase in renal impairment.[50] Overall, available real-world studies confirm the excellent efficacy and safety profile of both EBR/GZR and GLE/PIB in the treatment of patients with HCV with CKD and ESRD.

Decompensated Cirrhosis

DAAs have revolutionized HCV treatment in patients with decompensated cirrhosis, who were traditionally excluded from therapy during the interferon era. Studies have shown that patients with decompensated cirrhosis are able to achieve an SVR, but at rates lower than those with compensated cirrhosis. Treatment of HCV offers many potential benefits in decompensated cirrhosis; the SVR in this context has been associated with a decreased risk for HCC, decreased need for liver transplantation, lower risk for HCV recurrence after transplantation, improved measures for hepatic decompensation such as Model for End-Stage Liver Disease, Child-Pugh stage, and hepatic venous pressure gradient, and improvement in transplant-free survival.[51] However, the timing of treatment in liver transplant candidates remains a subject of debate, particularly owing to concerns for lost access to HCV-positive donor organs and potential for delay to transplant owing to transient improvements in Model for End-Stage Liver Disease, which has been described as "Model for End-Stage Liver Disease purgatory." Ideally, HCV treatment in patients with decompensated cirrhosis should be managed at a liver transplant center with expertise in the management of this population, with caution to avoid protease inhibitor-based regimens owing to a risk for hepatotoxicity and liver failure.[28]

Real-world studies have shown variable efficacy in patients with decompensated cirrhosis depending on type of regimen and genotype. The HCV-TARGET group reported a high SVR 90% to 97% in patients with GT1 HCV and decompensated cirrhosis who were treated with SOF/LDV with or without RBV, and for 12 or 24 weeks. Foster and colleagues[52] also reported a high overall SVR of 89.5% in 409 patients with GT1 HCV decompensated cirrhosis treated with SOF/LDV or SOF/DCV, with a higher SVR observed in patients with than without RBV (91.9% vs 84.6%), although RBV dose reduction and/or discontinuation was required in 6% and 20% of patients, respectively. Data from the European Compassionate Use Protocol group revealed a variable SVR by Child-Pugh class, including an SVR of 94%, 86%, and 76% for patients with Child-Pugh classes A, B, and C, respectively;[17] similar to observations from Foster and colleagues,[52] RBV was associated with an improved SVR in patients with Child-Pugh class B and C disease (SVR of 79%–88%). These data support current guideline recommendations for the use of RBV with SOF/LDV in the treatment of patients with GT1 HCV and decompensated cirrhosis.

Patients with GT3 HCV experience the lowest reported SVR rates in context of decompensated cirrhosis. Foster and colleagues[52] reported an overall SVR of 68.8% with SOF/LDV or SOF/DCV for GT3, although was higher with versus without RBV (72.8% vs 61.2%). The French ATU study group reported an overall SVR of 63% with SOF/DCV with or without RBV for 12 or 24 weeks in patients with Child class B/C decompensated cirrhosis (vs 83% with Child A compensated cirrhosis); a trend for a higher SVR was observed with extended 24-week treatment, but was not statistically significant in the context of the small sample size.[19] Finally, Belperio and colleagues[16] reported an overall SVR of 80.4% and 83.3% in US veterans with GT3 disease with decompensated cirrhosis who were treated with SOF/DCV or SOF/VEL, respectively, with or without RBV; no difference in the SVR was observed with the addition of RBV.

Direct-Acting Antiviral Experienced Patients

Although the treatment of HCV infection has been revolutionized by well-tolerated DAAs, 5% to 10% of patients experience DAA treatment failure for various reasons, including poor drug adherence, drug–drug interactions, advanced liver cirrhosis, virologic factors, reinfection, and resistance-associated amino acid substitutions (RAS).[53,54] Retreatment options are limited and currently SOF/VEL/VOX represents the first-line therapy for all genotypes with consideration for RBV in patients with cirrhosis or risk factors for treatment failure.[28,29] For patients in infected with GT1 or GT2, SOF/VEL and GLE/PIB can be used in individuals who have been previously treated with protease and non-NS5A inhibitors.[28] Routine testing for RAS before treatment with SOF/VEL/VOX is not recommended because the treatment outcomes were not associated with the presence of RAS in clinical trials.

The largest real-world study evaluating treatment efficacy in DAA-experienced patients was reported by Belperio and colleagues.[22] In this cohort, 573 GT1-4 patients within the US VHA who failed prior oral DAA regimens (98.9% NS5A experienced, 87.8% NS5B experienced) were treated with SOF/VEL/VOX for 12 weeks. The overall SVR rates were greater than 90% across GT1 to GT4 HCV, including 91.4% in those with prior NS5A and NS5B experience, although a lower SVR (78.9%–86.7%) was observed in patients who failed prior SOF/VEL. Preliminary data from the DHC-R and Trio cohort groups presented at the 2019 International Liver Congress suggest a similarly high SVR of greater than 99% among DAA-experienced patients, the majority of whom were previously treated with SOF/LDV with or without RBV.[55,56] Available real-world data suggest that SOF/VEL/VOX was well-tolerated overall; the most common reported adverse events were fatigue and headache.[55]

SUMMARY

Overall, real-world studies have largely confirmed that oral DAA regimens are associated with outstanding safety and efficacy profiles which are comparable to results reported in phase III trials. This has now been validated across diverse patient populations across geography, HCV genotype, and special populations including patients with HIV/HCV coinfection, CKD, and decompensated cirrhosis. Generic DAA formulations represent an important if not essential component of HCV elimination programs, and the available data suggest equivalent efficacy as results reported with their originator drugs. Real-world studies have additionally provided important clarification of predictors for treatment response across patient subgroups, although additional studies with adequate power are needed to further inform the development of optimal regimens for populations, which continue to experience a lower SVR, including patients with GT3 HCV, decompensated cirrhosis, and those who failed prior DAA regimens.[21] Significant evidence gaps remain in other populations that have been under-represented in clinical trials, such as patients who have undergone liver transplantation, are immunosuppressed, or have substance use disorders. Finally, although treatment failure of SOF/VEL/VOX in DAA-experienced patients is expected to be uncommon, additional salvage strategies will be needed to address those who fail to achieve an SVR for which real-world evidence will play an essential role in guiding clinicians and informing treatment guidelines.

DISCLOSURE

A. Tran reports no relevant conflicts of interest. J.K. Lim reports clinical trial contracts (to institution) from AbbVie and Gilead and consulting honoraria from Gilead.

REFERENCES

1. Organization, W.H. Global hepatitis report 2017. 2017.
2. Blonde L, Khunti K, Harris SB, et al. Interpretation and impact of real-world clinical data for the practicing clinician. Adv Ther 2018;35(11):1763–74.
3. Afdhal NH, Serfaty L. Effect of registries and cohort studies on HCV treatment. Gastroenterology 2016;151(3):387–90.
4. Messina JP, Humphreys I, Flaxman A, et al. Global distribution and prevalence of Hepatitis C Virus genotypes. Hepatology 2015;61(1):77–87.

5. Terrault NA, Zeuzem S, Di Bisceglie AM, et al. Effectiveness of Ledipasvir-Sofosbuvir combination in patients with Hepatitis C Virus infection and factors associated with sustained virologic response. Gastroenterology 2016;151(6): 1131–40.e5.
6. Lim JK, Liapakis AM, Shiffman ML, et al. Safety and effectiveness of Ledipasvir and Sofosbuvir, with or without ribavirin, in treatment-experienced patients with genotype 1 Hepatitis C Virus infection and cirrhosis. Clin Gastroenterol Hepatol 2018;16(11):1811–9.e4.
7. Ioannou GN, Beste LA, Chang M, et al. Effectiveness of Sofosbuvir, Ledipasvir/Sofosbuvir and Paritaprevir/Ritonavir/Ombitasvir and Dasabuvir-based antiviral regimens for Hepatitis C in 17,847 patients in the Veterans Affairs National Healthcare System. Hepatology 2016;64:11a.
8. Backus LI, Belperio PS, Shahoumian TA, et al. Real-world effectiveness of ledipasvir/sofosbuvir in 4,365 treatment-naive, genotype 1 hepatitis C-infected patients. Hepatology 2016;64(2):405–14.
9. Curry MP, Tapper EB, Bacon B, et al. Effectiveness of 8- or 12-weeks of ledipasvir and sofosbuvir in real-world treatment-naive, genotype 1 hepatitis C infected patients. Aliment Pharmacol Ther 2017;46(5):540–8.
10. Buggisch P, Vermehren J, Mauss S, et al. Real-world effectiveness of 8-week treatment with ledipasvir/sofosbuvir in chronic hepatitis C. J Hepatol 2018; 68(4):663–71.
11. Pol S, Bourliere M, Lucier S, et al. Safety and efficacy of daclatasvir-sofosbuvir in HCV genotype 1-mono-infected patients. J Hepatol 2017;66(1):39–47.
12. Kramer JR, Puenpatom A, Erickson KF, et al. Real-world effectiveness of elbasvir/grazoprevir In HCV-infected patients in the US veterans affairs healthcare system. J Viral Hepat 2018;25(11):1270–9.
13. Flamm SL, Bacon B, Curry MP, et al. Real-world use of elbasvir-grazoprevir in patients with chronic hepatitis C: retrospective analyses from the TRIO network. Aliment Pharmacol Ther 2018;47(11):1511–22.
14. D'Ambrosio R, Pasulo L, Puoti M, et al. Real-world effectiveness and safety of glecaprevir/pibrentasvir in 723 patients with chronic hepatitis C. J Hepatol 2019; 70(3):379–87.
15. Berg T, Naumann U, Stoehr A, et al. Real-world effectiveness and safety of glecaprevir/pibrentasvir for the treatment of chronic hepatitis C infection: data from the German Hepatitis C-Registry. Aliment Pharmacol Ther 2019;49(8):1052–9.
16. Belperio PS, Shahoumian TA, Loomis TP, et al. Real-world effectiveness of daclatasvir plus sofosbuvir and velpatasvir/sofosbuvir in hepatitis C genotype 2 and 3. J Hepatol 2019;70(1):15–23.
17. Welzel TM, Petersen J, Herzer K, et al. Daclatasvir plus sofosbuvir, with or without ribavirin, achieved high sustained virological response rates in patients with HCV infection and advanced liver disease in a real-world cohort. Gut 2016;65(11): 1861–70.
18. Nelson DR, Cooper JN, Lalezari JP, et al. All-oral 12-week treatment with daclatasvir plus sofosbuvir in patients with hepatitis C virus genotype 3 infection: ALLY-3 phase III study. Hepatology 2015;61(4):1127–35.
19. Hézode C, Lebray P, De Ledinghen V, et al. Daclatasvir plus sofosbuvir, with or without ribavirin, for hepatitis C virus genotype 3 in a French early access programme. Liver Int 2017;37(9):1314–24.
20. Cornberg M, Petersen J, Schober A, et al. Real-world use, effectiveness and safety of anti-viral treatment in chronic hepatitis C genotype 3 infection. Aliment Pharmacol Ther 2017;45(5):688–700.

21. Hezode C. Treatment of hepatitis C: results in real life. Liver Int 2018;38(Suppl 1):21–7.
22. Belperio PS, Shahoumian TA, Loomis TP, et al. Real-world effectiveness of sofosbuvir/velpatasvir/voxilaprevir in 573 direct-acting antiviral experienced hepatitis C patients. J Viral Hepat 2019;26(8):980–90.
23. Di Biagio A, Taramasso L, Cenderello G. Treatment of hepatitis C virus genotype 4 in the DAA era. Virol J 2018;15(1):180.
24. Crespo J, Calleja JL, Fernandez I, et al. Real-world effectiveness and safety of oral combination antiviral therapy for Hepatitis C Virus genotype 4 infection. Clin Gastroenterol Hepatol 2017;15(6):945–9.e1.
25. Sanai FM, Altraif IH, Alswat K, et al. Real life efficacy of ledipasvir/sofosbuvir in hepatitis C genotype 4-infected patients with advanced liver fibrosis and decompensated cirrhosis. J Infect 2018;76(6):536–42.
26. Hezode C, Abergel A, Chas J, et al. Sustained virologic response to daclatasvir and sofosbuvir, with or without ribavirin, among patients in the French Daclatasvir ATU Programme infected with HCV genotypes 4, 5, and 6. J Hepatol 2016; 64(Suppl 2):S755.
27. Asselah T, Hassanein T, Waked I, et al. Eliminating hepatitis C within low-income countries – The need to cure genotypes 4, 5, 6. J Hepatol 2018;68(4):814–26.
28. AASLD-IDSA. Recommendations for testing, managing, and treating hepatitis C. Available at: http://www.hcvguidelines.org. Accessed on July 2, 2019.
29. European Association for the Study of the Liver. Electronic address: easloffice@easloffice.eu, European Association for the Study of the Liver. EASL recommendations on treatment of hepatitis C 2018. J Hepatol 2018;69(2):461–511.
30. Organization, W.H. Progress report on access to hepatitis C treatment: focus on overcoming barriers in low- and middle-income countries. 2018.
31. Baumert TF, Berg T, Lim JK, et al. Status of direct-acting antiviral therapy for Hepatitis C Virus infection and remaining challenges. Gastroenterology 2019;156(2): 431–45.
32. Omar H, El Akel W, Elbaz T, et al. Generic daclatasvir plus sofosbuvir, with or without ribavirin, in treatment of chronic hepatitis C: real-world results from 18 378 patients in Egypt. Aliment Pharmacol Ther 2018;47(3):421–31.
33. Premkumar M, Grover GS, Dhiman RK. Chronic hepatitis C: do generics work as well as branded drugs? J Clin Exp Hepatol 2017;7(3):253–61.
34. Hlaing NKT, Nangia G, Tun KT, et al. High sustained virologic response in genotypes 3 and 6 with generic NS5A inhibitor and sofosbuvir regimens in chronic HCV in myanmar. J Viral Hepat 2019;26(10):1186–99.
35. Liu CH, Huang YJ, Yang SS, et al. Generic sofosbuvir-based interferon-free direct acting antiviral agents for patients with chronic hepatitis C virus infection: a real-world multicenter observational study. Sci Rep 2018;8(1):13699.
36. Liu CH, Sun HY, Liu CJ, et al. Generic velpatasvir plus sofosbuvir for hepatitis C virus infection in patients with or without human immunodeficiency virus coinfection. Aliment Pharmacol Ther 2018;47(12):1690–8.
37. Freeman J, Khwairakpam G, Dragunova J, et al. Sustained virological response for 94% of people treated with low-cost, legally imported generic direct acting antivirals for hepatitis C: analysis of 1087 patients in 4 treatment programmes. J Hepatol 2017;66(1):S55–6.
38. Hill A, Khwairakpam G, Wang J, et al. High sustained virological response rates using imported generic direct acting antiviral treatment for hepatitis C. J Virus Erad 2017;3(4):200–3.

39. Lashen SA, Shamseya MM, Madkour MA, et al. Tolerability and effectiveness of generic direct-acting antiviral drugs in eradication of hepatitis C genotype 4 among Egyptian patients. Liver Int 2019;39(5):835–43.
40. Wyles DL, Sulkowski MS, Dieterich D. Management of hepatitis C/HIV coinfection in the era of highly effective hepatitis C virus direct-acting antiviral therapy. Clin Infect Dis 2016;63(Suppl 1):S3–11.
41. Schlabe S, Rockstroh JK. Advances in the treatment of HIV/HCV coinfection in adults. Expert Opin Pharmacother 2018;19(1):49–64.
42. Pineda JA, Garcia-Garcia JA, Aguilar-Guisado M, et al. Clinical progression of hepatitis C virus-related chronic liver disease in human immunodeficiency virus-infected patients undergoing highly active antiretroviral therapy. Hepatology 2007;46(3):622–30.
43. Bhattacharya D, Belperio PS, Shahoumian TA, et al. Effectiveness of all-oral antiviral regimens in 996 human immunodeficiency virus/Hepatitis C Virus genotype 1-coinfected patients treated in routine practice. Clin Infect Dis 2017;64(12):1711–20.
44. Piroth L, Wittkop L, Lacombe K, et al. Efficacy and safety of direct-acting antiviral regimens in HIV/HCV-co-infected patients - French ANRS CO13 HEPAVIH cohort. J Hepatol 2017;67(1):23–31.
45. Ingiliz P, Christensen S, Kimhofer T, et al. Sofosbuvir and Ledipasvir for 8 weeks for the treatment of chronic Hepatitis C Virus (HCV) infection in HCV-monoinfected and HIV-HCV-coinfected individuals: results from the german Hepatitis C cohort (GECCO-01). Clin Infect Dis 2016;63(10):1320–4.
46. Berenguer J, Gil-Martin A, Jarrin I, et al. Reinfection by hepatitis C virus following effective all-oral direct-acting antiviral drug therapy in HIV/hepatitis C virus coinfected individuals. AIDS 2019;33(4):685–9.
47. Ladino M, Pedraza F, Roth D. Hepatitis C virus infection in chronic kidney disease. J Am Soc Nephrol 2016;27(8):2238–46.
48. Saxena V, Koraishy FM, Sise ME, et al. Safety and efficacy of sofosbuvir-containing regimens in hepatitis C-infected patients with impaired renal function. Liver Int 2016;36(6):807–16.
49. Butt AA, Ren Y, Puenpatom A, et al. Effectiveness, treatment completion and safety of sofosbuvir/ledipasvir and paritaprevir/ritonavir/ombitasvir + dasabuvir in patients with chronic kidney disease: an ERCHIVES study. Aliment Pharmacol Ther 2018;48(1):35–43.
50. Aglitti A, Caruso R, Calvanese G, et al. Real-life effectiveness and safety of Glecaprevir/Pibrentasvir in HCV infected patients with chronic kidney disease. Dig Liver Dis 2019;51:e66.
51. Kwo P, Agrawal S. Treating hepatitis C virus in patients with decompensated cirrhosis: why is it so difficult and does a sustained response rate rescue the patient from liver transplantation? Clin Liver Dis (Hoboken) 2015;6(6):133–5.
52. Foster GR, Irving WL, Cheung MC, et al. Impact of direct acting antiviral therapy in patients with chronic hepatitis C and decompensated cirrhosis. J Hepatol 2016;64(6):1224–31.
53. Sagnelli E, Starace M, Minichini C, et al. Resistance detection and re-treatment options in hepatitis C virus-related chronic liver diseases after DAA-treatment failure. Infection 2018;46(6):761–83.
54. Heo YA, Deeks ED. Sofosbuvir/velpatasvir/voxilaprevir: a review in chronic hepatitis C. Drugs 2018;78(5):577–87.
55. Vermehren J, Stoehr A, Wiesch JSZ, et al. THU-188-retreatment with sofosbuvir/velpatasvir/voxilaprevir in patients with chronic hepatitis C virus infection and

prior DAA failure: an analysis from the German hepatitis C registry (DHC-R). J Hepatol 2019;70(1):e245.

56. Bacon B, Curry M, Flamm S, et al. THU-116-Effectiveness of the salvage therapy sofosbuvir-velpatasvir-voxilaprevir (SOF-VEL-VOX) in chronic hepatitis C: clinical practice experience from the TRIO network. J Hepatol 2019;70(1):e209.

57. Afdhal N, Zeuzem S, Kwo P, et al. Ledipasvir and sofosbuvir for untreated HCV genotype 1 infection. N Engl J Med 2014;370(20):1889–98.

58. Afdhal N, Reddy KR, Nelson DR, et al. Ledipasvir and sofosbuvir for previously treated HCV genotype 1 infection. N Engl J Med 2014;370(16):1483–93.

59. Kowdley KV, Gordon SC, Reddy KR, et al. Ledipasvir and sofosbuvir for 8 or 12 weeks for chronic HCV without cirrhosis. N Engl J Med 2014;370(20):1879–88.

60. Feld JJ, Jacobson IM, Hezode C, et al. Sofosbuvir and Velpatasvir for HCV Genotype 1, 2, 4, 5, and 6 infection. N Engl J Med 2015;373(27):2599–607.

61. Foster GR, Afdhal N, Roberts SK, et al. Sofosbuvir and Velpatasvir for HCV genotype 2 and 3 infection. N Engl J Med 2015;373(27):2608–17.

62. Curry MP, O'Leary JG, Bzowej N, et al. Sofosbuvir and Velpatasvir for HCV in patients with decompensated cirrhosis. N Engl J Med 2015;373(27):2618–28.

63. Leroy V, Angus P, Bronowicki JP, et al. Daclatasvir, sofosbuvir, and ribavirin for hepatitis C virus genotype 3 and advanced liver disease: a randomized phase III study (ALLY-3+). Hepatology 2016;63(5):1430–41.

64. Bourliere M, Gordon SC, Flamm SL, et al. Sofosbuvir, Velpatasvir, and Voxilaprevir for previously treated HCV infection. N Engl J Med 2017;376(22):2134–46.

65. Jacobson IM, Lawitz E, Gane EJ, et al. Efficacy of 8 weeks of Sofosbuvir, Velpatasvir, and Voxilaprevir in patients with chronic HCV infection: 2 phase 3 randomized trials. Gastroenterology 2017;153(1):113–22.

66. Zeuzem S, Ghalib R, Reddy KR, et al. Grazoprevir-Elbasvir combination therapy for treatment-naive cirrhotic and noncirrhotic patients with chronic Hepatitis C virus genotype 1, 4, or 6 infection: a randomized trial. Ann Intern Med 2015; 163(1):1–13.

67. Kwo P, Gane EJ, Peng CY, et al. Effectiveness of Elbasvir and Grazoprevir combination, with or without ribavirin, for treatment-experienced patients with chronic Hepatitis C infection. Gastroenterology 2017;152(1):164–175 e4.

68. Wei L, Jia JD, Wang FS, et al. Efficacy and safety of elbasvir/grazoprevir in participants with hepatitis C virus genotype 1, 4, or 6 infection from the Asia-Pacific region and Russia: Final results from the randomized C-CORAL study. J Gastroenterol Hepatol 2019;34(1):12–21.

69. Forns X, Lee SS, Valdes J, et al. Glecaprevir plus pibrentasvir for chronic hepatitis C virus genotype 1, 2, 4, 5, or 6 infection in adults with compensated cirrhosis (EXPEDITION-1): a single-arm, open-label, multicentre phase 3 trial. Lancet Infect Dis 2017;17(10):1062–8.

70. Zeuzem S, Foster GR, Wang S, et al. Glecaprevir-Pibrentasvir for 8 or 12 Weeks in HCV genotype 1 or 3 infection. N Engl J Med 2018;378(4):354–69.

71. Wyles D, Poordad F, Wang S, et al. Glecaprevir/pibrentasvir for hepatitis C virus genotype 3 patients with cirrhosis and/or prior treatment experience: a partially randomized phase 3 clinical trial. Hepatology 2018;67(2):514–23.

72. Asselah T, Kowdley KV, Zadeikis N, et al. Efficacy of Glecaprevir/Pibrentasvir for 8 or 12 weeks in patients with Hepatitis C virus genotype 2, 4, 5, or 6 infection without cirrhosis. Clin Gastroenterol Hepatol 2018;16(3):417–26.

73. Tapper EB, Bacon BR, Curry MP, et al. Real-world effectiveness for 12 weeks of ledipasvir-sofosbuvir for genotype 1 hepatitis C: the Trio Health study. J Viral Hepat 2017;24(1):22–7.

74. Honer Zu Siederdissen C, Buggisch P, Boker K, et al. Treatment of hepatitis C genotype 1 infection in Germany: effectiveness and safety of antiviral treatment in a real-world setting. United European Gastroenterol J 2018;6(2):213–24.
75. Calleja JL, Crespo J, Rincon D, et al. Effectiveness, safety and clinical outcomes of direct-acting antiviral therapy in HCV genotype 1 infection: Results from a Spanish real-world cohort. J Hepatol 2017;66(6):1138–48.
76. Wehmeyer MH, Ingiliz P, Christensen S, et al. Real-world effectiveness of sofosbuvir-based treatment regimens for chronic hepatitis C genotype 3 infection: Results from the multicenter German hepatitis C cohort (GECCO-03). J Med Virol 2018;90(2):304–12.
77. Goel A, Bhargava R, Rai P, et al. Treatment of chronic genotype-3 hepatitis C virus infection using direct-acting antiviral agents: an Indian experience. Indian J Gastroenterol 2017;36(3):227–34.
78. Zeng QL, Xu GH, Zhang JY, et al. Generic ledipasvir-sofosbuvir for patients with chronic hepatitis C: a real-life observational study. J Hepatol 2017;66(6):1123–9.
79. Hajarizadeh B. Generic direct acting antiviral treatment: the first step towards elimination of hepatitis C in Iran. Hepat Mon 2017;17(1):e45788.
80. Abozeid M, Alsebaey A, Abdelsameea E, et al. High efficacy of generic and brand direct acting antivirals in treatment of chronic hepatitis C. Int J Infect Dis 2018;75:109–14.
81. Ahmed OA, Safwat E, Khalifa MO, et al. Sofosbuvir plus daclatasvir in treatment of chronic Hepatitis C genotype 4 infection in a cohort of Egyptian patients: an experiment the size of Egyptian village. Int J Hepatol 2018;2018:9616234.
82. El-Nahaas SM, Fouad R, Elsharkawy A, et al. High sustained virologic response rate using generic directly acting antivirals in the treatment of chronic hepatitis C virus Egyptian patients: single-center experience. Eur J Gastroenterol Hepatol 2018;30(10):1194–9.
83. Marciano S, Haddad L, Reggiardo MV, et al. Effectiveness and safety of original and generic sofosbuvir for the treatment of chronic hepatitis C: a real world study. J Med Virol 2018;90(5):951–8.
84. Gupta S, Rout G, Patel AH, et al. Efficacy of generic oral directly acting agents in patients with hepatitis C virus infection. J Viral Hepat 2018;25:771–8.

Hepatitis C
Does Successful Treatment Alter the Natural History and Quality of Life?

Humberto C. Gonzalez, MD[a,b], Stuart C. Gordon, MD[a,b],*

KEYWORDS

- Sustained virologic response • SVR • Mortality • Survival
- Extrahepatic manifestations • Quality of life • Antiviral therapy

KEY POINTS

- Hepatitis C cure with antiviral therapy reduces all-cause mortality.
- Sustained virologic response (SVR) is associated with improvement in liver-related outcomes. SVR reduces risk of liver failure, hepatocellular carcinoma, and fibrosis progression.
- SVR improves the course of extrahepatic manifestations, mixed cryoglobulinemia, non-Hodgkin lymphoma, cardiovascular disease, diabetes mellitus, and quality of life.

INTRODUCTION

The consequences of chronic hepatitis C virus (HCV) infection, both liver related and extrahepatic, are well documented. Untreated HCV viremia can lead not only to impaired quality of life and end-stage liver disease but also to a host of nonliver disorders, ranging from lymphoproliferative to dermatologic to metabolic. Only more recently have the downstream benefits of viral eradication become clearer. In a landmark 2012 article, van der Meer and colleagues[1] showed that sustained virologic response (SVR) reduces all-cause mortality among HCV patients with advanced fibrosis. More recently, Kanwal and colleagues[2] showed that although HCV eradication reduces subsequent risk of hepatocellular carcinoma (HCC), these benefits diminish if treatment is started too late (evolution to more advanced fibrosis). In 2018, Mahale and colleagues[3] likewise showed that various HCV extrahepatic manifestations in fact lessen in incidence after SVR, but again such benefits are best seen among patients treated early in their disease course with antiviral therapy.

[a] Department of Gastroenterology and Hepatology, Henry Ford Hospital, 2799 West Grand Boulevard, Detroit, MI 48202, USA; [b] Wayne State University School of Medicine, 42 W Warren Ave, Detroit, MI 48202, USA
* Corresponding author. Henry Ford Health System, 2799 West Grand Boulevard, Detroit, MI 48202.
E-mail address: sgordon3@hfhs.org

Gastroenterol Clin N Am 49 (2020) 301–314
https://doi.org/10.1016/j.gtc.2020.01.007

An analysis of whether successful HCV treatment alters the natural history of HCV or quality of life also depends on whether such treatment was interferon (IFN) based or direct-acting antiviral (DAA) based, inasmuch as selection bias prevented many HCV patients from receiving IFN-based treatment owing largely to its adverse side-effect profile. In addition, once DAA therapy became available, the birth cohort of HCV patients was much older and with more age-related comorbid conditions. As more DAA-treated patients can be followed longitudinally and compared with their untreated counterparts, literature is emerging showing the unique benefits of DAA-based SVR as it relates to the subsequent incidence of hepatic and nonhepatic conditions. This review outlines the role that both IFN-based and DAA-based HCV treatment play on the natural history and quality of life among patients with chronic HCV infection.

MORTALITY
Interferon-Based Treatment

The benefit of SVR on overall and liver-related mortality has been demonstrated in large cohort studies. Five-year mortality rates for 22,942 IFN/ribavirin-treated patients in a US Department of Veterans Affairs (USVA) study were 6.7% versus 14.4% (HCV genotype 1); 7.3% versus 15.9% (genotype 2); and 8.0% versus 24.4% (genotype 3) for SVR versus non-SVR, respectively ($P<.0001$ for all).[4] A longitudinal, international multicenter study of 530 patients with advanced HCV fibrosis or cirrhosis treated with IFN plus or minus ribavirin reported a 10-year overall morality of 9% for those who achieved SVR versus 26% for those who did not.[1] Additionally, a prospective study derived from the Hepatitis C Antiviral Long-Term Treatment Against Cirrhosis (HALT-C) cohort analyzed 526 patients with advanced fibrosis who were previously treated with peginterferon and ribavirin with the compound endpoint of mortality or liver transplant. At 7.5 years of follow-up, 2% of individuals with SVR versus 21% without SVR met the endpoint. Viral eradication resulted in a more than 5-fold reduction in the risk of death or liver transplant (hazard ratio [HR] 0.17; 95% CI, 0.06–0.46) in those who achieved viral eradication.[5]

Direct-Acting Antiviral Regimens

Given the relatively recent introduction of DAAs, there are fewer studies investigating long-term outcomes among patients who achieve SVR. In a prospective observational study of HCV patients (ANRS CO12 CirVir) with biopsy-proved compensated cirrhosis (N = 1323), 50% achieved SVR after treatment with IFN-based or DAA regimens. SVR was associated with decrease in 5 year mortality (95.2% vs 84.5%; HR, 0.27 95% CI, 0.18-0.42; P<.001) from both liver-related and all causes.[6] This is consistent with findings from a larger prospective study (ANRS CO22 Hepather; N = 9.895) of DAA-treated patients, which found that SVR was associated with decreased all-cause mortality (adjusted HR 0.48; 95% CI, 0.33–0.70) after approximately 3 years of follow-up.[7] Likewise, among a large cohort of USVA patients with advanced liver disease (N = 15.059), incidence of mortality was 2.6/100 patient-years and 12.3/100 patient-years (for SVR vs non-SVR, respectively) after 1.6-year of follow-up, a reduction of 78.9%[8] (Table 1).[1,4–14]

HEPATIC MORBIDITY
Cirrhosis

Among HCV patients with cirrhosis, achievement of SVR appears to reduce progression of liver disease and decompensation. Studies of HCV patients with biopsy-proved advanced fibrosis/cirrhosis have reported a significant reduction in the

Table 1
Benefits of sustained virologic response in chronic hepatitis C

Clinical Scenario		Sustained Virologic Response	Nonsustained Virologic Response	Follow-up (y)	Treatment	Reference	Notes
Overall mortality		6.7%	14.4%	5	IFN/RBV	Backus et al,[4] 2011	F3–F4
		9%	26%	10	IFN/RBV	van der Meer et al,[1] 2012	Ishak ≥3
		2.2%	21.3%	7.5	IFN/RBV	Morgan et al,[5] 2010	F4
		4.8%	15.5%	4.85	IFN or DAA	Nahon et al,[6] 2017	F4 = 42%
		57% risk reduction		2.7	DAA	Carrat et al,[7] 2019	FIB-4 >3.25
		4.2%	18.3%	1.6	DAA	Backus et al,[8] 2019	
Hepatocellular carcinoma		1.5%	6.2%	2–14	IFN	Morgan et al,[9] 2013	All fibrosis stages
		0.9/100 person-years	3.45/100 person-years	0.5	DAA	Kanwal et al,[10] 2017	39% cirrhotics
		0.43/100 person-years	1.15/100 person-years	6.1	IFN, IFN/DAA, or DAA	Ioannou et al,[11] 2018	16% cirrhotics
Portal hypertension	Incident liver failure	0%	13%	2.1	IFN	Veldt et al,[12] 2007	Ishak 4–6
		2.1%	29.9%	8.4	IFN	van der Meer et al,[1] 2012	Ishak 4–6
	De novo varices	0%	15.5%	11.4	IFN	Bruno et al,[13] 2010	CTP class A
		3.5%	31.8%	5.6	IFN	D'Ambrosio et al,[14] 2011	CTP class A

Abbreviations: F, fibrosis; IFN, interferon-based treatment; RBV, ribavirin.
Data from Refs.[1,4–14]

incidence of liver failure (defined as ascites, variceal bleeding, hepatic encephalopathy, or elevated bilirubin) among IFN-treated patients who achieved SVR versus those who did not (0%–2% vs 13%–30%, respectively).[1,12] Development of de novo esophageal varices in subjects with compensated cirrhosis treated with IFN-based therapies also was lower among patients who achieved SVR (0%–3.5%) versus non-SVR (15.1%–31.8%).[13,14] SVR also appears to reduce portal hypertension, because studies have shown that SVR patients demonstrated significantly lower hepatic venous portal gradient than nonresponders[15] (see **Table 1**).

IFN-based treatment of patients with decompensated cirrhosis was rare, given the risk of further decompensation[16]; hence, there is paucity of data in this setting. The available studies do indicate that achievement of SVR among patients with decompensated cirrhosis is associated with significantly decreased rates of liver decompensating events and death.[17,18]

Among HCV patients with cirrhosis and clinically significant portal hypertension (N = 226), treatment with IFN-free regimens was associated with a statistically significant reduction in hepatic venous portal gradient after SVR (2 mm Hg ± 3.2 mm Hg), but clinically significant portal hypertension persisted in 78% of the cohort. Albumin less than 3.5 mg/dL was noted to have a negative impact on reduction in portal hypertension.[19]

Several studies have shown reductions in Child-Turcotte-Pugh (CTP) and Model for End-stage Liver Disease (MELD) score after treatment with DAA regimens. In the SOLAR-1 trial, patients with decompensated cirrhosis CTP class B and C were randomized to 12 weeks or 24 weeks of sofosbuvir and ledipasvir with ribavirin. Four weeks after the end of treatment, MELD scores improved by 2 points to 2.7 points in a majority of patients.[20] In the ASTRAL-4 study, patients with CTP class B were treated with sofosbuvir and velpatasvir. Approximately half of those with MELD scores less than 15 had improved scores; more than 80% of those with scores over 15 improved.[21] In the ALLY-1 study, patients treated with sofosbuvir, daclatasvir, and ribavirin had reductions in CTP scores in 70% of class B and 62% of class C as well as improvement in MELD scores among approximately 40% to 50% of patients.[22] A retrospective study found, however, that the presence of ascites, encephalopathy, albumin less than 3.5 g/dL, alanine aminotransferase less than 60 U/L, and a body mass index greater than 25 kg/m^2 at baseline was associated with increased risk of not achieving a reduction of CTP to class A, independent of SVR.[23]

Liver Transplant Waitlist

There are only limited data on the effect of SVR on patients treated with IFN-based regimens while on the liver transplant waitlist, and those studies included only small numbers of patients and were characterized by reports of severe side effects, drug discontinuation, and low SVR rates.[24,25] Conversely, the widespread use of DAAs in decompensated cirrhosis has translated into major changes to the characteristics of patients on liver transplant waitlists. One study of the US Scientific Registry of Transplant Recipients database found that compared with the IFN era (2003–2011), the proportion of patients waitlisted due to HCV-related causes decreased by 5% in 2011 to 2013 (protease inhibitors) and by 32% in 2014 to 2015 (DAAs).[26] Another study found that use of DAAs among waitlisted patients with decompensated cirrhosis has led to a delisting rate of 19% to 25%[27,28] and identified change in MELD score between baseline and end of treatment as the more important predictor of delisting,[28] although follow-up of delisted patients (1.5–2 years) indicates that a majority of patients were able to remain off the transplant waitlist, with only 7% to 9% relisted for decompensation or de novo HCC.[28,29]

Hepatocellular Carcinoma

Viral hepatitis–induced cirrhosis increases the risk of HCC[30] and the reported incidence of HCC among HCV patients, with cirrhosis ranges from 2% to 8%, depending on the duration of follow-up, sample size, and cohort characteristics.[31] A meta-analysis of 30 observational studies (primarily from the IFN era of treatment) from 17 countries (N = 32,528) found that SVR was associated with reduced risk of HCC (relative risk 0.24; 95% CI, 0.18–0.32).[9] The Evaluation of Pegintron in Control of Hepatitis C Cirrhosis and HALT-C trials enrolled patients who had previously failed antiviral treatment to receive maintenance IFN versus placebo; they found no reduction in HCC incidence with maintenance therapy in the absence of SVR, suggesting that viral eradication likely is the factor responsible for the reduced risk of HCC.[32,33]

Two small studies initially raised concern when they reported incident cases of HCC arising shortly after successful treatment with DAAs.[34,35] A large USVA study of DAA patients (N = 22,500), however, found that SVR was associated with a 76% reduction in risk of HCC compared with non-SVR; the effect was evident early after SVR and continued to increase over time.[10] Another USVA study considered risk of HCC after SVR for antiviral regimens with and without IFN (N = 62,354). Incidence of HCC after IFN-free DAA treatment was 1.32/100 patient-years versus 1.06/100 patient-years for DAA regimens that included IFN and 0.81/100 patient-years for IFN-only regimens; after adjustment for confounders, there were no significant differences between the groups.[11] The overall risk of developing HCC after SVR is 0.33% per year, however, and the main risk factors include the presence of cirrhosis, SVR after age 64, and diabetes[36] (see **Table 1**). Recently, the importance of determining the fibrosis-4 (FIB-4) score before and after antiviral therapy has been suggested. Incidence of HCC was approximately twice as high among patients with cirrhosis and high FIB-4 scores (>3.25) prior to treatment compared with those with low (<3.25) FIB-4 scores. Decreases in high FIB-4 score to low post-SVR score were associated with reduction in HCC risk of approximately 50%. Rates of HCC also were higher among noncirrhotics with high FIB-4 scores before or after SVR compared with those with lower scores.[37]

Fibrosis Regression

SVR is associated with regression of liver fibrosis and cirrhosis.[16,38] Combined data from 4 randomized clinical trials (N = 153) showed that 49% of patients achieving SVR after receiving IFN-based treatment demonstrated reversal of biopsy-proved cirrhosis at 20-month intervals between biopsies; age (<40 years) and body mass index (<27 kg/m^2) also were associated with cirrhosis regression.[39] A meta-analysis comparing SVR versus non-SVR patients with cirrhosis found that the likelihood of observing regression of cirrhosis was associated with SVR and time of follow-up. The relative risk for regression of cirrhosis was 4.33 (CI, 1.1–17.0; $P<.04$) when the mean or median time for the follow-up liver biopsy was greater than 36 months versus to 1.79 (CI, 1.26–2.29; $P<.01$) when less than 36 months.[40] In a 10-year large cohort observational study, patients who achieved SVR had significant lower FIB-4 scores than untreated counterparts, indicating long-term fibrosis regression.[41]

In the DAA era, data on cirrhosis regression with DAA are scarce and generally limited to transient elastography and serologic markers.[42] Improvements in liver stiffness have been reported in a few studies. In 1 study (N = 48), 24% of patients had cirrhosis regression after reaching SVR after DAA therapy.[43] In another study of patients with advanced fibrosis/cirrhosis (N = 304; median liver stiffness of 16.9 kPa; interquartile range [IQR] 11.8–27.7), liver stiffness was reduced to 11.9 kPa (IQR

8.2–20.9) at 24 weeks post-treatment.[44] A study with longer follow-up (40 weeks after SVR; N = 392) found that median liver stiffness decreased from 12.65 kPa (IQR 9.45–19.2) to 8.55 kPa (IQR 5.93–15.25); the investigators also found that median FIB-4 score was reduced from 2.54 (IQR 1.65–4.43) to 1.80 (IQR 1.23–2.84) and the aspartate aminotransferase–to–platelet ratio index decreased from 1.10 (IQR 0.65–2.43) to 0.43 (IQR 0.3–0.79).[45] The validity of liver stiffness cutoffs for aviremic patients, however, has been questioned. Among HCV patients with cirrhosis who underwent paired biopsies (preantiviral and postantiviral therapy) and transient elastography at the time of the post-treatment biopsy, the sensitivity and specificity of liver stiffness to detect cirrhosis after viral eradication were 61% and 95%, respectively.[46] It is possible this is a reflection of the decrease in liver stiffness that results from resolution of hepatic inflammation after SVR.[42] For this reason, data on cirrhosis resolution after DAA treatment are still limited.

EXTRAHEPATIC MANIFESTATIONS

Although HCV primarily infects the hepatocytes, a wide variety of manifestations involving other organs, including the central nervous system, endocrine system, peripheral nerves, blood vessels, joints, and skin, have been described. The exact pathophysiologic mechanism of extrahepatic manifestations in HCV is not always clear.[47]

Mixed Cryoglobulinemia

Mixed cryoglobulinemia (MC)—a B-cell disorder that causes systemic vasculitis leading to immune complex formation and deposits resulting in renal, cutaneous, musculoskeletal, and neurologic complications[48]—has been reported in up to 50% of patients with HCV, although only 15% are symptomatic.[47] MC is characterized by fatigue, palpable purpura, arthralgias, and detectable serum immunoglobulins that precipitate at low temperature.[49]

The link between HCV and MC was reported in a randomized crossover-controlled clinical trial where the use of IFN-α reduced cryoglobulins, with rebound observed when therapy was withdrawn.[50] SVR achieved through the use of pegylated IFN and ribavirin eliminated HCV-induced MC vasculitis manifestations; clinical relapse of MC was paired with the return of viremia.[51] A USVA study of patients treated with an IFN-based regimen (N = 160,875) demonstrated that SVR reduced the future risk of MC, in addition to glomerulonephritis, diabetes, porphyria cutanea tarda, stroke, and non-Hodgkin lymphoma (NHL).[3]

DAAs have been shown to be safe and effective in the setting of MC, although there seems to be a lag between SVR and clinical improvement in MC symptoms. At 12 weeks after DAA therapy, at least partial resolution of vasculitis symptoms was reported in 61% of patients.[52] Longer follow-up is associated with continued clinical improvement. Cutaneous and musculoskeletal manifestations improve most consistently, with renal and neurologic symptoms improving in a less reliable manner.[16,52,53] A USVA study indicates that DAA-induced SVR significantly reduced the future risk of development of MC and glomerulonephritis but not NHL or diabetes.[54] Relapse of MC after SVR may be transient but can be associated with B-cell NHL.[55]

Non-Hodgkin Lymphoma

The association between HCV and NHL was first reported in 1994.[56] Later this relationship was validated by a large retrospective USVA study showing that HCV infection is associated with a 20% to 30% increase in risk of NHL.[57] HCV is associated with both low-grade and high-grade NHL, but this association is stronger with particular subtypes, including lymphoplasmacytic lymphoma, marginal zone lymphoma, and diffuse large B-cell lymphoma.[58] The pathophysiologic mechanism of HCV in lymphoma development is not clear but thought to be similar to the process that drives development of MC. Antigen-driven clonal B-cell lymphoproliferation may progress to NHL, likely as a result of continued antigen stimulation.[47]

Further evidence of the relationship between HCV and NHL has been derived from studies that reveal regression and cure of low-grade NHL after SVR.[59] Complete responders to antineoplastic treatment who received antivirals had longer disease-free survival; moreover, the rate of relapse was less than 1% among patients who achieved SVR versus 29% of non-SVR patients.[60]

Evidence for the effect of DAA treatment on NHL is less clear. One study (N = 46) found that despite a high rate of SVR among patients with indolent B-cell NHL or chronic lymphocytic leukemia, the lymphoproliferative disease response rate was only 67% (26% complete response and 41% partial response); responders seemed mainly represented by marginal zone lymphomas.[61]

Cardiovascular Disease

HCV is associated with insulin resistance and can lead to hyperlipidemia, hepatic steatosis, endothelial dysfunction, and a systemic inflammatory state, all of which contribute to vascular injury.[62,63] In addition, HCV individuals have higher levels of proinflammatory cytokines than their noninfected counterparts.[64]

Although early studies evaluating the relationship between HCV and cardiovascular disease (CVD) have reported conflicting data regarding this association,[65,66] more recently it has become clear that HCV increases the risk of CVD. Increased risk of coronary artery disease events (HR 1.27; 95% CI, 1.2–1.31) has been reported in a large USVA cohort comparing HCV-infected versus noninfected subjects.[67] In the IFN era, results of studies on the impact of SVR were mixed; some reported no CVD benefit,[68] whereas others reported a reduction in risk,[69] and still others found improvement in rates of stroke but not coronary artery disease.[3]

Recently, a large USVA study (N = 242,000) of HCV patients without prior CVD events compared treated patients (IFN + ribavirin or DAA) to untreated controls. Incidence of CVD events in the treated group was 7.2% versus 13.8% in the untreated group. Furthermore, among the control group, incidence of CVD events was 30.4/1000 patient-years (95% CI, 29.2–31.7) in the control group, 23.5/1000 patient-years (95% CI, 21–25.3) in the IFN-based treatment group, and 16.3/1000 patient-years (95% CI, 14.7–18.0) in the DAA-treated group. SVR was associated with lower risk of CVD events (HR 0.87; 95% CI, 0.77–0.98).[70] Treatment with DAA and attainment of SVR has been shown to improve intimal media thickness and carotid thickening but not carotid plaque, in individuals with advanced liver fibrosis or compensated cirrhosis.[71]

Diabetes

HCV impairs glucose metabolism and contributes to insulin resistance.[72] In patients with risk factors for metabolic syndrome, presence of HCV increases by 11-fold the risk of type 2 diabetes mellitus.[73] Additionally, cirrhosis, Child-Pugh class, and advancing age are associated with higher rates of type 2 diabetes mellitus among HCV patients.[74] IFN-based studies suggest that achieving SVR is associated with improved insulin resistance and reduced risk of type 2 diabetes mellitus.[75,76] This information should be interpreted, however, with caution because IFN treatment may cause weight loss, which may have an impact on insulin resistance, and ribavirin may cause hemolytic anemia, which can affect the interpretation of hemoglobin A_{1C}.[16,77]

A USVA study of DAA-treated patients (N = 2400) found that patients who achieved SVR had lower hemoglobin A_{1C} and insulin requirements at 3 months to 15 months of follow-up, compared with their treatment failure counterparts.[78] Data from the Chronic Hepatitis Cohort Study comparing untreated, treatment failure, and SVR patients, however, found that an initial decline in hemoglobin A_{1C} among SVR patients was not maintained over a longer period of follow-up, rebounding to pretreatment levels by 30 months post-treatment initiation, even after controlling for changes in body mass index.[79]

QUALITY OF LIFE

Several neuropsychiatric symptoms have been described among HCV-infected patients, including fatigue, depression, and defects in attention and verbal reasoning. There is evidence that up to 50% of HCV individuals develop mild neurocognitive impairment, which is not fully attributable to liver dysfunction or psychosocial factors. Magnetic resonance spectroscopy has shown neuroinflammation in HCV, likely related to the virus crossing the blood-brain barrier.[80,81]

Patient-reported outcomes (PROs) are defined as measurements based on reports directly from patients about their health status without interpretation of clinicians. PROs are substantially impaired in HCV individuals compared with the general population.[82] In addition, health-related quality of life is lower prior to initiation of antiviral therapy. This impairment can be influenced by stigmatization and may affect a patient's experience and adherence to treatment.[83]

IFN-based regimens were associated with severely impaired PROs, likely due to the number of treatment side effects—anemia, flulike symptoms, cytopenias, fatigue, and depression.[84] Adjuvant ribavirin also is associated with moderate, but reversible, PRO impairment.[85] Placebo followed by IFN-free and ribavirin-free regimen (sofosbuvir/velpatasvir/voxilaprevir) resulted in improved PROs.[84]

A placebo-controlled study (N = 931) investigated PROs among patients receiving several different treatment regimens, including IFN-based and DAA regimens with and without ribavirin. Baseline PROs were similar and did not change significantly among placebo-treated patients. Despite differences in on-treatment PROs, overall PROs improved with SVR, regardless of the regimen.[86] A post hoc analysis of phase 3 clinical trials of sofosbuvir-based regimens (ASTRAL-1, ASTRAL-2, and ASTRAL-3 and ASTRAL-4; N = 1701) found that patients with cirrhosis had the most profound PRO impairment at baseline and that all patients had improvements in PROs at the end of treatment. The largest gains were among patients with decompensated cirrhosis, both during antiviral therapy and after achieving SVR. PRO improvement likely is related to viral eradication but also might be attributed to improved hepatic function.[85]

SUMMARY

After the discovery of HCV came the realization that this human pathogen mediated not only progressive liver disease and HCC but also a host of other disease states, including neurocognitive, renal, endocrine, cardiovascular, dermatologic, and neoplastic. The answer to the question of whether SVR either improves or prevents the subsequent risk of these conditions, including morbidity and mortality, recently has been clarified. Now, with more long-term follow-up of both IFN-treated and DAA-treated patients, via longitudinal and cross-sectional analyses, has come clarity that HCV viral eradication unquestionably improves quality of life; favorably alters the natural history of HCV, including mortality; and mitigates the development of a variety of extrahepatic manifestations. Early treatment is essential, and attempts to limit antiviral therapy to patients with advanced fibrosis is shortsighted. One recent meta-analysis that suggested a lack of long-term benefit[87] was methodologically flawed and misguided.[88] The overwhelming evidence for this beneficial role of SVR supports the goal of the World Health Organization of global HCV eradication by the year 2030.[89]

DISCLOSURE

S.C. Gordon receives grant/research support from AbbVie Pharmaceuticals, Conatus, CymaBay, Gilead Pharmaceuticals, Intercept Pharmaceuticals, and Merck. H.C. Gonzalez has served as a consultant/advisor for Gilead Pharmaceuticals. He also received grant/research support from Celenge.

REFERENCES

1. van der Meer AJ, Veldt BJ, Feld JJ, et al. Association between sustained virological response and all-cause mortality among patients with chronic hepatitis C and advanced hepatic fibrosis. JAMA 2012;308(24):2584–93.
2. Kanwal F, Kramer JR, Asch SM, et al. Long-term risk of hepatocellular carcinoma in HCV patients treated with direct acting antiviral agents. Hepatology 2020; 71(1):44–55.
3. Mahale P, Engels EA, Li R, et al. The effect of sustained virological response on the risk of extrahepatic manifestations of hepatitis C virus infection. Gut 2018; 67(3):553–61.
4. Backus LI, Boothroyd DB, Phillips BR, et al. A sustained virologic response reduces risk of all-cause mortality in patients with hepatitis C. Clin Gastroenterol Hepatol 2011;9(6):509–16.e1.
5. Morgan TR, Ghany MG, Kim HY, et al. Outcome of sustained virological responders with histologically advanced chronic hepatitis C. Hepatology 2010; 52(3):833–44.
6. Nahon P, Bourcier V, Layese R, et al. Eradication of hepatitis C virus infection in patients with cirrhosis reduces risk of liver and non-liver complications. Gastroenterology 2017;152(1):142–56.e2.
7. Carrat F, Fontaine H, Dorival C, et al. Clinical outcomes in patients with chronic hepatitis C after direct-acting antiviral treatment: a prospective cohort study. Lancet 2019;393(10179):1453–64.
8. Backus LI, Belperio PS, Shahoumian TA, et al. Impact of sustained virologic response with direct-acting antiviral treatment on mortality in patients with advanced liver disease. Hepatology 2019;69(2):487–97.
9. Morgan RL, Baack B, Smith BD, et al. Eradication of hepatitis C virus infection and the development of hepatocellular carcinoma: a meta-analysis of observational studies. Ann Intern Med 2013;158(5 Pt 1):329–37.
10. Kanwal F, Kramer J, Asch SM, et al. Risk of hepatocellular cancer in HCV patients treated with direct-acting antiviral agents. Gastroenterology 2017;153(4): 996–1005.e1.
11. Ioannou GN, Green PK, Berry K. HCV eradication induced by direct-acting antiviral agents reduces the risk of hepatocellular carcinoma. J Hepatol 2018;68(1): 25–32.

12. Veldt BJ, Heathcote EJ, Wedemeyer H, et al. Sustained virologic response and clinical outcomes in patients with chronic hepatitis C and advanced fibrosis. Ann Intern Med 2007;147(10):677–84.
13. Bruno S, Crosignani A, Facciotto C, et al. Sustained virologic response prevents the development of esophageal varices in compensated, Child-Pugh class A hepatitis C virus-induced cirrhosis. A 12-year prospective follow-up study. Hepatology 2010;51(6):2069–76.
14. D'Ambrosio R, Aghemo A, Rumi MG, et al. The course of esophageal varices in patients with hepatitis C cirrhosis responding to interferon/ribavirin therapy. Antivir Ther 2011;16(5):677–84.
15. Roberts S, Gordon A, McLean C, et al. Effect of sustained viral response on hepatic venous pressure gradient in hepatitis C-related cirrhosis. Clin Gastroenterol Hepatol 2007;5(8):932–7.
16. Ioannou GN, Feld JJ. What are the benefits of a sustained virologic response to direct-acting antiviral therapy for hepatitis C virus infection? Gastroenterology 2019;156(2):446–60.e2.
17. Iacobellis A, Perri F, Valvano MR, et al. Long-term outcome after antiviral therapy of patients with hepatitis C virus infection and decompensated cirrhosis. Clin Gastroenterol Hepatol 2011;9(3):249–53.
18. Iacobellis A, Siciliano M, Perri F, et al. Peginterferon alfa-2b and ribavirin in patients with hepatitis C virus and decompensated cirrhosis: a controlled study. J Hepatol 2007;46(2):206–12.
19. Lens S, Alvarado-Tapias E, Marino Z, et al. Effects of all-oral anti-viral therapy on HVPG and systemic hemodynamics in patients with hepatitis c virus-associated cirrhosis. Gastroenterology 2017;153(5):1273–83.e1.
20. Charlton M, Everson GT, Flamm SL, et al. Ledipasvir and sofosbuvir plus ribavirin for treatment of HCV infection in patients with advanced liver disease. Gastroenterology 2015;149(3):649–59.
21. Curry MP, O'Leary JG, Bzowej N, et al. Sofosbuvir and velpatasvir for HCV in patients with decompensated cirrhosis. N Engl J Med 2015;373(27):2618–28.
22. Poordad F, Schiff ER, Vierling JM, et al. Daclatasvir with sofosbuvir and ribavirin for hepatitis C virus infection with advanced cirrhosis or post-liver transplantation recurrence. Hepatology 2016;63(5):1493–505.
23. El-Sherif O, Jiang ZG, Tapper EB, et al. Baseline factors associated with improvements in decompensated cirrhosis after direct-acting antiviral therapy for hepatitis C virus infection. Gastroenterology 2018;154(8):2111–21.e8.
24. Crippin JS, McCashland T, Terrault N, et al. A pilot study of the tolerability and efficacy of antiviral therapy in hepatitis C virus-infected patients awaiting liver transplantation. Liver Transpl 2002;8(4):350–5.
25. Annicchiarico BE, Siciliano M, Avolio AW, et al. Treatment of chronic hepatitis C virus infection with pegylated interferon and ribavirin in cirrhotic patients awaiting liver transplantation. Transplant Proc 2008;40(6):1918–20.
26. Flemming JA, Kim WR, Brosgart CL, et al. Reduction in liver transplant wait-listing in the era of direct-acting antiviral therapy. Hepatology 2017;65(3):804–12.
27. Belli LS, Berenguer M, Cortesi PA, et al. Delisting of liver transplant candidates with chronic hepatitis C after viral eradication: a European study. J Hepatol 2016;65(3):524–31.
28. Pascasio JM, Vinaixa C, Ferrer MT, et al. Clinical outcomes of patients undergoing antiviral therapy while awaiting liver transplantation. J Hepatol 2017;67(6):1168–76.

29. Perricone G, Duvoux C, Berenguer M, et al. Delisting HCV-infected liver transplant candidates who improved after viral eradication: outcome 2 years after delisting. Liver Int 2018;38(12):2170–7.
30. West J, Card TR, Aithal GP, et al. Risk of hepatocellular carcinoma among individuals with different aetiologies of cirrhosis: a population-based cohort study. Aliment Pharmacol Ther 2017;45(7):983–90.
31. Goodgame B, Shaheen NJ, Galanko J, et al. The risk of end stage liver disease and hepatocellular carcinoma among persons infected with hepatitis C virus: publication bias? Am J Gastroenterol 2003;98(11):2535–42.
32. Bruix J, Poynard T, Colombo M, et al. Maintenance therapy with peginterferon alfa-2b does not prevent hepatocellular carcinoma in cirrhotic patients with chronic hepatitis C. Gastroenterology 2011;140(7):1990–9.
33. Lok AS, Everhart JE, Wright EC, et al. Maintenance peginterferon therapy and other factors associated with hepatocellular carcinoma in patients with advanced hepatitis C. Gastroenterology 2011;140(3):840–9 [quiz: e812].
34. Ravi S, Axley P, Jones D, et al. Unusually high rates of hepatocellular carcinoma after treatment with direct-acting antiviral therapy for hepatitis C related cirrhosis. Gastroenterology 2017;152(4):911–2.
35. Conti F, Buonfiglioli F, Scuteri A, et al. Early occurrence and recurrence of hepatocellular carcinoma in HCV-related cirrhosis treated with direct-acting antivirals. J Hepatol 2016;65(4):727–33.
36. El-Serag HB, Kanwal F, Richardson P, et al. Risk of hepatocellular carcinoma after sustained virological response in Veterans with hepatitis C virus infection. Hepatology 2016;64(1):130–7.
37. Ioannou GN, Beste LA, Green PK, et al. Increased risk for hepatocellular carcinoma persists up to 10 years after HCV eradication in patients with baseline cirrhosis or high FIB-4 scores. Gastroenterology 2019;157(5):1264–78.e4.
38. Gonzalez HC, Duarte-Rojo A. Virologic cure of hepatitis C: impact on hepatic fibrosis and patient outcomes. Curr Gastroenterol Rep 2016;18(7):32.
39. Poynard T, McHutchison J, Manns M, et al. Impact of pegylated interferon alfa-2b and ribavirin on liver fibrosis in patients with chronic hepatitis C. Gastroenterology 2002;122(5):1303–13.
40. Akhtar E, Manne V, Saab S. Cirrhosis regression in hepatitis C patients with sustained virological response after antiviral therapy: a meta-analysis. Liver Int 2015; 35(1):30–6.
41. Lu M, Li J, Zhang T, et al. Serum biomarkers indicate long-term reduction in liver fibrosis in patients with sustained virological response to treatment for HCV infection. Clin Gastroenterol Hepatol 2016;14(7):1044–55.e3.
42. Grgurevic I, Bozin T, Madir A. Hepatitis C is now curable, but what happens with cirrhosis and portal hypertension afterwards? Clin Exp Hepatol 2017;3(4):181–6.
43. Pineda JA, Merchante N, Mancebo M, et al. Short-term effect of DAA IFN-free regimens on liver stiffness [abstract]. J Hepatol 2017;66(1 Suppl):S525.
44. Dolmazashvili E, Abutidze A, Chkhartishvili N, et al. Regression of liver fibrosis over a 24-week period after completing direct-acting antiviral therapy in patients with chronic hepatitis C receiving care within the national hepatitis C elimination program in Georgia: results of hepatology clinic HEPA experience. Eur J Gastroenterol Hepatol 2017;29(11):1223–30.
45. Bachofner JA, Valli PV, Kroger A, et al. Direct antiviral agent treatment of chronic hepatitis C results in rapid regression of transient elastography and fibrosis markers fibrosis-4 score and aspartate aminotransferase-platelet ratio index. Liver Int 2017;37(3):369–76.

46. D'Ambrosio R, Aghemo A, Fraquelli M, et al. The diagnostic accuracy of Fibroscan for cirrhosis is influenced by liver morphometry in HCV patients with a sustained virological response. J Hepatol 2013;59(2):251–6.
47. Jacobson IM, Cacoub P, Dal Maso L, et al. Manifestations of chronic hepatitis C virus infection beyond the liver. Clin Gastroenterol Hepatol 2010;8(12):1017–29.
48. Ramos-Casals M, Stone JH, Cid MC, et al. The cryoglobulinaemias. Lancet 2012; 379(9813):348–60.
49. Pozzato G, Mazzaro C, Gattei V. Hepatitis C virus-associated non-hodgkin lymphomas: biology, epidemiology, and treatment. Clin Liver Dis 2017;21(3): 499–515.
50. Ferri C, Marzo E, Longombardo G, et al. Interferon-alpha in mixed cryoglobulinemia patients: a randomized, crossover-controlled trial. Blood 1993;81(5):1132–6.
51. Cacoub P, Comarmond C, Domont F, et al. Cryoglobulinemia vasculitis. Am J Med 2015;128(9):950–5.
52. Emery JS, Kuczynski M, La D, et al. Efficacy and safety of direct acting antivirals for the treatment of mixed cryoglobulinemia. Am J Gastroenterol 2017;112(8): 1298–308.
53. Comarmond C, Garrido M, Pol S, et al. Direct-acting antiviral therapy restores immune tolerance to patients with hepatitis c virus-induced cryoglobulinemia vasculitis. Gastroenterology 2017;152(8):2052–62.e2.
54. El-Serag HB, Christie IC, Puenpatom A, et al. The effects of sustained virological response to direct-acting anti-viral therapy on the risk of extrahepatic manifestations of hepatitis C infection. Aliment Pharmacol Ther 2019;49(11):1442–7.
55. Landau DA, Saadoun D, Halfon P, et al. Relapse of hepatitis C virus-associated mixed cryoglobulinemia vasculitis in patients with sustained viral response. Arthritis Rheum 2008;58(2):604–11.
56. Ferri C, Caracciolo F, Zignego AL, et al. Hepatitis C virus infection in patients with non-Hodgkin's lymphoma. Br J Haematol 1994;88(2):392–4.
57. Giordano TP, Henderson L, Landgren O, et al. Risk of non-Hodgkin lymphoma and lymphoproliferative precursor diseases in US veterans with hepatitis C virus. JAMA 2007;297(18):2010–7.
58. de Sanjose S, Benavente Y, Vajdic CM, et al. Hepatitis C and non-Hodgkin lymphoma among 4784 cases and 6269 controls from the International Lymphoma Epidemiology Consortium. Clin Gastroenterol Hepatol 2008;6(4):451–8.
59. Hermine O, Lefrere F, Bronowicki JP, et al. Regression of splenic lymphoma with villous lymphocytes after treatment of hepatitis C virus infection. N Engl J Med 2002;347(2):89–94.
60. La Mura V, De Renzo A, Perna F, et al. Antiviral therapy after complete response to chemotherapy could be efficacious in HCV-positive non-Hodgkin's lymphoma. J Hepatol 2008;49(4):557–63.
61. Arcaini L, Besson C, Frigeni M, et al. Interferon-free antiviral treatment in B-cell lymphoproliferative disorders associated with hepatitis C virus infection. Blood 2016;128(21):2527–32.
62. Adinolfi LE, Restivo L, Guerrera B, et al. Chronic HCV infection is a risk factor of ischemic stroke. Atherosclerosis 2013;231(1):22–6.
63. Targher G, Bertolini L, Padovani R, et al. Differences and similarities in early atherosclerosis between patients with non-alcoholic steatohepatitis and chronic hepatitis B and C. J Hepatol 2007;46(6):1126–32.
64. Oliveira CP, Kappel CR, Siqueira ER, et al. Effects of hepatitis C virus on cardiovascular risk in infected patients: a comparative study. Int J Cardiol 2013;164(2): 221–6.

65. Arcari CM, Nelson KE, Netski DM, et al. No association between hepatitis C virus seropositivity and acute myocardial infarction. Clin Infect Dis 2006;43(6):e53–6.
66. Vassalle C, Masini S, Bianchi F, et al. Evidence for association between hepatitis C virus seropositivity and coronary artery disease. Heart 2004;90(5):565–6.
67. Butt AA, Xiaoqiang W, Budoff M, et al. Hepatitis C virus infection and the risk of coronary disease. Clin Infect Dis 2009;49(2):225–32.
68. Leone S, Prosperi M, Costarelli S, et al. Incidence and predictors of cardiovascular disease, chronic kidney disease, and diabetes in HIV/HCV-coinfected patients who achieved sustained virological response. Eur J Clin Microbiol Infect Dis 2016;35(9):1511–20.
69. Innes HA, McDonald SA, Dillon JF, et al. Toward a more complete understanding of the association between a hepatitis C sustained viral response and cause-specific outcomes. Hepatology 2015;62(2):355–64.
70. Butt AA, Yan P, Shuaib A, et al. Direct-acting antiviral therapy for hcv infection is associated with a reduced risk of cardiovascular disease events. Gastroenterology 2019;156(4):987–96.e8.
71. Petta S, Adinolfi LE, Fracanzani AL, et al. Hepatitis C virus eradication by direct-acting antiviral agents improves carotid atherosclerosis in patients with severe liver fibrosis. J Hepatol 2018;69(1):18–24.
72. White DL, Ratziu V, El-Serag HB. Hepatitis C infection and risk of diabetes: a systematic review and meta-analysis. J Hepatol 2008;49(5):831–44.
73. Mehta SH, Brancati FL, Strathdee SA, et al. Hepatitis C virus infection and incident type 2 diabetes. Hepatology 2003;38(1):50–6.
74. Caronia S, Taylor K, Pagliaro L, et al. Further evidence for an association between non-insulin-dependent diabetes mellitus and chronic hepatitis C virus infection. Hepatology 1999;30(4):1059–63.
75. Delgado-Borrego A, Jordan SH, Negre B, et al. Reduction of insulin resistance with effective clearance of hepatitis C infection: results from the HALT-C trial. Clin Gastroenterol Hepatol 2010;8(5):458–62.
76. Arase Y, Suzuki F, Suzuki Y, et al. Sustained virological response reduces incidence of onset of type 2 diabetes in chronic hepatitis C. Hepatology 2009;49(3):739–44.
77. Greenberg PD, Rosman AS, Eldeiry LS, et al. Decline in haemoglobin A1c values in diabetic patients receiving interferon-alpha and ribavirin for chronic hepatitis C. J Viral Hepat 2006;13(9):613–7.
78. Hum J, Jou JH, Green PK, et al. Improvement in glycemic control of type 2 diabetes after successful treatment of hepatitis C virus. Diabetes Care 2017;40(9):1173–80.
79. Li J, Gordon SC, Rupp LB, et al. Sustained virological response does not improve long-term glycaemic control in patients with type 2 diabetes and chronic hepatitis C. Liver Int 2019;39(6):1027–32.
80. Yarlott L, Heald E, Forton D. Hepatitis C virus infection, and neurological and psychiatric disorders - a review. J Adv Res 2017;8(2):139–48.
81. Barreira DP, Marinho RT, Bicho M, et al. Psychosocial and neurocognitive factors associated with hepatitis C - implications for future health and wellbeing. Front Psychol 2018;9:2666.
82. Younossi ZM, Guyatt G, Kiwi M, et al. Development of a disease specific questionnaire to measure health related quality of life in patients with chronic liver disease. Gut 1999;45(2):295–300.

83. Younossi Z, Henry L. Systematic review: patient-reported outcomes in chronic hepatitis C--the impact of liver disease and new treatment regimens. Aliment Pharmacol Ther 2015;41(6):497–520.
84. Younossi ZM, Stepanova M, Reddy R, et al. Viral eradication is required for sustained improvement of patient-reported outcomes in patients with hepatitis C. Liver Int 2019;39(1):54–9.
85. Younossi ZM, Stepanova M, Feld J, et al. Sofosbuvir and velpatasvir combination improves patient-reported outcomes for patients with HCV infection, without or with compensated or decompensated cirrhosis. Clin Gastroenterol Hepatol 2017;15(3):421–30.e6.
86. Cacoub P, Bourliere M, Asselah T, et al. French patients with hepatitis C treated with direct-acting antiviral combinations: the effect on patient-reported outcomes. Value Health 2018;21(10):1218–25.
87. Jakobsen JC, Nielsen EE, Feinberg J, et al. Direct-acting antivirals for chronic hepatitis C. Cochrane Database Syst Rev 2017;(9):CD012143.
88. European Association for the Study of the Liver. Response to the Cochrane systematic review on DAA-based treatment of chronic hepatitis C. J Hepatol 2017; 67(4):663–4.
89. Ward JW, Hinman AR. What is needed to eliminate hepatitis B virus and hepatitis C virus as global health threats. Gastroenterology 2019;156(2):297–310.

Hepatitis E

Epidemiology, Clinical Course, Prevention, and Treatment

Amit Goel, MD, DM[a], Rakesh Aggarwal, MD, DM[b],*

KEYWORDS

• Hepatitis E • Transmission • Prevention • Vaccination

KEY POINTS

- Hepatitis E is caused by infection with hepatitis E virus (HEV), belonging most often to genotypes 1 to 4; of these, genotypes 1 and 2 can cause infection only in humans, whereas genotypes 3 and 4 circulate freely in many mammalian animals, with occasional transmission to humans.
- Most of the disease burden of hepatitis E worldwide is related to infection with genotype 1 or 2 HEV in resource-constrained parts of the world, mainly Asia and Africa, caused by human-to-human, fecal-oral transmission, usually through contamination of drinking water supplies.
- By comparison, genotype 3 or 4 infection has been reported more commonly from the developed world (Europe, North America, Far East), and is related to zoonotic transmission from an animal source through eating undercooked/uncooked meat or close contact with animals.
- The clinical consequences of HEV infection can vary from complete absence of symptoms, through acute viral hepatitis–like illness, to acute liver failure, with severe forms being more common when genotype 1 or 2 HEV infection occurs during pregnancy. Genotype 3 or 4 HEV infection can cause persistent infection in immunosuppressed persons.

INTRODUCTION

The term hepatitis E refers to clinical consequences associated with infection with hepatitis E virus (HEV), the most recently discovered of the 5 currently known hepatotropic viruses. The existence of HEV as a cause of liver disease was first suspected in the early 1980s when patients in large outbreaks of acute hepatitis in India (in Delhi during 1955–1956[1] and in the Kashmir Valley during 1978[2]) were detected to lack serologic markers of hepatitis A and B virus infection. Epidemiologic features of these outbreaks fitted a

a Department of Gastroenterology, Sanjay Gandhi Postgraduate Institute of Medical Sciences, Lucknow, India; b Department of Gastroenterology, Jawaharlal Institute of Postgraduate Medical Education and Research, Puducherry, India
* Corresponding author.
E-mail address: aggarwal.ra@gmail.com

Gastroenterol Clin N Am 49 (2020) 315–330
https://doi.org/10.1016/j.gtc.2020.01.011
0889-8553/20/© 2020 Elsevier Inc. All rights reserved.

fecal-oral route of transmission. Hence, the causative agent for these outbreaks was putatively named as enterically transmitted non-A, non-B hepatitis virus.

Soon thereafter, viruslike particles (VLPs) were identified in stools collected during acute hepatitis that developed in a Russian scientist who voluntarily ingested a suspension prepared from stools of patients during a similar non-A, non-B hepatitis outbreak in Afghanistan.[3] This was followed by demonstration of liver injury and fecal excretion of similar VLPs in primates inoculated with stool suspensions from similar human cases or from experimentally infected animals, partially fulfilling the Koch's postulates.[4] Sequencing and cloning of the viral genome followed,[5] and the agent was named HEV to indicate its enteric route of transmission, disease occurrence in form of epidemics, and the fact that this was the fifth hepatotropic virus to be recognized (after hepatitis A, B, C, and D viruses).

Initially, the virus was thought to have a limited geographic and host niche, causing acute infection only among humans residing in low-income countries of Asia and Africa, with only occasional travel-related cases in developed countries of Europe and North America. However, in the last 2 decades, understanding about HEV has undergone a sea change, with identification of a broad host range with zoonotic transmission, of indigenous cases worldwide, of chronic infection, and of transmission through blood transfusion. However, several aspects of HEV pathogenesis, including mechanism of liver injury, determinants of disease severity, and the reason for its propensity to cause serious disease in pregnant women, remain unexplained.

This article summarizes the current information about epidemiology, routes of transmission, clinical manifestations, prevention, and treatment of HEV infection.

HEPATITIS E VIRUS

HEV virions are small (27–34 nm diameter) particles, consisting of an icosahedral protein capsid that encloses an approximately 7.2-kilobase long, single-stranded, positive-sense RNA genome. The virions were initially thought to be nonenveloped. However, HEV is now known to exist in 2 forms: as naked particles in the stools of infected persons and as enveloped virions in blood circulation; in the latter, the envelope seems to protect the virions from inactivation by circulating specific antibodies.[6]

Viruses with genomic sequences similar to HEV have been identified in several mammalian species (including pigs, deer, wild boars, mongoose, rabbits, rats, ferrets, and bats), birds, and fish. These viruses are all placed together with human HEV in family Hepeviridae, with 2 genera, namely Piscihepevirus, which infect fish, and Orthohepevirus, which infect mammals and birds. The latter genus is further subdivided into 4 species, namely Orthohepevirus A, B, and C, which infect mammals, and Orthohepevirus D, which infects birds.

All the isolates that are known to cause human infection are placed in genus Orthohepevirus A. Based on phylogenetic relatedness, the members of this genus are currently organized into 8 genotypes (GT1–GT8).[7] Of these, GT1 and GT2 are known to infect only humans, GT3 to GT6 infect several mammalian species, and GT7 and GT8 circulate among camels. Most of the human infections are related to GT1 to GT4, with occasional cases caused by GT7.[8]

EPIDEMIOLOGY
Geographic Distribution of Hepatitis E Virus Genotypes

Human infection
Each HEV genotype that causes disease in humans has a distinct geographic distribution. GT1 HEV has been isolated from patients with acute hepatitis in several parts of

Asia (in particular South Asia and Central Asia) and Africa, where hepatitis E disease is very common. GT2 HEV was originally identified in Mexico in early 1980s, and was subsequently reported from western Africa (Nigeria and Chad), but has not been reported from other parts of the world. Cases with GT3 HEV infection have been reported mainly from developed countries, predominantly those in Europe and North America but also in the Asia-Pacific region (eg, Australia, Japan). GT4 HEV has been reported almost exclusively from countries in Southeast Asia, including China, Taiwan, Japan, and Vietnam, with an occasional case report from Europe. GT7 HEV has been reported in humans only as occasional case reports from the Mediterranean region; no cases have been reported from outside this region.

Infection in Animal species

GT1 and GT2 HEV seem incapable of causing infection in animals. GT3 and GT4 HEV circulate freely in many mammalian species, in particular pigs, wild boar, and deer. These genotypes infect pig populations, nearly universally, in all parts of the world, irrespective of the frequency of HEV infection or disease in local human populations. Infection in pigs occurs early in life, and is associated with transient viremia, viral excretion, and seroconversion, without any clinical manifestations.[9] In geographic regions where infection with GT1 and GT2 HEV is infrequent, HEV infection in both humans and pigs seems to be caused by isolates belonging to the same genotype; for example, GT3 in Europe, the United States, Australia, and Japan, and GT4 in Taiwan, China, and Japan.[10] However, in regions where human disease is caused predominantly by GT1/GT2 HEV, which cannot infect animals, the genotypes circulating among swine and humans are different. For instance, in India, human cases of HEV disease are caused almost exclusively by GT1 HEV,[11] whereas the swine HEV isolates have been found to belong to GT4.[12]

Epidemiologic Patterns of Hepatitis E Virus Infection and Disease

The epidemiologic characteristics of HEV infection vary by HEV genotype, with 2 distinct patterns – for GT1 and GT2, and for GT3 and GT4 (**Table 1**).

The disease caused by GT1 and GT2 HEV accounts for a large proportion of the disease burden, and is highly endemic in Asia and Africa. In many of these areas, HEV infection is associated with outbreaks of acute hepatitis. These outbreaks are of variable size, with some affecting several thousand persons, and are usually related to fecal contamination of drinking water supplies. During the outbreaks, young adults in the age group of 15 to 40 years are affected more often, with fewer cases among children and the elderly. In Africa, outbreaks have frequently been reported in areas with humanitarian crises and among refugee populations, with poor access to sanitation and clean water. A characteristic feature of HEV outbreaks is the occurrence of more severe disease and an unusually high mortality among pregnant women; this is described in greater detail later in relation to clinical manifestations.

In addition, in these areas, HEV infection accounts for a large proportion of sporadic cases with acute hepatitis. In some areas, such as the Middle East and South America, although sporadic cases occur, outbreaks have not been reported. The age distribution, clinical features, and propensity for severe disease in pregnant women in sporadic cases are similar to those observed during epidemics. Also, these cases seem to be related to waterborne transmission, albeit at a lower scale than that in outbreaks.

By comparison, the disease associated with GT3 or GT4 infection is encountered primarily in developed countries of Europe or the United States, and less frequently from developed countries in Asia (eg, Japan, Hong Kong, Singapore, Australia). This disease occurs in occasional sporadic patients, most of whom are elderly. Liver injury

Table 1
Epidemiologic patterns of human hepatitis E virus infection

Feature	Genotype 1 and 2 Endemic Regions	Genotype 3 and 4 Endemic Regions
Geographic distribution	Developing countries in Asia, Africa, and parts of Latin America	Predominantly in developed countries: Europe, United States, Australia, and developed countries in Asia (eg, Japan, Taiwan, Hong Kong)
Transmission	Fecal-oral route, mostly through contamination of drinking water supplies	Consumption of undercooked animal meat; animal contact; transfusion of viremic blood units
Reservoir	Humans	Primarily animals
Epidemiologic patterns	Outbreaks, frequent sporadic cases	Only occasional sporadic cases
Seasonal pattern	Yes	No
Characteristics of affected persons	Usually healthy, with no prior illness	Often have coexistent illness, including immunocompromised states (eg, solid organ transplant)
Age	Mostly young adults	Mostly elderly
Clinical presentations	Acute hepatitis, acute liver failure	Acute hepatitis, chronic hepatitis
Probability to develop icteric illness	High	Very low
Severity of hepatitis	Mild to severe	Mostly mild to moderate
Associations of infection in pregnant women	Illness more likely and more severe; increased risk of poor fetal outcome	No association with disease frequency, severity, or outcomes has been observed
Persistent infection	Not reported	Occurs among immunosuppressed persons and is thought to progress to hepatic fibrosis including liver cirrhosis
Nonhepatic clinical manifestations	Pancreatitis reported; others uncommon	More common; primarily neurologic illnesses
Specific treatment	None	Ribavirin or pegylated interferon in persons with chronic infection
Preventive measure	Safe drinking water, good sanitation and hygiene	Avoid contact with animals; adequate cooking of meat; nucleic acid testing of the donated blood units

in them is milder, and HEV infection comes to attention in many of them only during laboratory investigations. Many of the cases are in people with an immunocompromised state, such as organ transplant recipients.[13] The exact mode of infection is unclear. The available evidence suggests that most of these cases are related to zoonotic transmission from animals through ingestion of infected animal meat. This view is based on frequent history of ingestion of undercooked or uncooked meat in these patients and demonstration of HEV RNA in pig meat (in particular, pig liver and sausages made from it) meant for human consumption in these areas. The association with pregnancy, which is so characteristic of GT1/GT2 disease, is not observed with GT3 or GT4 infection.

The epidemiology of HEV infection in Egypt does not seem to fit into these patterns. In that country, despite a very high anti-HEV seroprevalence, clinical disease caused by HEV or severe acute hepatitis in pregnant women is very infrequent.[14] The reason for this is unclear.

Routes of Transmission and Reservoirs of Infection

The primary route of entry of HEV into a naive host is enteric, irrespective of viral genotype, although the source or reservoir of infection differs by genotype.

The transmission of GT1 and GT2 HEV is human to human, through contamination of drinking water supplies, and possibly food, with the virus excreted in feces of HEV-infected persons. Transmission through close person-to-person contact has been found to be infrequent. Also, in GT1-predominant regions, transplacental transmission of HEV infection from infected pregnant women to their newborns has been shown to occur, through detection of HEV RNA or immunoglobulin (Ig) M anti-HEV antibodies in cord blood collected at childbirth.

By contrast, for GT3 and GT4 HEV, the transmission is predominantly zoonotic, through consumption of uncooked or undercooked meat, in particular livers, from HEV-infected pigs or other animals, or through close contact with such animals.[15,16]

In recent years, transfusion of contaminated blood or blood product has emerged as another avenue for transmission of HEV infection. A proportion of healthy blood donors in developed countries of Europe and North America have been shown to have asymptomatic HEV viremia. Further, some of the recipients of blood and blood products from such donors have been shown to develop HEV infection.[17] Most of these data have been related to GT3 HEV, and, to a smaller extent, to GT4 HEV. The contribution of this route to the overall HEV disease burden remains unclear.

Global Burden of Disease

A modeling study estimated that, in the year 2005, 73% of the world's population lived in countries where HEV GT1 and GT2 circulation is common. Further, it was estimated that GT1/GT2 HEV caused approximately 20 million new infections, 3.4 million symptomatic cases of acute hepatitis, 70,000 deaths, and 3000 stillbirths annually in these regions.[18] A more recent estimate from the Global Burden of Disease Study 2017 estimated that annually nearly 19.44 million (95% confidence interval = 17.33 million to 21.84 million) cases of acute hepatitis E occur worldwide.[19]

No estimates for the illness caused by HEV GT3 and GT4 are available, because these genotypes do not cause easily identifiable acute illness, and the disease has been recognized only in certain high-risk groups, such as those with an immunocompromised state.

Seroprevalence Data

HEV infection, irrespective of whether symptomatic or not, induces production of specific antibodies, initially of IgM isotype, followed within a few days by IgG antibodies. IgM anti-HEV antibodies disappear by around 6 months postinfection, whereas the IgG anti-HEV antibodies seem to persist for at least a few years. Thus, detection of IgM anti-HEV antibodies indicates recent HEV infection, whereas that of IgG anti-HEV indicates past exposure to HEV. Antibodies to the 4 genotypes cross react, with a common serotype.

Seroprevalence rates of anti-HEV antibodies vary widely between as well as within countries and regions.[20] These differences are thought to be at least partially attributable to extraneous factors, such as differences in performance characteristics of the assays used, differences in age distribution between the subjects studied in various studies, and the subpopulations studied. However, overall, the seroprevalence rates are higher in resource-poor countries, ranging up to 70%,[21] compared with high-income countries (usually <20%).[22] In addition, in all populations, the seroprevalence rates are lower among children and increase with age, with estimated cumulative incidence rates of HEV infection of 0.5% to 1.0% per year in persons aged 0 to 15 years, 1.0% to 1.4% per year in those 15 to 30 years old, and about 0.2% or lower per year after 30 years.[18]

CLINICAL MANIFESTATIONS

Clinical consequences of human HEV infection vary widely. Globally, in high-endemicity as well as low-endemicity regions, most patients who have detectable anti-HEV antibodies cannot recall having had liver disease in the past, indicating that the HEV infection in them had been asymptomatic. Further, during disease outbreaks, a proportion of those infected have mild liver injury with nonspecific features of an infectious disease and laboratory evidence of liver injury in the form of increased levels of serum aminotransferases but no jaundice (anicteric hepatitis).

Overall, it has been estimated that fewer than 20% of those infected with HEV develop symptomatic disease.[18] The syndrome most often associated with HEV infection is that of acute icteric hepatitis. The clinical course of this presentation of HEV infection is more severe, and the prognosis is much worse, when the disease occurs in pregnant women. Occasionally, the infection is associated with involvement of body organ systems other than the liver.

Acute Icteric Hepatitis

Acute icteric hepatitis E usually begins as a nonspecific illness (the so-called prodromal phase or prodrome) with malaise, fever, anorexia, nausea, and vomiting, which is often indistinguishable from other viral illnesses; sometimes, marked anorexia, prominent vomiting, dark-colored urine, or right upper abdominal discomfort may provide a clue to the hepatic origin. These symptoms last for a few days to a week, and are followed by appearance of yellow discoloration of eyes (jaundice). With the onset of jaundice, prodromal symptoms and appetite usually improve. The illness is associated with a marked increase (usually >8–10 times the upper limit of normal) of serum transaminase levels, and a variable degree of hyperbilirubinemia.

Clinical disease is most common among otherwise-healthy young adults, with very few children or elderly being affected.[23] Men are affected more often than women, possibly because of their greater risk of exposure.

The symptoms as well as the biochemical abnormalities most often resolve spontaneously in 4 to 6 weeks. A small proportion (0.5%–4%) of patients with icteric hepatitis may progress to acute liver failure, a severe form of disease. It is characterized by alteration of sensorium (hepatic encephalopathy) coupled with abnormal coagulation, and carries a high risk of mortality if facilities for intensive care support and/or liver transplant are not available.

Occasional patients with acute icteric hepatitis have prominent cholestasis, manifesting as intense pruritus and deep jaundice, which persists for several weeks during the convalescent phase. Systemic symptoms during this phase are minimal and the person often otherwise feels well. The condition usually has a benign course and resolves completely in a few weeks to months without any specific therapy or sequelae.

Acute Icteric Hepatitis in Pregnant Women

During outbreaks of hepatitis E in disease-endemic areas, pregnant women, particularly in the second and third trimesters, are at a higher risk of developing icteric acute viral hepatitis compared with men and nonpregnant women. Further, in them, the disease is more severe, with a larger proportion of pregnant women with acute hepatitis E progressing to acute liver failure, and a higher risk of mortality.[24] In some studies, the case fatality rate among pregnant women with acute hepatitis E has been 15% to 25%, compared with less than 1% overall. In addition, these women are at an increased risk of miscarriage, preterm delivery, still birth, and perinatal mortality.[25] Their newborns, besides being at risk of HEV infection through vertical maternofetal transmission, are more prone to anicteric or even icteric hepatitis, hypoglycemia, and neonatal death.[26]

The reason for this increased susceptibility and enhanced liver injury during pregnancy remains unknown. Immunologic and hormonal factors are suspected to be responsible. The available studies have implicated changes in immune regulation, zinc and vitamin D deficiency, specific viral mutations, higher viral load, and reduced expression of progesterone receptor and progesterone-induced binding factor; however, the relative contributions of these various factors are not yet known.[27]

The association of severity of hepatitis E with pregnancy has not been reported from developed countries with GT3/GT4 disease. This lack of association may be related to a low frequency of HEV infection among young people in such regions or to a real difference in the pathogenesis of disease caused by the different HEV genotypes.

Chronic Hepatitis E

HEV infection was initially thought to be a self-limited condition, with the virus being cleared from the host's body within a few weeks. However, it was later found that, in some immunosuppressed persons, in particular solid-organ transplant recipients who are receiving immunosuppressive drugs, HEV can persist in the host for a long duration, extending over months to years. Such patients have persistent liver inflammation and can progress to cirrhosis.

Chronic hepatitis E, defined empirically as detection of HEV RNA in serum or stool of a person for longer than 6 months, is observed mostly among persons with impaired immune response. Most of these patients have been solid-organ transplant recipients receiving immunosuppressive drugs,[28] and a few were receiving anticancer chemotherapy for a hematological malignancy or had human immunodeficiency virus infection. Recently, some cases have also been identified among those receiving milder immunosuppressive regimens for rheumatologic or connective tissue disorders.[29]

Although the risk of exposure to HEV in such groups is possibly no higher than in the general population resident in the same geographic area, they are apparently less likely to clear the virus and hence more prone to develop persistent infection.[30] All patients with chronic hepatitis E have had GT3 HEV infection, except 1 who had GT4 virus.[31] Chronic HEV infection seems to be extremely infrequent with GT1 infection; in studies of renal transplant recipients with increased serum transaminase levels in India, none had evidence of chronic HEV infection.[32,33]

The prevalence of HEV infection in organ transplant recipients in Europe has ranged from 2.3% to 43.9% and 0.9% to 3.5%, depending on whether serologic test or HEV RNA, respectively, is used for the diagnosis. Among solid-organ transplant recipients, use of tacrolimus (as opposed to other immunosuppressive drugs) and thrombocytopenia have been found to be associated with a higher risk of persistent HEV infection.[30]

The clinical spectrum of chronic HEV infection is broad, including asymptomatic increase in transaminase level, acute hepatitis, chronic hepatitis and subacute liver failure. In a large series, the commonest symptoms were fatigue, diarrhea, arthralgia, weight loss, abdominal pain, jaundice, itching, fever, and nausea.[30] Persons with chronic HEV infection often have a persistent increase of serum transaminase levels and histologic evidence of chronic hepatitis. It has been estimated that up to 10% of such patients may progress to liver cirrhosis.[34] Chronic HEV infection in persons with prior liver transplant has particularly severe adverse outcomes, such as post-transplant hepatitis, rapid progression to liver cirrhosis or liver failure, and need for liver retransplant; also, the HEV infection may recur following liver retransplant.[35]

Initial suspicion of HEV infection in the general population is usually based on the detection of HEV IgM and IgG antibodies. However, these tests may have a limited sensitivity in patients with chronic HEV infection, because of coexistent immunosuppression, which may delay or preclude seroconversion. Hence, diagnosis of HEV infection in such patients needs HEV RNA testing in serum and/or stool.[36]

Hepatitis E Virus Superinfection in Patients with Preexisting Chronic Liver Disease

People with cirrhosis have a reduced liver functional reserve. Hence, in them, even a mild additional liver injury, regardless of the cause, may tip the balance leading to liver decompensation.

In several countries with predominance of GT1 HEV as the cause of human disease, HEV has been shown to be an important cause of superimposed injury in patients with preexisting chronic liver disease, and to present as acute-on-chronic liver disease.[37] These patients have a higher mortality than those with stable compensated cirrhosis.[38] Similar cases have more recently been described from China too, where GT4 HEV is predominant.[39,40] By contrast, although HEV superinfection in patients with cirrhosis has also been reported from Europe, an association with increased mortality has not been found[41]; this may be because of the milder liver injury caused by the GT3 HEV prevalent in these areas.

HEV infection in a person with underlying chronic liver disease usually begins as an illness resembling typical acute hepatitis. However, within a few days, ascites, encephalopathy, or both appear, suggesting decompensated liver disease. Diagnosis of underlying chronic liver disease may first become apparent only when imaging or endoscopic examination reveal findings characteristic of chronic liver damage or portal hypertension. The mortality is higher than that following HEV infection in previously healthy persons.

Extrahepatic Manifestations

Involvement of body organs other than liver has been reported in some persons with HEV infection (**Table 2**). Of these, involvement of the nervous system, pancreas, and kidneys has been the most common, with occasional reports of hematological and autoimmune manifestations.[42] Most of the reports of extrahepatic manifestations of HEV infection have been from low-endemicity regions, raising the possibility that these are specific to the HEV genotype prevalent there (GT3), but this could also reflect the availability of better medical and investigative facilities.

The pathogenesis of these manifestations remains unclear and it is uncertain whether these result from viral multiplication in nonhepatic tissues, an immune complex-mediated bystander injury secondary to liver dysfunction, worsening of a

Table 2 Extrahepatic manifestations of hepatitis E virus infection	
Neurologic syndromes	*Central nervous system* • Acute transverse myelitis • Acute meningoencephalitis • Aseptic meningitis • Neuralgic amyotrophy • Pseudotumor cerebri • Bilateral pyramidal syndrome *Peripheral nervous system* • Guillain-Barré syndrome • Cranial nerve palsies • Peripheral neuropathy
Pancreas	Acute pancreatitis
Renal	Membranous glomerulonephritis Membranoproliferative glomerulonephritis IgA nephropathy Nephroangiosclerosis Reduced glomerular filtration rate Cryoglobulinemia
Biliary tree	Acalculous cholecystitis
Hematological	Thrombocytopenia Hemolysis Aplastic anemia Pure red cell aplasia Hemophagocytic syndrome
Heart	Myocarditis
Miscellaneous	Henoch-Schönlein purpura Skin rash Arthralgia Thyroiditis Myasthenia gravis Monoclonal gammopathy of uncertain significance

preexisting abnormality of nonhepatic organ caused by liver disease, or an incidental coexisting illness.

In cases in whom such nonhepatic manifestations are not accompanied by a hepatic illness, and HEV infection is identified only on laboratory testing, the pathogenetic significance of HEV infection may be uncertain, particularly when the diagnosis of HEV infection is based on detection of anti-HEV IgM antibodies, rather than of HEV RNA.

Acute pancreatitis
Several case reports and case series have documented the occurrence of acute pancreatitis in patients with hepatitis E.[43] These reports have mostly been from disease-endemic areas where GT1 HEV infection is common. The features of pancreatic involvement often appear in the second or third week of hepatic illness, and mostly resolve over time.

Neurologic illness
Several abnormalities in central or peripheral nervous systems have been attributed to HEV infection (see **Table 2**).[44] These abnormalities have been associated with acute as well as chronic HEV infection, and seem to occur irrespective of whether the person is

immunocompromised or immunocompetent. Most such cases have had infection with GT3 HEV; however, this finding may be related to the easier availability of facilities for molecular testing for HEV RNA and nucleic acid sequencing in areas where this genotype is frequent. In some reports, HEV RNA was detected in cerebrospinal fluid of the affected persons, strengthening the role of HEV in the causation of neurologic injury. In a renal transplant recipient with chronic HEV, viral genomic sequences recovered from serum and cerebrospinal fluid were different, indicating compartmentalization of HEV quasispecies between these body fluids, and suggesting HEV neurotropism.[45]

Kidney injury

Recent data suggest that kidneys are often involved in HEV infection. HEV capsid protein and HEV RNA have been detected in urine of experimental animals as well as in patients with acute or chronic hepatitis caused by HEV GT4.[46] This renal excretion of HEV capsid or RNA has not been shown to induce any renal injury in humans. A small experimental study has shown active involvement of kidneys by showing evidence of virus replication and viral protein–induced kidney injury in the form of inflammatory cell infiltration of the renal interstitium.[47]

PREVENTION

Prevention of Food-Borne and Water-Borne Transmission

Because HEV infection is transmitted primarily through fecal contamination of food and water, the most effective measures for its prevention include ensuring good personal hygiene, provision of clean public water supplies, proper disposal of human excreta, and general measures for food safety.[48] These measures are of particular importance for people who are at a higher risk of acquiring HEV infection or an increased risk of severe disease or chronic infection if HEV infection occurs, such as travelers to developing countries, solid-organ transplant recipients, persons on immunosuppressive drugs or anticancer chemotherapy, pregnant women, and persons with chronic liver disease. Isolation of infected persons has a limited role because person-to-person transmission is infrequent.[49] These measures should be effective against all HEV genotypes.

HEV is inactivated by heating at 70°C;[50] hence, the use of boiled water and adequate cooking of food should help markedly reduce or eliminate the risk of its transmission. In regions with zoonotic transmission of GT3 and GT4, adequate cooking of meat before consumption should be particularly useful.

Prevention of Transmission Through Blood Transfusion

Numerous reports, in particular from the developed world, over the last 10 to 15 years have convincingly showed the presence of HEV viremia in a proportion of blood units collected from healthy donors. This finding has led to the recognition of HEV as a transfusion-transmittable infection and the adoption in several countries of screening of donated blood for HEV RNA. Such screening needs nucleic acid testing, which is costly, and needs specialized equipment and trained manpower. Hence, some countries have adopted a policy of selectively screening screening only blood products that are to be transfused to specific groups that are deemed at a high risk of HEV infection; for example, organ transplant recipients or immunosuppressed persons.

Hepatitis E Vaccine

Inability of HEV to grow well in culture systems precludes the development of a live attenuated or inactivated vaccine. However, attempts at developing recombinant subunit vaccines have been highly successful.

The open reading frame 2 in the HEV genome codes for the viral capsid protein, which plays a key role in virus assembly and its attachment to host cells. It is also highly immunogenic, and contains neutralization epitopes, antibodies to which render it incapable of infecting the host cells. This work has led to several recombinant HEV capsid proteins expressed in different prokaryotic or eukaryotic systems being tried as candidate HEV vaccines.[51] Two of these candidate vaccines have undergone clinical trials and have both shown excellent safety and efficacy. One of these has been commercially developed. It has been approved for use in persons in the age group of 16 to 65 years for prevention of HEV infection, and is marketed in China as Hecolin. Three intramuscular doses at 0, 1, and 6 months are recommended. In a large community trial, it had an efficacy rate of ~95% and was associated with only minor local adverse events.[52] However, it has not yet been approved in any other country.

In 2013, the World Health Organization's Strategic Advisory Group of Experts on Immunization set up a Hepatitis E Vaccine Working Group to assess the status of this hepatitis E vaccine. **Table 3** summarizes the potential role of this vaccine in various settings and populations, based on the available information on HEV epidemiology and the available HEV vaccine, as identified by this group.[53]

TREATMENT OF HEPATITIS E
Acute Hepatitis

Most patients with acute hepatitis E have a mild illness with spontaneous recovery without any residual damage. Hence, they do not need any specific treatment beyond counseling about the benign nature of their illness and periodic monitoring for signs of progression to severe disease. They can continue their daily routines, including light physical activity, until symptoms resolve. Antipyretic, antiemetic, and mild analgesic drugs are helpful for symptom relief. Strict bed rest, vitamin preparations (including vitamin K), appetite stimulants, antibiotics and hepatoprotective agents have no role. Dietary restrictions do not provide any benefit and may lead to diminution of overall food intake.

Altered sleep pattern, excessive irritability, or prolongation of prothrombin time may predict advent of severe disease. Degree of increase in liver enzyme levels has no relation with disease severity; hence, frequent repetition of liver function tests is of limited value. Antiviral drugs have not been systematically evaluated in patients with severe acute hepatitis E.

Chronic Hepatitis

No controlled studies are available for treatment of chronic HEV infection, and hence the current practice is based on uncontrolled observational data. In persons with chronic hepatitis E who are receiving immunosuppressive drugs, reduction of dose or discontinuation of the drug is associated with clearance of viremia in around one-third of cases, and hence should be the first-line intervention.[30] If this fails, ribavirin monotherapy (for at least 3 months, and preferably 6 months) is recommended; this treatment is associated with a sustained virological response (absence of detectable HEV RNA in serum at 3–6 months after stopping treatment) in around 78% of the subjects treated.[54] Occasional cases of ribavirin resistance have been reported, and are thought to be related to a specific genetic variation in the viral genome. Attempts have been made to increase the effectiveness of the ribavirin through the addition of sofosbuvir, a direct-acting inhibitor specifically of hepatitis C virus replication. However, the results are still inconclusive.[55]

Table 3
Current status of the use of hepatitis E virus vaccine in various settings or population subgroups

Population Group	Recommendation	Explanations and Comments
General population residing in high-endemicity regions	No recommendation. However, national authorities may decide to use the vaccine based on the local epidemiology	• Limited data on HEV-related morbidity and mortality in high-endemicity regions, making it impossible to calculate absolute effectiveness and cost-effectiveness • No safety and efficacy data for age <16 y or >65 y • No efficacy data beyond 4.5 y after vaccination • Efficacy and safety data are limited to 1 country • Vaccine efficacy proved directly only against genotype 4 HEV, whereas the disease in high-endemicity areas is caused by genotype 1 or 2 • Role of vaccine in reducing fecal viral excretion or transmission of infection is unknown
Pregnant women or women of childbearing age	No clear recommendation is possible	• No population-based data on incidence of or mortality related to hepatitis E among pregnant women or neonates in any region of the world • No data on safety and efficacy of vaccine during pregnancy • Not clear whether vaccine would protect against severe hepatitis E observed during pregnancy • Difficult to identify and vaccinate women of childbearing age in high-endemicity areas
Patients with preexisting chronic liver disease		• No data on immunogenicity in such patients • Limited data on absolute risk of disease or death caused by HEV infection in such patients
Immunosuppressed groups		• No data on immunogenicity in such patients • Most such patients have genotype 3 HEV infection, efficacy of vaccine against which is unclear
Travelers from low-endemic to high-endemic areas	Not recommended routinely. May be recommended for travelers at a higher risk of HEV infection (such as humanitarian relief workers traveling to an	• The absolute risk of hepatitis E among travelers is low • Risk can be reduced by precautions related to water and food

(continued on next page)

Population Group	Recommendation	Explanations and Comments
	outbreak area) or of serious disease following HEV infection (eg, pregnant women)	• Vaccination time schedule (0, 1, 6 mo) is too long for a travel vaccine
Prevention and control of HEV outbreaks	Use of vaccine to mitigate outbreaks of hepatitis E should be considered	• No data on efficacy of vaccine when given postexposure • No data on whether vaccination reduces fecal shedding or transmission of HEV • Vaccine time schedule is too prolonged (0, 1, 6 mo), with only limited data for 2 doses (0 and 1 mo)

Table 3
(continued)

In a few small case series, pegylated interferon alfa was found to be useful in those who could not tolerate or failed to respond to prolonged ribavirin treatment;[56] however, this treatment is not suited for solid-organ transplant recipients because it is associated with an increased risk of rejection of the transplanted organ.

DISCLOSURE

Nothing to disclose.

REFERENCES

1. Viswanathan R. Infectious hepatitis in Delhi (1955-56): a critical study: epidemiology. Indian J Med Res 1957;45(Suppl 1):1–29.
2. Khuroo MS. Study of an epidemic of non-A, non-B hepatitis. Possibility of another human hepatitis virus distinct from post-transfusion non-A, non-B type. Am J Med 1980;68(6):818–24.
3. Balayan MS, Andjaparidze AG, Savinskaya SS, et al. Evidence for a virus in non-A, non-B hepatitis transmitted via the fecal-oral route. Intervirology 1983;20(1): 23–31.
4. Bradley DW, Krawczynski K, Cook EH Jr, et al. Enterically transmitted non-A, non-B hepatitis: serial passage of disease in cynomolgus macaques and tamarins and recovery of disease-associated 27- to 34-nm viruslike particles. Proc Natl Acad Sci U S A 1987;84(17):6277–81.
5. Reyes GR, Purdy MA, Kim JP, et al. Isolation of a cDNA from the virus responsible for enterically transmitted non-A, non-B hepatitis. Science 1990;247(4948): 1335–9.
6. Takahashi M, Tanaka T, Takahashi H, et al. Hepatitis E Virus (HEV) strains in serum samples can replicate efficiently in cultured cells despite the coexistence of HEV antibodies: characterization of HEV virions in blood circulation. J Clin Microbiol 2010;48(4):1112–25.
7. Purdy MA, Harrison TJ, Jameel S, et al. ICTV virus taxonomy profile: hepeviridae. J Gen Virol 2017;98(11):2645–6.
8. Aggarwal R, Goel A. Advances in hepatitis E - I: virology, pathogenesis and diagnosis. Expert Rev Gastroenterol Hepatol 2016;10(9):1053–63.

9. Meng XJ, Purcell RH, Halbur PG, et al. A novel virus in swine is closely related to the human hepatitis E virus. Proc Natl Acad Sci U S A 1997;94(18):9860–5.

10. Lu L, Li C, Hagedorn CH. Phylogenetic analysis of global hepatitis E virus sequences: genetic diversity, subtypes and zoonosis. Rev Med Virol 2006; 16(1):5–36.

11. Gupta N, Sarangi AN, Dadhich S, et al. Acute hepatitis E in India appears to be caused exclusively by genotype 1 hepatitis E virus. Indian J Gastroenterol 2018; 37(1):44–9.

12. Shukla P, Chauhan UK, Naik S, et al. Hepatitis E virus infection among animals in northern India: an unlikely source of human disease. J Viral Hepat 2007;14(5): 310–7.

13. Goel A, Aggarwal R. Advances in hepatitis E - II: epidemiology, clinical manifestations, treatment and prevention. Expert Rev Gastroenterol Hepatol 2016;10(9): 1065–74.

14. Kamel MA, Troonen H, Kapprell HP, et al. Seroepidemiology of hepatitis E virus in the Egyptian Nile Delta. J Med Virol 1995;47(4):399–403.

15. Doceul V, Bagdassarian E, Demange A, et al. Zoonotic hepatitis E virus: classification, animal reservoirs and transmission routes. Viruses 2016;8(10) [pii:E270].

16. Pavio N, Meng XJ, Renou C. Zoonotic hepatitis E: animal reservoirs and emerging risks. Vet Res 2010;41(6):46.

17. Hewitt PE, Ijaz S, Brailsford SR, et al. Hepatitis E virus in blood components: a prevalence and transmission study in southeast England. Lancet 2014; 384(9956):1766–73.

18. Rein DB, Stevens GA, Theaker J, et al. The global burden of hepatitis E virus genotypes 1 and 2 in 2005. Hepatology 2012;55(4):988–97.

19. GBD 2017 Disease and Injury Incidence and Prevalence Collaborators. Global, regional, and national incidence, prevalence, and years lived with disability for 354 diseases and injuries for 195 countries and territories, 1990-2017: a systematic analysis for the Global Burden of Disease Study 2017. Lancet 2018; 392(10159):1789–858.

20. Aggarwal R. The global prevalence of hepatitis E virus infection and susceptibility: a systematic review. Geneva (Switzerland): World Health Organization; 2010. Available at: http://whqlibdoc.who.int/hq/2010/WHO_IVB_10.14_eng.pdf.

21. Kmush B, Wierzba T, Krain L, et al. Epidemiology of hepatitis E in low- and middle-income countries of Asia and Africa. Semin Liver Dis 2013;33(1):15–29.

22. Engle RE, Kuniholm MH, Nelson KE, et al. Hepatitis E virus seroprevalence in the National Health and Nutrition Examination Survey: facts trump opinion. Hepatology 2015;61(4):1442.

23. Naik SR, Aggarwal R, Salunke PN, et al. A large waterborne viral hepatitis E epidemic in Kanpur, India. Bull World Health Organ 1992;70(5):597–604.

24. Khuroo MS, Teli MR, Skidmore S, et al. Incidence and severity of viral hepatitis in pregnancy. Am J Med 1981;70(2):252–5.

25. Patra S, Kumar A, Trivedi SS, et al. Maternal and fetal outcomes in pregnant women with acute hepatitis E virus infection. Ann Intern Med 2007;147(1):28–33.

26. Khuroo MS, Kamili S, Khuroo MS. Clinical course and duration of viremia in vertically transmitted hepatitis E virus (HEV) infection in babies born to HEV-infected mothers. J Viral Hepat 2009;16(7):519–23.

27. Navaneethan U, Al Mohajer M, Shata MT. Hepatitis E and pregnancy: understanding the pathogenesis. Liver Int 2008;28(9):1190–9.

28. Kamar N, Selves J, Mansuy JM, et al. Hepatitis E virus and chronic hepatitis in organ-transplant recipients. N Engl J Med 2008;358(8):811–7.

29. Pischke S, Peron JM, von Wulffen M, et al. Chronic hepatitis E in rheumatology and internal medicine patients: a retrospective Multicenter European Cohort Study. Viruses 2019;11(2) [pii:E186].
30. Kamar N, Garrouste C, Haagsma EB, et al. Factors associated with chronic hepatitis in patients with hepatitis E virus infection who have received solid organ transplants. Gastroenterology 2011;140(5):1481–9.
31. Geng Y, Zhang H, Huang W, et al. Persistent hepatitis E virus genotype 4 infection in a child with acute lymphoblastic leukemia. Hepat Mon 2014;14(1):e15618.
32. Munjal S, Gupta N, Sharma RK, et al. Lack of persistent hepatitis E virus infection as a cause for unexplained transaminase elevation in renal transplant recipients in India. Indian J Gastroenterol 2014;33(6):550–3.
33. Naik A, Gupta N, Goel D, et al. Lack of evidence of hepatitis E virus infection among renal transplant recipients in a disease-endemic area. J Viral Hepat 2013;20(4):e138–40.
34. Kamar N, Rostaing L, Izopet J. Hepatitis E virus infection in immunosuppressed patients: natural history and therapy. Semin Liver Dis 2013;33(1):62–70.
35. Haagsma EB, van den Berg AP, Porte RJ, et al. Chronic hepatitis E virus infection in liver transplant recipients. Liver Transpl 2008;14(4):547–53.
36. Te H, Doucette K. Viral hepatitis: guidelines by the American Society of Transplantation Infectious Disease Community of Practice. Clin Transplant 2019; 33(9):e13514.
37. Acharya SK, Sharma PK, Singh R, et al. Hepatitis E virus (HEV) infection in patients with cirrhosis is associated with rapid decompensation and death. J Hepatol 2007;46(3):387–94.
38. Radha Krishna Y, Saraswat VA, Das K, et al. Clinical features and predictors of outcome in acute hepatitis A and hepatitis E virus hepatitis on cirrhosis. Liver Int 2009;29(3):392–8.
39. Zhang S, Chen C, Peng J, et al. Investigation of underlying comorbidities as risk factors for symptomatic human hepatitis E virus infection. Aliment Pharmacol Ther 2017;45(5):701–13.
40. Ke WM, Li XJ, Yu LN, et al. Etiological investigation of fatal liver failure during the course of chronic hepatitis B in southeast China. J Gastroenterol 2006;41(4): 347–51.
41. Blasco-Perrin H, Madden RG, Stanley A, et al. Hepatitis E virus in patients with decompensated chronic liver disease: a prospective UK/French study. Aliment Pharmacol Ther 2015;42(5):574–81.
42. Bazerbachi F, Haffar S, Garg SK, et al. Extra-hepatic manifestations associated with hepatitis E virus infection: a comprehensive review of the literature. Gastroenterol Rep (Oxf) 2016;4(1):1–15.
43. Bhagat S, Wadhawan M, Sud R, et al. Hepatitis viruses causing pancreatitis and hepatitis: a case series and review of literature. Pancreas 2008;36(4):424–7.
44. Cheung MC, Maguire J, Carey I, et al. Review of the neurological manifestations of hepatitis E infection. Ann Hepatol 2012;11(5):618–22.
45. Kamar N, Izopet J, Cintas P, et al. Hepatitis E virus-induced neurological symptoms in a kidney-transplant patient with chronic hepatitis. Am J Transplant 2010;10(5):1321–4.
46. Geng Y, Zhao C, Huang W, et al. Detection and assessment of infectivity of hepatitis E virus in urine. J Hepatol 2016;64(1):37–43.
47. Wang L, Xia J, Wang L, et al. Experimental infection of rabbits with genotype 3 hepatitis E virus produced both chronicity and kidney injury. Gut 2017;66(3): 561–2.

48. Goel A, Aggarwal R. Prevention of hepatitis E: another step forward. Future Microbiol 2011;6(1):23–7.
49. Aggarwal R, Naik SR. Hepatitis E: intrafamilial transmission versus waterborne spread. J Hepatol 1994;21(5):718–23.
50. Emerson SU, Arankalle VA, Purcell RH. Thermal stability of hepatitis E virus. J Infect Dis 2005;192(5):930–3.
51. Aggarwal R, Jameel S. Hepatitis E vaccine. Hepatol Int 2008;2(3):308–15.
52. Zhu FC, Zhang J, Zhang XF, et al. Efficacy and safety of a recombinant hepatitis E vaccine in healthy adults: a large-scale, randomised, double-blind placebo-controlled, phase 3 trial. Lancet 2010;376(9744):895–902.
53. Hepatitis E vaccine: WHO position paper, May 2015. Wkly Epidemiol Rec 2015; 90(18):185–200.
54. Kamar N, Izopet J, Tripon S, et al. Ribavirin for chronic hepatitis E virus infection in transplant recipients. N Engl J Med 2014;370(12):1111–20.
55. Dao Thi VL, Debing Y, Wu X, et al. Sofosbuvir inhibits hepatitis E virus replication in vitro and results in an additive effect when combined with ribavirin. Gastroenterology 2016;150(1):82–5.e4.
56. Peters van Ton AM, Gevers TJ, Drenth JP. Antiviral therapy in chronic hepatitis E: a systematic review. J Viral Hepat 2015;22(12):965–73.

Epstein-Barr Virus and Cytomegalovirus Infections of the Liver

Chalermrat Bunchorntavakul, MD[a], K. Rajender Reddy, MD[b],*

KEYWORDS

- Cytomegalovirus • Epstein-Barr virus • Infectious mononucleosis • Liver
- Transplantation • Hepatitis

KEY POINTS

- Epstein-Barr virus (EBV) and cytomegalovirus (CMV) infections are common in humans.
- EBV and CMV can be associated with a variety of liver manifestations.
- In the setting of liver transplantation, CMV is the most common infectious complication.
- EBV is the major cause of post-transplant lymphoproliferative disorders.

INTRODUCTION

Epstein-Barr virus (EBV) and cytomegalovirus (CMV) are human herpesviruses (HHV) that are common in humans. Primary EBV and CMV infections mostly are asymptomatic but can be associated with infectious mononucleosis (IM) syndrome, including fever, tonsillar pharyngitis, and lymphadenopathy.[1–3] Like other herpesviruses, they are characterized by their ability to maintain lifelong latent infections, particularly for CMV, which then can reactivate later, in an immunocompromised state. Both EBV and CMV infections can be associated with a variety of clinical syndromes, including liver disorders.[1–3] The most common liver disorder associated with EBV and CMV in immunocompetent hosts is acute hepatitis, in which the severity varies from asymptomatic alanine aminotransferase (ALT) and aspartate aminotransferase (AST) elevations, self-limited icteric hepatitis to acute liver failure (ALF). In addition, atypical manifestations, such as cholestasis, chronic hepatitis, precipitation of acute-on-chronic liver failure (ACLF), and autoimmune hepatitis (AIH), also can occur in association with EBV infection[2–6] (**Table 1**). The recognition of EBV and CMV as the cause of liver

a Division of Gastroenterology and Hepatology, Department of Medicine, Rajavithi Hospital, College of Medicine, Rangsit University, 2 Phayathai Road, Ratchathewi, Bangkok 10400, Thailand; b Division of Gastroenterology and Hepatology, Department of Medicine, University of Pennsylvania, 2 Dulles, 3400 Spruce Street, Philadelphia, PA 19104, USA
* Corresponding author.
E-mail address: rajender.reddy@uphs.upenn.edu

Gastroenterol Clin N Am 49 (2020) 331–346
https://doi.org/10.1016/j.gtc.2020.01.008
0889-8553/20/© 2020 Elsevier Inc. All rights reserved.

Table 1 Liver disorders associated with Epstein-Barr virus infections	
Acute liver disorders	Acute hepatitis (with or without features of IM) Cholestasis or cholestatic hepatitis ALF
Chronic liver disorders	Chronic active hepatitis (may mimic AIH) Granulomatous hepatitis Vanishing bile duct syndrome Precipitation of AIH Precipitation of acute-on-chronic-liver failure
Liver transplant setting	PTLDs Non-PTLD EBV syndromes

disorders seems to be underestimated. Based on limited data, it is estimated that EBV and CMV infections account for 1% to 4% of adult patients presenting with acute hepatitis in population-based studies from developed countries[7,8] and account for up to 29% and 2% of adult patients with acute sporadic viral hepatitis and ACLF in India, respectively.[9] In the setting of liver transplantation (LT), CMV is the most common infectious complication among LT recipients, which then is associated with significant morbidity and thus requires prophylactic measures[10]; EBV is the major cause of post-transplant lymphoproliferative disorders (PTLDs), accounting for up to 85% of cases.[11]

EPSTEIN-BARR VIRUS INFECTIONS
Virology and Transmission

EBV is a double-stranded DNA virus with an envelope and a member of the herpesvirus family (HHV-4). It is one of the more common viruses in humans, affecting greater than 90% of the adult population.[1,12] Like other herpesviruses, EBV has a tendency for establishing a latency phase in the host. It infects B cells of the immune system and epithelial cells.[12] The EBV receptor on human cells is the B-cell surface molecule CD21, which is the receptor for the C3d component of complement.[12] Primary infection elicits a strong cellular immune response and, once brought under control, EBV latency persists in the resting memory B cells for the rest of a person's life in which the infected (transformed) B cells are shielded from the immune system and also are capable of indefinite growth.[1,12] Viral latency is characterized by 3 distinct processes, including viral persistence, restricted viral gene expression, and potential to reactivate due to lytic replication.[12]

EBV infection usually occurs in individuals of a young age, in particular those with low socioeconomic status or poor hygienic standards. By their third decade of life, 80% to 100% of these individuals become carriers of the infection.[13] The oral route is the primary route of transmission and the virus can persistently shed in the oropharynx of patients with IM for up to 18 months after clinical recovery.[14] Transmission via blood transfusion also has been documented; however, transmission through sexual intercourse and breastfeeding are unclear, although EBV has been isolated from the genital fluid and breast milk.[14]

Manifestations and Diagnosis of Epstein-Barr Virus Infection

Acute and chronic EBV infections in adults can be associated with a variety of manifestations (eg, IM, oral hairy leukoplakia, and chronic active EBV infection), lymphoproliferative disorders (hemophagocytic lymphohistiocytosis, lymphomatoid granulomatosis, and PTLDs), and malignancies (eg, Burkitt lymphoma, Hodgkin lymphoma, T-cell lymphoma, and nasopharyngeal carcinoma).[1,3,12,14] Although most EBV infections in young children are asymptomatic or have nonspecific symptoms, infections of adolescents and adults commonly result in IM.[1,3,14] IM typically begins with malaise, headache, and low-grade fever before development of the more specific signs of tonsillitis and/or pharyngitis (>80%), cervical lymphadenopathy (>90%), and moderate to high fever (>90%).[1,3,14] On physical examination, splenomegaly and hepatomegaly are present in greater than 50% and greater than 10% of patients, respectively.[1,3,14] Less common complications of IM include hemolytic anemia, thrombocytopenia, aplastic anemia, hemophagocytosis, myocarditis, severe hepatitis, splenic rupture, rash, and neurologic complications. Most symptoms of IM are attributed to the activation of immune response against EBV.[1]

Most patients with IM have leukocytosis with an absolute increase in the number of peripheral mononuclear cells, elevated ALT levels, and atypical lymphocytes.[1,3,12] The atypical lymphocytes are primary T cells, many of which are as a response to the EBV-infected B cells.[1] Activation of B cells by EBV, with resultant production of polyclonal antibodies, causes elevated titers of heterophile antibodies and occasionally causes increases in cold agglutinins, cryoglobulins, antinuclear antibodies, or rheumatoid factor.[1] Reactive heterophile antibodies in a patient with a compatible syndrome are highly specific for EBV infection, although false-negative results during the early phase of clinical symptoms can occur.[14,15] EBV-specific antibodies directed against the EBV capsid antigen usually present at the onset of clinical illness and are reliable markers of EBV infection; Immunoglobulin(Ig)M levels wane approximately 3 months later (indicating acute infection), whereas IgG levels persist for life.[14,15] Approximately 10% of IM-like illness may be caused by infectious agents other than EBV, such as CMV, human immunodeficiency virus (HIV), toxoplasma, HHV-6 and viral hepatitis B.[14]

EPSTEIN-BARR VIRUS HEPATITIS
Incidence and Clinical Features of Epstein-Barr Virus Hepatitis

Acute EBV infection typically is associated with hepatocellular hepatitis. In patients presenting with features of IM, mild hepatitis has been observed in up to 70% to 90%.[4,16] Furthermore, patients with acute pharyngitis and hepatitis may trigger a diagnosis of acute EBV infection. The EBV hepatitis usually is mild (ALT rarely exceeds 1000 U/L), unrecognized, and resolves spontaneously, although jaundice is present in 5% to 10% of cases.[4,6,16,17] EBV hepatitis also can present in patients without classical features of IM. In a retrospective review from the Jaundice Hotline service at the Royal Cornwall Hospital, United Kingdom, EBV hepatitis was diagnosed in 17 patients (0.9%) among 1995 patients presenting with jaundice and/or hepatitis over a 13-year study period, and only 2 patients had associated features of IM.[8] Compared with IM, non-IM EBV hepatitis tended to affect an older age group (the median age was 40 years with approximately half ages >60 years) and the diagnosis is suggested by the presence of a lymphocytosis and/or splenomegaly (noted in 88% of cases).[8] In a prospective study in Iceland on the causes of markedly elevated ALT greater than 500 U/L, EBV and CMV were the causes of viral hepatitis in approximately 4% and 1% of cases, respectively.[7] The median age of patients with EBV hepatitis was 17 (15–20) years and splenomegaly was reported in 12% of cases.[7] Taken together, the diagnosis of EBV hepatitis should be considered in patients with unexplained hepatitis, especially in young adults but also in older patients, particularly in the presence of other suggestive features for example, viral-illness features and/or splenomegaly.

Although a majority of cases present with hepatocellular injury, features of mixed or cholestatic injury are not uncommon in EBV hepatitis (reported in up to 10%–50% of cases).[6,8,16–19] The mechanism for the cholestatic component is unknown; it is assumed to be related to a mildly swollen bile duct rather than a direct infection of the biliary epithelial cells.[17] It also has been suggested that the virus increases the production of inflammatory cytokines, which affect sinusoid and canalicular transport.[6] The major biochemical difference between EBV and CMV hepatitis was the more pronounced mixed cholestatic pattern observed in EBV.[7,20] Importantly, because cholestatic feature is not typical for EBV infection, other or concurrent diagnosis of liver disease, such as drug-induced, sepsis, or bile duct disorders, should be excluded.

Although rare, cases of severe hepatitis and ALF-complicated IM resulting in death or LT have been reported anecdotally.[4,16,17,21–24] In a literature review of 16 case reports during 1949 to 1993, overall mortality of IM-associated ALF was 87% without LT.[21] More recently, in the US Acute Liver Failure Study Group, EBV-related ALF was rare and accounted for less than 1% of ALF cases (4 among 1887 consecutive adult ALF patients) but was associated with a high mortality rate.[25] Median patient age was 30 (18–44) years; 75% were male, and only 25% were immunosuppressed. The median presenting ALT was 504 (156–4920) IU/mL, alkaline phosphatase (ALP) was 431 (136–1009) IU/mL, and bilirubin was 17 (13–22) mg/dL. Although all of the patients were treated with an antiviral agent, 2 died of ALF, 1 underwent LT, and 1 survived with supportive care.[25]

Diagnosis and Management of Epstein-Barr Virus Hepatitis

In general, heterophile and EBV-specific antibodies are helpful for the diagnosis of EBV infection. Cross-reacting antibodies may be present, however, and cases of acute EBV hepatitis with cross-reacting antibodies to other herpesviruses, in particular CMV and hepatitis E virus (HEV), have been frequently reported (likely because of polyclonal B-cell stimulation).[26–29] Serologic cross-reactivity to EBV and CMV causes problems in the diagnosis of acute hepatitis E virus infection.[30,31] In a 3-year retrospective study from London, HEV IgM was positive or equivocal in 61 of 1423 samples tested for HEV serology.[31] Only 13.3% of samples with positive HEV IgM were HEV polymerase chain reaction (PCR) positive. A high degree of EBV and CMV cross-reactivity was noted, with 33.3% and 24.2% of HEV IgM–positive samples also testing positive for EBV and CMV IgM, respectively.[31] EBV DNA PCR using blood, plasma, or tissue is more reliable than serology. Taken together, the diagnosis of EBV, CMV, and HEV hepatitis should be based on a combination of clinical features, serology, and confirmatory PCR testing.

Liver biopsy may be required to confirm the diagnosis of EBV hepatitis in highly selected cases. Characteristic histopathologic findings in EBV hepatitis include a diffuse lymphocytic sinusoidal infiltrate in a string of beads pattern, expansion of portal tracts by a predominantly lymphocytic infiltrate, and intact lobular architecture.[25,32] Centrilobular cholestasis is uncommon but possible.[6] In severe cases, massive hepatic necrosis can be seen.[25,33] In situ hybridization of EBV-encoded RNA (EBER) is a helpful ancillary test.[25,32,34] Correlation of clinical history, laboratory findings, and histopathologic features is essential to distinguish EBV hepatitis from autoimmune liver diseases, transplant rejection, lymphomas, and drug-induced liver injury.[32] Notably, 2 hypotheses have been proposed to explain the pathogenesis of EBV hepatitis; either due to the direct damage of the hepatocytes, because viral particles have been found inside liver cells along with intracellular inclusions, or to the indirect liver damage by inflammatory mediators, such as cytokines, interferon, tumor necrosis factor (TNF), and Fas ligand, that are produced after the activation of CD8$^+$ T cells.[6,35,36]

Most cases of EBV hepatitis are mild and resolve spontaneously, and only supportive treatment is needed.[6] In cases of severe EBV hepatitis, antiviral medications (eg, ganciclovir and valganciclovir), with or without corticosteroids, have been beneficial.[37–39] For those with ALF, LT can be considered a rescue option and has had good outcomes.[21,25]

EPSTEIN-BARR VIRUS INFECTION AND CHRONIC LIVER DISEASE

EBV infection has been a well-known trigger agent for AIH, both for type 1 and for type 2.[4,40–42] The time elapsing between EBV infection and clinical presentation of AIH ranges from 3 months to 5 months.[40,42] Chronic active hepatitis by EBV itself mimicking AIH also has been reported, including mortality in a case.[4,40,43–45] The differential diagnosis between EBV-triggered AIH and chronic EBV hepatitis with features of autoimmunity is challenging but is important because the latter could have negative effect after immunosuppressive therapy, whereas in EBV-triggered AIH, the immunosuppressive therapy could be beneficial.[42] The latent time between EBV infection and clinical presentation of AIH along with the decrease of IgM anti-EBV levels at the time of the onset of the autoantibodies, the absence of EBV-DNA in the peripheral mononuclear cells, the typical histologic features of AIH with negativity of EBER favor the diagnosis of AIH rather than EBV hepatitis.[40,42]

Apart from AIH-like features, EBV infection has been linked to chronic active hepatitis,[46–48] granulomatous hepatitis,[49] and vanishing bile duct syndrome.[50] In addition, cases of EBV reactivation with chronic hepatitis after anti-TNF therapies have been reported.[51,52] Although EBV has been implicated for causing various chronic liver diseases, the role of EBV infection in this context is still unclear and further studies are needed to delineate whether EBV is only an innocent bystander or a true causative agent.[4,53,54] Additionally, EBV and CMV infections account for 2% of viral-precipitated ACLF cases in India.[9] In a study of 100 patients with ACLF due to hepatitis B in China, EBV-DNA and CMV-DNA were concomitantly present in 23% and 5% of cases, respectively.[55] The presence of EBV-DNA was observed more commonly in older age, particularly greater than 60 years old, and was associated with increased liver disease severity (whereas the presence of CMV-DNA did not affect the prognosis).[55]

EPSTEIN-BARR VIRUS INFECTION AND HEPATOCELLULAR CARCINOMA

EBV was the first human virus implicated directly in carcinogenesis (such as in cancers of stomach, nasopharyngeal, breast, and lymphomas) and currently accounts for 1% of the global cancer burden (5.6% of all infection-attributable cancers).[4,54] In a meta-analysis of 918 hepatobiliary cancer cases from 15 studies, the pooled EBV prevalence (detection of EBV-DNA in tissue samples) was 23%.[56] Thus, a pooled odds ratio was 9.35 among 5 case-control studies, suggesting that EBV potentially is a risk factor in the development of hepatobiliary cancers.[56] The prevalence of EBV among hepatocellular carcinomas seems somewhat varied among countries, with a higher prevalence among studies from China and Japan compared with studies from the United States.[56–60] The role of EBV as a causative or facilitating agent, however, in the pathogenesis of hepatocellular carcinoma is unclear and remains to be further explored.

EPSTEIN-BARR VIRUS IN LIVER TRANSPLANTATION
Post-transplant Lymphoproliferative Disorders

PTLDs are heterogeneous lymphoid disorders ranging from indolent polyclonal proliferations to aggressive lymphomas (approximately 85% are of B-cell origin) that complicate solid organ or hematopoietic transplantation.[11,61] It is recognized as potentially one of the more devastating complications of organ transplantation. The incidence of PTLDs in adults is variable and is based on the transplanted organ: 2% to 5% in kidney or liver, 1% to 6% in heart, 4% to 10% in lung, and up to 20% in small intestine transplants.[61] In an adult LT series, the cumulative incidence was 0.5% at 6 months, 1.1% at 18 months, 2.1% at 5 years, and 4.7% at 15 years post-LT, with the highest incidence being during the first 18 months.[62] The pathogenesis of PTLDs in most cases (60%–85%) relates to EBV-driven B-cell proliferations in the setting of chronic T-cell immunosuppression.[11,61,62] Through unclear pathogenetic mechanisms, however, EBV-negative tumors and T-cell tumors (approximately 30% also positive for EBV) also can occur.[61,63] In addition, recent epidemiologic studies report a decrease in early EBV-positive PTLDs and an increase in late EBV-negative PTLDs (which is associated with poorer prognosis).[64,65] Risk factors for PTLDs include viral infections (eg, pretransplant EBV seronegativity, hepatitis C virus infection, and CMV mismatch), degree of immunosuppression (eg, intensive immunosuppression; anti–T-cell antibody use, such as OKT3; and antithymocyte globulins), recipient age (younger age), allograft type (small intestine), and host genetic variations.[11,61–63,66] EBV-related PTLD commonly is localized extranodally (>90%), and patients therefore often present with symptoms related to the site of the disease and the type of organ(s) involved.[67] The clinical manifestations of PTLDs can vary from asymptomatic state to localized signs (eg, lymphadenopathy, abdominal mass, and swelling in the oral cavity) to IM-like syndrome and to a very aggressive disease with rapid evolution to multiorgan failure.[11,61,68]

According to the World Health Organization pathology classification of 2017, tissue biopsy remains the current gold standard for PTLD diagnosis.[11,69] Localization patterns of PTLDs are variable according to the transplanted organ. For nonliver solid organ transplant recipients, PTLDs localized to the liver are uncommon and seen in 5% of PTLDs that occur after kidney and lung transplant and in 9% of PTLDs that occur after heart transplant.[70] PTLDs in LT recipients have preference, however, for localization to the liver.[11] Post-transplant lymphomas are more likely than general lymphomas to have extranodal involvement, be high grade, have aggressive clinical behavior, and have poor outcomes.[68,71] Poor prognostic factors for PTLDs include high-grade histology, poor performance status, EBV negativity, and graft involvement.[68,71] Based on the Collaborative Transplant Study, which included 165 LT recipients with post-transplant lymphomas, 21.8%, 12.1%, 9.7%, 4.2%, and 4.2% had disease localized to the liver, gastrointestinal tract, lymph node, central nervous system, and lung, respectively, whereas 13.3% demonstrated multifocal disease. The 5-year survival rates were 33% for liver disease, 62% for nodal disease and 21% for disseminated disease.[70]

High index of suspicion and early diagnosis of PTLDs are important to facilitate prompt initiation of treatment and prevent evolution to more aggressive variants.[11] Although diagnosis can be assumed based on clinical presentation and the measurement of quantitative EBV viral load in the peripheral blood, the gold standard for diagnosis remains tissue biopsy with histopathologic and immunohistochemical examination (**Fig. 1**). EBV viral load is highly sensitive for predicting PTLDs, but the specificity in LT recipients is approximately only 50%.[11,68] In high-risk

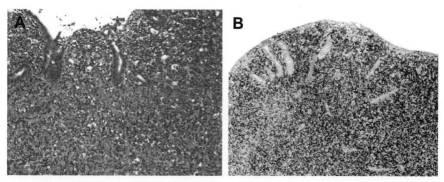

Fig. 1. EBV-positive monomorphic PTLD, diffuse large B-cell lymphoma, in an LT recipient. (A) The colonic mucosa is densely infiltrated by large-sized atypical lymphoid cells (hematoxylin-eosin, ×200). (B) The atypical lymphoid cells are positive for EBV in situ hybridization study (EBV in situ hybridization, ×200). (*Courtesy of* Dr. Napat Angkathunyakul, MD, Ramathibodi Hospital, Mahidol University; with permission.)

populations, such as those who are EBV-seronegative, EBV viral load monitoring for PTLD prevention is recommended: weekly monitoring over the initial high-risk period (EBV doubling times is as short as 49–56 hours) and then less frequently by increasing increments until set point is achieved.[69] Data to support this approach of prospective surveillance in populations at low risk of PTLDs, such as adult transplant recipients seropositive for EBV before LT, are lacking and thus not recommended.[69] Once diagnosis of early PTLD is made, reduction in immunosuppression to the lowest tolerated levels (often by 25%–50% of baseline, depending on the severity of disease and concern for graft rejection) should be initiated.[68,69,71] Early lesions and polymorphic PTLDs (usually EBV-positive) often respond well (typically seen in 2–4 weeks) to immunosuppression reduction.[11,69] In those patients with progressive disease after reduction of immunosuppression, rituximab alone or in combination with cytotoxic chemotherapy (sequential approach) is recommended for the treatment of CD20+ PTLDs.[69] There are insufficient data on the use of antiviral agents and immunoglobulins as routine prophylaxis for PTLD prevention in EBV-mismatched patients and thus their use as adjunctive treatment of PTLDs cannot be recommended for or againt.[69]

Non–post-transplant Lymphoproliferative Disorder Epstein-Barr Virus Syndromes

The features of non-PTLD EBV disease after LT include the manifestations of IM; organ-specific diseases, such as hepatitis; pneumonitis; gastrointestinal symptoms; and hematological manifestations, such as leukopenia, thrombocytopenia, hemolytic anemia, and hemophagocytosis.[69]

CYTOMEGALOVIRUS INFECTION OF THE LIVER
Virology and Transmission

Like EBV, CMV is an enveloped double-stranded DNA virus, a member of the herpesvirus family (HHV-5), and is one of the most common chronic viral infections in humans. It establishes latent infection after the resolution of primary infection where T cells (both CD4+ and CD8+) play an important role in controlling viral replication and disease but do not eliminate the virus completely.[2] Initial infection occurs in mucosal epithelial cells, and viral dissemination occurs via infected circulating CD14+ monocytes with a tropism within the human body that includes parenchymal, connective tissue, and hematopoietic cells.[5,72] In the liver, CMV most frequently infects hepatocytes and macrophages, whereas stromal and vascular endothelial cells are the primary targets in the gastrointestinal tract.[5] Secondary symptomatic disease may present later in the life of the host, reflecting 1 of 2 possibilities: reactivation of latent CMV and reinfection with a novel exogenous strain.[2]

The seroprevalence rates of prior CMV infection increase gradually with age and range between 40% and 100% in adult population.[2] In population-based studies in the United States, CMV seroprevalence has increased from 36% to 40% in 6 year olds to 11 year olds to 54% to 60% in 30 year olds to 50 year olds and then to 91% in those ages greater than 80 years.[73,74] In addition, CMV seropositivity was independently associated with female sex, foreign birthplace, high household crowding, and low household socioeconomic status.[73,74] CMV has been cultured from multiple sites and body fluids, including urine, blood, saliva, genital fluid, stool, tears, and breast milk.[2,5] Transmission can occur via multiple routes, such as kissing, sexual exposure, blood and tissue exposure, close contact (more common in children), and perinatal and occupational exposure.[2,5] There is evidence that CMV can survive in saliva on environmental surfaces for 1 hours to 6 hours, depending on the surfaces.[75]

Manifestations of Cytomegalovirus Infection

The spectrum of human illness caused by CMV is diverse and mostly dependent on the host.[2,6,76,77] CMV infection is defined as evidence of CMV replication regardless of symptoms.[10] CMV disease is defined as evidence of CMV infection with attributable symptoms, which can be categorized further as a viral syndrome with fever, malaise, leukopenia, and/or thrombocytopenia or as tissue-invasive disease.[10] CMV infection in immunocompromised individuals (usually infected via reactivation and reinfection along with the primary acquisition of the virus) causes substantial morbidity and mortality, especially among transplant recipients and those infected with the HIV.[2,6] Whereas primary CMV infection in the immunocompetent host generally is asymptomatic or may present as an IM-like syndrome in approximately 10% of cases, severe organ-specific complications have been reported.[2,6,76,77] Compared with EBV, CMV-associated IM tends to occur in older individuals and less commonly has associated exudative tonsillitis, cervical lymphadenopathy, and splenomegaly.[2,78] In immunocompromised hosts, CMV infection or reactivation typically is present as CMV disease and occasionally may manifest as tissue-invasive disease, which mainly involves the gastrointestinal tract.[5,79–81]

CYTOMEGALOVIRUS HEPATITIS
Incidence and Clinical Features

Hepatic biochemical test abnormalities frequently are encountered (30%–80%) in patients with symptomatic primary CMV infection, in both immunocompetent and immunocompromised individuals.[2,6,20,76–78] Subclinical transaminitis is the most common finding among immunocompetent individuals (ALT tends to be higher than AST) whereas elevations of ALP and total bilirubin are less typical (jaundice presents in 3%–9%).[2,6,20,76–78] Occasionally, patients may present with more severe hepatic dysfunction, including ALF requiring LT[82,83] and severe cholestasis (with or without biliary tract involvement).[84,85] In addition, acute pancreatitis (with or without cholangitis),[86,87] portal vein thrombosis,[88,89] and Budd-Chiari syndrome[89] have been reported in associated with acute CMV infection in immunocompetent hosts. Approximately 6% to 8% of CMV hepatitis cases were detected during pregnancy and might be explained by immunosuppression associated with pregnancy.[20,90]

Among immunocompromised patients, CMV hepatitis commonly is associated with disseminated CMV but rarely may be isolated to the liver.[91] Unlike other immunocompromised settings, CMV hepatitis in LT recipients often manifests with isolated liver disease (disseminated disease is uncommon) in which the symptoms may be clinically indistinguishable from acute cellular rejection.[79,92,93]

Diagnosis and Management of Cytomegalovirus Hepatitis

Diagnosis of CMV infection is based on clinical suspicion and CMV-specific tests, such as serology, to detect IgG and IgM antibodies, CMV-DNA, and CMV antigenemia (pp65) assays.[10] Serologic tests may be helpful but sometimes unreliable because cases of acute CMV hepatitis with cross-reacting antibodies to EBV and HEV have been reported (discussed previously). Although no universal cutoff is accepted, quantitative PCR for CMV-DNA is the standard method for the early detection and management of CMV infections and almost entirely has replaced the isolation and culture of the virus.[10]

Liver biopsy is not imperative for initiating antiviral therapy but may be required in selected cases where diagnosis is uncertain while there are confounding clinical features.[6] CMV hepatitis is characterized histologically by the classic CMV viral cytopathic effect in hepatocytes, biliary epithelium, endothelial cells, and Kupffer cells. Infected cells have both cytoplasmic and nuclear enlargement with cytoplasmic and intranuclear inclusion bodies. Other nonspecific changes include mild lobular hepatitis, hepatocellular necrosis, patchy portal mononuclear infiltrate, and microabscesses[6] (**Fig. 2**). In immunosuppressed hosts, CMV cytopathic effect typically is observed; however, in immunocompetent individuals with CMV hepatitis, cytopathic cells and immunohistochemical staining may not be seen on liver biopsy because a strong immune response often destroys the infected cells.[6,91] Because CMV infection is a risk factor for liver graft rejection and vice versa, a liver biopsy generally is performed to distinguish between CMV hepatitis and acute cellular rejection in LT recipients.[5,79] Immunohistochemistry and/or in situ DNA hybridization are helpful to confirm and to increase sensitivity for the diagnosis of CMV hepatitis.[10,91]

There are several agents available for the systemic antiviral therapy for CMV infection by targeting CMV DNA polymerase, and these include ganciclovir, valganciclovir, foscarnet, and cidofovir.[2] The efficacy of these agents has been proved extensively

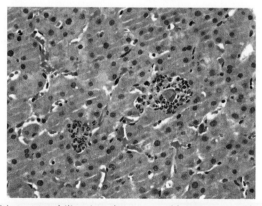

Fig. 2. CMV hepatitis: neutrophilic microabscesses and hepatocyte with CMV cytopathic effect (cytomegaly with intracytoplasmic inclusions) (hematoxylin-eosin, ×400). (*Courtesy of* Dr. Napat Angkathunyakul, MD, Ramathibodi Hospital, Mahidol University; with permission.)

and, therefore, they are recommended for the treatment of CMV hepatitis in immuno-compromised patients.[10,79] Among immunocompetent patients with symptomatic CMV infection and transaminitis, especially with IM syndrome, the illness is self-limited, and antiviral therapy usually is not indicated.[2] With limited data and without controlled studies, however, antiviral therapy is suggested in those immunocompetent patients with severe CMV hepatitis.[20,85,94] In the vast majority of cases of CMV hepatitis, the prognosis is good, although mortality and need for LT from ALF due to CMV have been reported.[20,82,83]

PREVENTION OF CYTOMEGALOVIRUS IN LIVER TRANSPLANTATION

Despite recent advances in the diagnosis and treatment, CMV infections remain one of the more common infectious complications affecting solid organ transplant recipients carrying higher risks of complications.[10,79–81] In addition to the direct effects of CMV infection and disease, there also are indirect effects, both general and transplant-specific, that include higher rates of all types of infections, acute and chronic graft rejection, vascular thrombosis, graft loss, PTLDs, new-onset diabetes mellitus, and mortality.[10,79–81]

In the absence of prevention strategy, overall, 18% to 29% of all LT recipients will develop CMV disease, which occurs most commonly during the first 3 months after transplantation.[79] CMV serostatus of donor and of recipient (D/R) are key risk factors of CMV disease after LT and they direct CMV preventive strategy: the incidence is as high as 44% to 65% in CMV D+/R−, 8% to 18% among CMV D+/R+ or D−/R+, and

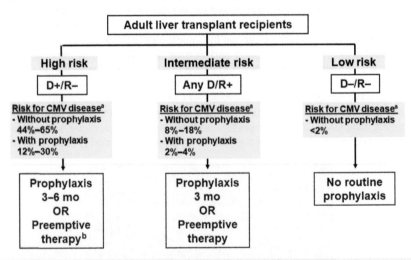

Prophylaxis:
- eg, valganciclovir (not FDA approved), valaciclovir, oral ganciclovir or IV ganciclovir
- Starting within 10 d after transplant and continuing for a finite period

Preemptive therapy:
- Monitoring at least once weekly for 3–4 mo after transplant
- Anti-CMV treatment when CMV-DNA or pp65 Ag assay is at a positive threshold

Fig. 3. Approach to CMV prophylaxis in adult LT recipients. [a] Estimated incidence of CMV disease during the first 12 months after LT; [b] Many authorities prefer to use prophylaxis especially for programs or patients unable to meet the stringent logistic requirements required with a preemptive therapy. Ag, antigen; FDA, The Food and Drug Administration of the United States; IV, intravenous.

1% to 2% among CMV D−/R−patients.[10,79–81] In addition, other risk factors include intensity and type of immunosuppressive regimens; certain associated infections, for example, HHV-6 and HHV-7; allograft rejection; and renal insufficiency.[80]

Both universal prophylactic and preemptive therapy are the recommended strategies to prevent CMV infection/reactivation in LT recipients with high and intermediate risks[10,79–81] **(Fig. 3)**. The International Consensus Guidelines on the Management of Cytomegalovirus in Solid-organ Transplantation recently have been published.[10] Apart from antiviral therapy, another important consideration in the treatment of CMV is the level of immunosuppression, because generally reducing immunosuppression facilitates better outcomes after treatment. In addition, the use of mammalian target of rapamycin inhibitors seems associated with decreased incidence of CMV infection.[95,96]

SUMMARY

EBV and CMV infections can be associated with a variety of hepatic manifestations, which often are overlooked by physicians. In immunocompetent hosts, they commonly manifest as acute hepatitis, with severity varying from asymptomatic, self-limited icteric hepatitis to, rarely, ALF. Atypical manifestations, such as cholestasis, chronic hepatitis, precipitation of ACLF, and AIH, have been reported with EBV infection, whereas cholestasis, portal vein thrombosis, and Budd-Chiari syndrome have been reported with CMV infection. In the setting of LT, CMV is the most common infectious complication and it carries significant morbidity necessitating proper preventive strategies, and EBV is the major cause of PTLDs.

CONFLICT OF INTEREST

None.

REFERENCES

1. Cohen JI. Epstein-Barr virus infection. N Engl J Med 2000;343(7):481–92.
2. Friel TJ. Epidemiology, clinical manifestations, and treatment of cytomegalovirus infection in immunocompetent adults. In: Bond S, editor. UpToDate; 2019. Available at: https://www.uptodate.com/contents/epidemiology-clinical-manifestations-and-treatment-of-cytomegalovirus-infection-in-immunocompetent-adults. Accessed March 11, 2019.
3. Sullivan JL. Clinical manifestations and treatment of Epstein-Barr virus infection. In: Mitty J, editor. UpToDate; 2019. Available at: https://www.uptodate.com/contents/clinical-manifestations-and-treatment-of-epstein-barr-virus-infection. Accessed May 20, 2019.
4. Petrova M, Kamburov V. Epstein-Barr virus: silent companion or causative agent of chronic liver disease? World J Gastroenterol 2010;16(33):4130–4.
5. Fakhreddine AY, Frenette CT, Konijeti GG. A Practical Review of Cytomegalovirus in Gastroenterology and Hepatology. Gastroenterol Res Pract 2019;2019: 6156581.
6. Noor A, Panwala A, Forouhar F, et al. Hepatitis caused by herpes viruses: a review. J Dig Dis 2018;19(8):446–55.
7. Bjornsson HK, Olafsson S, Bergmann OM, et al. A prospective study on the causes of notably raised alanine aminotransferase (ALT). Scand J Gastroenterol 2016;51(5):594–600.

8. Vine LJ, Shepherd K, Hunter JG, et al. Characteristics of Epstein-Barr virus hepatitis among patients with jaundice or acute hepatitis. Aliment Pharmacol Ther 2012;36(1):16–21.

9. Gupta E, Ballani N, Kumar M, et al. Role of non-hepatotropic viruses in acute sporadic viral hepatitis and acute-on-chronic liver failure in adults. Indian J Gastroenterol 2015;34(6):448–52.

10. Kotton CN, Kumar D, Caliendo AM, et al. The third international consensus guidelines on the management of cytomegalovirus in solid-organ transplantation. Transplantation 2018;102(6):900–31.

11. Bunchorntavakul C, Reddy KR. Hepatic manifestations of lymphoproliferative disorders. Clin Liver Dis 2019;23(2):293–308.

12. Sulivan JL. Virology of Epstein-Barr virus. In: Bond S, editor. UpToDate; 2019. Available at: https://www.uptodate.com/contents/virology-of-epstein-barr-virus. Accessed July 8, 2019.

13. Heath CW Jr, Brodsky AL, Potolsky AI. Infectious mononucleosis in a general population. Am J Epidemiol 1972;95(1):46–52.

14. Aronson MD, Auwaerter PG. Infectious mononucleosis. In: Bond S, editor. UpToDate; 2019. Available at: https://www.uptodate.com/contents/infectious-mononucleosis. Accessed July 9, 2019.

15. Evans AS, Niederman JC, Cenabre LC, et al. A prospective evaluation of heterophile and Epstein-Barr virus-specific IgM antibody tests in clinical and subclinical infectious mononucleosis: specificity and sensitivity of the tests and persistence of antibody. J Infect Dis 1975;132(5):546–54.

16. Crum NF. Epstein Barr virus hepatitis: case series and review. South Med J 2006;99(5):544–7.

17. Lawee D. Mild infectious mononucleosis presenting with transient mixed liver disease: case report with a literature review. Can Fam Physician 2007;53(8):1314–6.

18. Hinedi TB, Koff RS. Cholestatic hepatitis induced by Epstein-Barr virus infection in an adult. Dig Dis Sci 2003;48(3):539–41.

19. Salva I, Silva IV, Cunha F. Epstein-Barr virus-associated cholestatic hepatitis. BMJ Case Rep 2013;2013 [pii:bcr2013202213].

20. Leonardsson H, Hreinsson JP, Love A, et al. Hepatitis due to Epstein-Barr virus and cytomegalovirus: clinical features and outcomes. Scand J Gastroenterol 2017;52(8):893–7.

21. Feranchak AP, Tyson RW, Narkewicz MR, et al. Fulminant Epstein-Barr viral hepatitis: orthotopic liver transplantation and review of the literature. Liver Transpl Surg 1998;4(6):469–76.

22. Markin RS, Linder J, Zuerlein K, et al. Hepatitis in fatal infectious mononucleosis. Gastroenterology 1987;93(6):1210–7.

23. Papatheodoridis GV, Delladetsima JK, Kavallierou L, et al. Fulminant hepatitis due to Epstein-Barr virus infection. J Hepatol 1995;23(3):348–50.

24. Devereaux CE, Bemiller T, Brann O. Ascites and severe hepatitis complicating Epstein-Barr infection. Am J Gastroenterol 1999;94(1):236–40.

25. Mellinger JL, Rossaro L, Naugler WE, et al. Epstein-Barr virus (EBV) related acute liver failure: a case series from the US Acute Liver Failure Study Group. Dig Dis Sci 2014;59(7):1630–7.

26. Gupta E, Bhatia V, Choudhary A, et al. Epstein-Barr virus associated acute hepatitis with cross-reacting antibodies to other herpes viruses in immunocompetent patients: report of two cases. J Med Virol 2013;85(3):519–23.

27. Karadeniz A, Yesilbag Z, Kaya FO, et al. Acute hepatitis due to Epstein-Barr virus with cross-reacting antibodies to cytomegalovirus. Indian J Med Microbiol 2018; 36(1):143–4.

28. Fogeda M, de Ory F, Avellon A, et al. Differential diagnosis of hepatitis E virus, cytomegalovirus and Epstein-Barr virus infection in patients with suspected hepatitis E. J Clin Virol 2009;45(3):259–61.

29. Huang Q, Li XH, Zhu C, et al. Acute viral hepatitis presenting as cytomegalovirus, hepatitis E and Epstein-Barr virus IgM antibody positive. Antivir Ther 2016;21(2): 171–3.

30. Ghinoiu M, Naveau S, Barri-Ova N, et al. Acute hepatitis E infection associated with a false-positive serology against Epstein-Barr virus. Eur J Gastroenterol Hepatol 2009;21(12):1433–5.

31. Hyams C, Mabayoje DA, Copping R, et al. Serological cross reactivity to CMV and EBV causes problems in the diagnosis of acute hepatitis E virus infection. J Med Virol 2014;86(3):478–83.

32. Schechter S, Lamps L. Epstein-barr virus hepatitis: a review of clinicopathologic features and differential diagnosis. Arch Pathol Lab Med 2018;142(10):1191–5.

33. Adkins BJ, Steele RH. Death from massive hepatic necrosis in infectious mononucleosis. N Z Med J 1977;85(580):56–8.

34. Suh N, Liapis H, Misdraji J, et al. Epstein-Barr virus hepatitis: diagnostic value of in situ hybridization, polymerase chain reaction, and immunohistochemistry on liver biopsy from immunocompetent patients. Am J Surg Pathol 2007;31(9): 1403–9.

35. Chang MY, Campbell WG Jr. Fatal infectious mononucleosis. Association with liver necrosis and herpes-like virus particles. Arch Pathol 1975;99(4):185–91.

36. Kimura H, Nagasaka T, Hoshino Y, et al. Severe hepatitis caused by Epstein-Barr virus without infection of hepatocytes. Hum Pathol 2001;32(7):757–62.

37. Adams LA, Deboer B, Jeffrey G, et al. Ganciclovir and the treatment of Epstein-Barr virus hepatitis. J Gastroenterol Hepatol 2006;21(11):1758–60.

38. Cauldwell K, Williams R. Unusual presentation of Epstein-Barr virus hepatitis treated successfully with valganciclovir. J Med Virol 2014;86(3):484–6.

39. Pisapia R, Mariano A, Rianda A, et al. Severe EBV hepatitis treated with valganciclovir. Infection 2013;41(1):251–4.

40. Vento S, Guella L, Mirandola F, et al. Epstein-Barr virus as a trigger for autoimmune hepatitis in susceptible individuals. Lancet 1995;346(8975):608–9.

41. Zellos A, Spoulou V, Roma-Giannikou E, et al. Autoimmune hepatitis type-2 and Epstein-Barr virus infection in a toddler: art of facts or an artifact? Ann Hepatol 2013;12(1):147–51.

42. Peng H, Lim T, Nam J, et al. Autoimmune hepatitis following Epstein-Barr virus infection: a diagnostic dilemma. BMJ Case Rep 2019;12(7) [pii:e229615].

43. Chiba T, Goto S, Yokosuka O, et al. Fatal chronic active Epstein-Barr virus infection mimicking autoimmune hepatitis. Eur J Gastroenterol Hepatol 2004;16(2): 225–8.

44. Wada Y, Sato C, Tomita K, et al. Possible autoimmune hepatitis induced after chronic active Epstein-Barr virus infection. Clin J Gastroenterol 2014;7(1):58–61.

45. Yamashita H, Shimizu A, Tsuchiya H, et al. Chronic active Epstein-Barr virus infection mimicking autoimmune hepatitis exacerbation in a patient with systemic lupus erythematosus. Lupus 2014;23(8):833–6.

46. Sakamoto T, Uemura M, Fukui H, et al. Chronic active Epstein-Barr virus infection in an adult. Intern Med 1992;31(10):1190–6.

47. Yuge A, Kinoshita E, Moriuchi M, et al. Persistent hepatitis associated with chronic active Epstein-Barr virus infection. Pediatr Infect Dis J 2004;23(1):74–6.
48. Calkic L, Bajramovic-Omeragic L, Mujezinovic A. Infectious mononucleosis (Epstein-Barr virus infection) and chronic hepatitis. Med Glas (Zenica) 2019;16(2). https://doi.org/10.17392/1031-19.
49. Biest S, Schubert TT. Chronic Epstein-Barr virus infection: a cause of granulomatous hepatitis? J Clin Gastroenterol 1989;11(3):343–6.
50. Kikuchi K, Miyakawa H, Abe K, et al. Vanishing bile duct syndrome associated with chronic EBV infection. Dig Dis Sci 2000;45(1):160–5.
51. Cetkovska P, Lomicova I, Mukensnabl P, et al. Anti-tumour necrosis factor treatment of severe psoriasis complicated by Epstein-Barr Virus hepatitis and subsequently by chronic hepatitis. Dermatol Ther 2015;28(6):369–72.
52. Sondermann W, Baba HA, Korber A. Hepatitis due to EBV-reactivation under infliximab in a psoriasis patient. Dermatol Ther 2017;30(5). https://doi.org/10.1111/dth.12525.
53. Drebber U, Kasper HU, Krupacz J, et al. The role of Epstein-Barr virus in acute and chronic hepatitis. J Hepatol 2006;44(5):879–85.
54. Negro F. The paradox of Epstein-Barr virus-associated hepatitis. J Hepatol 2006;44(5):839–41.
55. Hu J, Zhao H, Lou D, et al. Human cytomegalovirus and Epstein-Barr virus infections, risk factors, and their influence on the liver function of patients with acute-on-chronic liver failure. BMC Infect Dis 2018;18(1):577.
56. Chen ZX, Peng XT, Tan L, et al. EBV as a potential risk factor for hepatobiliary system cancer: a meta-analysis with 918 cases. Pathol Res Pract 2019;215(2):278–85.
57. Sugawara Y, Makuuchi M, Takada K. Detection of Epstein-Barr virus DNA in hepatocellular carcinoma tissues from hepatitis C-positive patients. Scand J Gastroenterol 2000;35(9):981–4.
58. Sugawara Y, Mizugaki Y, Uchida T, et al. Detection of Epstein-Barr virus (EBV) in hepatocellular carcinoma tissue: a novel EBV latency characterized by the absence of EBV-encoded small RNA expression. Virology 1999;256(2):196–202.
59. Li W, Wu BA, Zeng YM, et al. Epstein-Barr virus in hepatocellular carcinogenesis. World J Gastroenterol 2004;10(23):3409–13.
60. Akhter S, Liu H, Prabhu R, et al. Epstein-Barr virus and human hepatocellular carcinoma. Cancer Lett 2003;192(1):49–57.
61. Al-Mansour Z, Nelson BP, Evens AM. Post-transplant lymphoproliferative disease (PTLD): risk factors, diagnosis, and current treatment strategies. Curr Hematol Malig Rep 2013;8(3):173–83.
62. Kremers WK, Devarbhavi HC, Wiesner RH, et al. Post-transplant lymphoproliferative disorders following liver transplantation: incidence, risk factors and survival. Am J Transplant 2006;6(5 Pt 1):1017–24.
63. Inayat F, Hassan GU, Tayyab GUN, et al. Post-transplantation lymphoproliferative disorder with gastrointestinal involvement. Ann Gastroenterol 2018;31(2):248–51.
64. Luskin MR, Heil DS, Tan KS, et al. The Impact of EBV Status on Characteristics and Outcomes of Posttransplantation Lymphoproliferative Disorder. Am J Transplant 2015;15(10):2665–73.
65. Peters AC, Akinwumi MS, Cervera C, et al. The changing epidemiology of post-transplant lymphoproliferative disorder in adult solid organ transplant recipients over 30 years: a single-center experience. Transplantation 2018;102(9):1553–62.

66. Lo RC, Chan SC, Chan KL, et al. Post-transplant lymphoproliferative disorders in liver transplant recipients: a clinicopathological study. J Clin Pathol 2013;66(5): 392–8.

67. Nijland ML, Kersten MJ, Pals ST, et al. Epstein-barr virus-positive posttransplant lymphoproliferative disease after solid organ transplantation: pathogenesis, clinical manifestations, diagnosis, and management. Transplant Direct 2016; 2(1):e48.

68. Kamdar KY, Rooney CM, Heslop HE. Posttransplant lymphoproliferative disease following liver transplantation. Curr Opin Organ Transplant 2011;16(3):274–80.

69. Allen UD, Preiksaitis JK. Post-transplant lymphoproliferative disorders, EBV infection and disease in solid organ transplantation: guidelines from the American Society of Transplantation Infectious Diseases Community of Practice. Clin Transplant 2019;33(9):e13652.

70. Opelz G, Dohler B. Lymphomas after solid organ transplantation: a collaborative transplant study report. Am J Transplant 2004;4(2):222–30.

71. Parker A, Bowles K, Bradley JA, et al. Management of post-transplant lymphoproliferative disorder in adult solid organ transplant recipients - BCSH and BTS guidelines. Br J Haematol 2010;149(5):693–705.

72. Collins-McMillen D, Buehler J. Molecular determinants and the regulation of human cytomegalovirus Latency and Reactivation. Viruses 2018;10(8) [pii:E444].

73. Bate SL, Dollard SC, Cannon MJ. Cytomegalovirus seroprevalence in the United States: the national health and nutrition examination surveys, 1988-2004. Clin Infect Dis 2010;50(11):1439–47.

74. Staras SA, Dollard SC, Radford KW, et al. Seroprevalence of cytomegalovirus infection in the United States, 1988-1994. Clin Infect Dis 2006;43(9):1143–51.

75. Stowell JD, Forlin-Passoni D, Din E, et al. Cytomegalovirus survival on common environmental surfaces: opportunities for viral transmission. J Infect Dis 2012; 205(2):211–4.

76. Bonnet F, Neau D, Viallard JF, et al. Clinical and laboratory findings of cytomegalovirus infection in 115 hospitalized non-immunocompromised adults. Ann Med Interne (Paris) 2001;152(4):227–35.

77. Wreghitt TG, Teare EL, Sule O, et al. Cytomegalovirus infection in immunocompetent patients. Clin Infect Dis 2003;37(12):1603–6.

78. Klemola E, Von Essen R, Henle G, et al. Infectious-mononucleosis-like disease with negative heterophil agglutination test. Clinical features in relation to Epstein-Barr virus and cytomegalovirus antibodies. J Infect Dis 1970;121(6): 608–14.

79. Yadav SK, Saigal S, Choudhary NS, et al. Cytomegalovirus infection in liver transplant recipients: current approach to diagnosis and management. J Clin Exp Hepatol 2017;7(2):144–51.

80. Marcelin JR, Beam E, Razonable RR. Cytomegalovirus infection in liver transplant recipients: updates on clinical management. World J Gastroenterol 2014;20(31): 10658–67.

81. Razonable RR. Cytomegalovirus infection after liver transplantation: current concepts and challenges. World J Gastroenterol 2008;14(31):4849–60.

82. Yu YD, Park GC, Park PJ, et al. Cytomegalovirus infection-associated fulminant hepatitis in an immunocompetent adult requiring emergency living-donor liver transplantation: report of a case. Surg Today 2013;43(4):424–8.

83. Shusterman NH, Frauenhoffer C, Kinsey MD. Fatal massive hepatic necrosis in cytomegalovirus mononucleosis. Ann Intern Med 1978;88(6):810–2.

84. Qian JY, Bai XY, Feng YL, et al. Cholestasis, ascites and pancytopenia in an immunocompetent adult with severe cytomegalovirus hepatitis. World J Gastroenterol 2015;21(43):12505–9.

85. Serna-Higuera C, Gonzalez-Garcia M, Milicua JM, et al. Acute cholestatic hepatitis by cytomegalovirus in an immunocompetent patient resolved with ganciclovir. J Clin Gastroenterol 1999;29(3):276–7.

86. Chan A, Bazerbachi F, Hanson B, et al. Cytomegalovirus hepatitis and pancreatitis in the immunocompetent. Ochsner J 2014;14(2):295–9.

87. Oku T, Maeda M, Waga E, et al. Cytomegalovirus cholangitis and pancreatitis in an immunocompetent patient. J Gastroenterol 2005;40(10):987–92.

88. Squizzato A, Ageno W, Cattaneo A, et al. A case report and literature review of portal vein thrombosis associated with cytomegalovirus infection in immunocompetent patients. Clin Infect Dis 2007;44(2):e13–6.

89. Spahr L, Cerny A, Morard I, et al. Acute partial Budd-Chiari syndrome and portal vein thrombosis in cytomegalovirus primary infection: a case report. BMC Gastroenterol 2006;6:10.

90. Eddleston M, Peacock S, Juniper M, et al. Severe cytomegalovirus infection in immunocompetent patients. Clin Infect Dis 1997;24(1):52–6.

91. McDonald GB, Sarmiento JI, Rees-Lui G, et al. Cytomegalovirus hepatitis after bone marrow transplantation: an autopsy study with clinical, histologic, and laboratory correlates. J Viral Hepat 2019;26(11):1344–50.

92. Paya CV, Hermans PE, Wiesner RH, et al. Cytomegalovirus hepatitis in liver transplantation: prospective analysis of 93 consecutive orthotopic liver transplantations. J Infect Dis 1989;160(5):752–8.

93. Seehofer D, Rayes N, Tullius SG, et al. CMV hepatitis after liver transplantation: incidence, clinical course, and long-term follow-up. Liver Transplant 2002; 8(12):1138–46.

94. Fernandez-Ruiz M, Munoz-Codoceo C, Lopez-Medrano F, et al. Cytomegalovirus myopericarditis and hepatitis in an immunocompetent adult: successful treatment with oral valganciclovir. Intern Med 2008;47(22):1963–6.

95. Andrassy J, Hoffmann VS, Rentsch M, et al. Is cytomegalovirus prophylaxis dispensable in patients receiving an mTOR inhibitor-based immunosuppression? a systematic review and meta-analysis. Transplantation 2012;94(12):1208–17.

96. Sheng L, Jun S, Jianfeng L, et al. The effect of sirolimus-based immunosuppression vs. conventional prophylaxis therapy on cytomegalovirus infection after liver transplantation. Clin Transplant 2015;29(6):555–9.

Extrahepatic Manifestations of Chronic Viral C Hepatitis

Salvatore Petta, MD, PhD*, Antonio Craxì, MD

KEYWORDS

- HCV • Extrahepatic complications • Cardiovascular disease
- Immune-related disorders • Diabetes • Kidney disease

KEY POINTS

- Hepatitis C virus (HCV) infection is a systemic disease associated with hepatic and extra-hepatic complications.
- Cross-sectional and cohort studies suggest that HCV infection increases the risk for mixed cryoglobulinemia, non-Hodgkin lymphoma, neuropsychiatric disorders, and cardiometabolic alterations, including diabetes, steatosis, kidney injury, and cardiovascular alterations.
- Experimental and clinical studies suggest that HCV infection can both directly and indirectly participate in the pathogenic mechanisms, leading to extrahepatic manifestations.
- Sustained virological eradication by both interferon and direct antiviral agents clearly has demonstrated a beneficial effect on occurrence and outcomes of extrahepatic comorbidities, suggesting that HCV infection must be eradicated in all infected individuals regardless of the severity of liver damage.
- Preliminary evidence suggests improvement of cardiovascular outcomes in patients in whom the virus is eradicated; however, large prospective studies are still needed to investigate this clinically relevant issue.

INTRODUCTION

Chronic infection by hepatitis C virus (HCV) has a worldwide distribution, with prevalence rates ranging from less than 1% to more than 5% depending on the geographic area, age of patients, and risk factors of studied populations.[1] Chronic hepatitis due to HCV infection is one of the most important causes of chronic liver disease, and consequently of morbidity and mortality related to liver disease, and this is mostly because of the development of liver cirrhosis and its complications such as hepatic decompensation and hepatocellular carcinoma.

Sezione di Gastroenterologia e Epatologia, PROMISE, Università di Palermo, Italia
* Corresponding author. Sezione di Gastroenterologia e Epatologia, PRMISE, Piazza delleCli-niche, 2, Palermo 90127, Italy.
E-mail address: salvatore.petta@unipa.it

Gastroenterol Clin N Am 49 (2020) 347–360
https://doi.org/10.1016/j.gtc.2020.01.012
0889-8553/20/© 2020 Elsevier Inc. All rights reserved.

When compared with studies assessing hepatitis B infection, several epidemiologic studies have documented a high prevalence of comorbidity in subjects with HCV infection. American Medicare data on a cohort of more than 400,000 HCV-infected individuals, 20% of them with liver cirrhosis, showed a prevalence of chronic renal injury and diabetes of 24% and 38% respectively, as well as of psychiatric disorders of about 15%.[2] Similar data have been reported in a cohort of more than 100,000 "Veterans" with HCV infection, where 21% of patients had diabetes, 53% arterial hypertension, 18% cardiovascular diseases, and 20% had psychiatric disorders.[3] When moving from United States to European data, Italian epidemiologic studies confirmed the high prevalence of comorbidity in subjects with HCV infection. Unpublished data from the PITER study (Italian Platform for the Study of Viral Hepatitis) noted a prevalence of diabetes of about 13%, cardiovascular diseases of 32%, renal damage of 3%, and neuropsychiatric disorders of 11%. Similar unpublished data arise from the HCV Sicilia Network (RESIST) in a cohort of more than 10,000 subjects: a prevalence of 13% of obesity, 25% diabetes, 42% hypertension, 5% cardiovascular disease, 4% chronic renal damage, and 12% neuropsychiatric disorders and lymphoproliferative disorders were reported in this population, with prevalence rates being much higher in the population older than 65 years.

The association between HCV infection and high prevalence of comorbidity has further clinical implications. The presence of extrahepatic comorbidities can adversely affect the prognosis in HCV-infected patients. Different cross-sectional and cohort studies well highlighted that the presence of metabolic risk factors namely hepatic steatosis, insulin resistance (IR), and diabetes are associated with the severity of liver disease and with a higher risk of developing hepatocellular carcinoma and hepatic decompensation.[4] Along this line, a Danish cohort study in a large cohort of patients with liver cirrhosis well reported that, as expected, the presence of comorbidity in this population increases the risk of mortality.[5] In line with these data, another large Australian population cohort study showed that HCV-infected patients have an increased risk of dying not only from causes related to liver disease but also from extrahepatic causes.[6]

Further, and consistent with the above-quoted epidemiologic data, emerging evidence also suggests that HCV infection does not have an exclusive hepatic pleiotropism and that it can be considered a systemic disease able to directly/indirectly participate in the occurrence of extrahepatic disorders, suggesting a bidiretional interplay between HCV infection and comorbidities. In this complex landscape, various studies have demonstrated a pathophysiologic link between HCV infection and immune-related disorders from cryoglobulinemia to B cell non-Hodgkin lymphoma, systemic autoimmune diseases, metabolic alterations including lipid profile alterations, fatty liver infiltration, IR and diabetes, cardiovascular alterations, and neurologic/psychiatric disorders[7] (**Fig. 1**). Beyond being useful from an epidemiologic and speculative point of view, a better understanding of this topic can have very relevant clinical implications, because of the availability of safe and highly effective direct antiviral regimens for the treatment of HCV infection[8] that can reduce the liver-related risks of HCV infection as well as improve extrahepatic prognosis.

HEPATITIS C VIRUS INFECTION AND IMMUNE-RELATED DISORDERS

Patients with HCV infection have an increased risk of developing immune-related diseases, such as mixed cryoglobulinemia (MC) and its complications, including non-Hodgkin lymphoma with B cells, and which are related to HCV lymphotropism.[7]

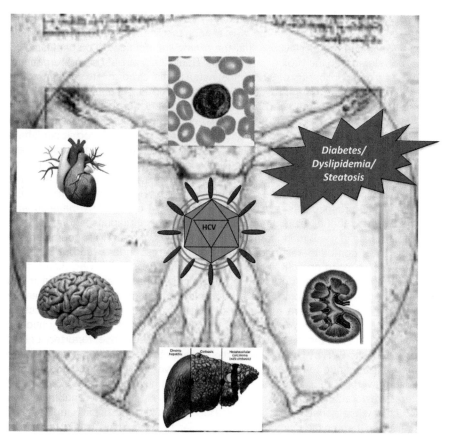

Fig. 1. HCV infection as a systemic disease. HCV infection can lead not only to hepatic complications but also to extrahepatic diseases such as immune-related disorders, neuropsychiatric diseases, and cardiometabolic alterations.

Cryoglobulinemia is defined as the presence of immunoglobulins precipitating in serum at a temperature of less than 37 °C, and patients with HCV infection have a high prevalence of MC (type II, monoclonal immunoglobulin (Ig) M-rheumatoid factor complexed with polyclonal IgG, and type III, polyclonal IgM-rheumatoid factor complexed with the corresponding antigen).[9] Specifically, circulating cryoglobulins are found in 40% to 60% of HCV-infected patients, even if only 5% to 10% of these patients will develop clinical consequences such as life-threatening systemic vasculitis, cutaneous vasculitis, renal involvement with membranoproliferative glomerulonephritis, neuropathy, and arthralgias.[9] From a pathophysiologic point of view, MC stems from the ability of the virus to infect and replicate in B cells, leading to clonal expansion of B lymphocytes through interaction of the HCV E2 glycoprotein with CD81 on the surface of B cells, production of rheumatoid factor–based immune complexes, and finally complement-driven vasculitis in different organs.[9]

Consistent with the direct link between cryoglobulinemic syndrome and HCV infection, various studies have tested the impact of virological eradication on the syndrome. Preliminary evidence arises from interferon (IFN)-based antiviral therapy in patients with HCV infection and MC. Gragnani and colleagues,[10] in a relatively large cohort of patients with HCV infection without MC or with symptomatic or asymptomatic MC, showed that the syndrome was a poor predictor of sustained virological response (SVR) and more relevantly that the clinical-immunological response in MC strongly correlated with the virological outcome. Specifically all but 2 out of 63 patients with SVR, at a mean follow-up of 92 months, had a partial or complete sustained clinical response, whereas no improvement was observed in patients without SVR.[10] These results underlined the need for treating this population of HCV-infected patients, even if it was not completely clear whether the clinical improvement was directly related to the virological eradication or also to the immunomodulatory effect of IFN. This uncertain mode of action of IFN based therapy, however, has been finally resolved in the era of the use of direct antiviral agents (DAA) that lead to a rapid virological clearance and without influencing the immune system. One of the earlier studies assessing the efficacy and clinical impact of SVR by DAA in patients with HCV-related MC prospectively evaluated a cohort of 44 consecutive patients who achieved SVR and that all patients at SVR 24 had a clinical response of vasculitis in terms of decrease in the Birmingham Vasculitis Activity Score (34% full complete responders, 32% complete responders, 27% partial responders, and 7% nonresponders) and in mean cryocrit value.[11] These impressive results were then further confirmed in a larger French study in a cohort of 148 patients where, at a mean follow-up of 15 months, cryoglobulins were no longer detected in blood samples in 53.1% of patients and where resolution of purpura, renal involvement, arthralgia, and neuropathy were observed in 97.2%, 91.5%, 85.7%, and 77.1% of patients, respectively.[12] All in all these studies, together with other evidence, reported a good clinical response to SVR by DAA, although it is important to recognize that a proportion of patients will continue to have MC manifestations even after virological clearance.

Consistent with the reported clinical improvement, it has been observed that after SVR there is restoration in immune response (increased numbers of T-regulatory cells, IgMDCD21-/low-memory B cells, CD4DCXCR5D interleukin (IL) 21D cells, and T-helper 17 cells and decreased numbers of T follicular helper cells), a rapid reverse in anergic features of B cells, whereas there is persistence for several months in phenotypic and functional features of virus-specific B-cell exhaustion.[13–15]

Another potential clinical consequence of HCV lymphotropism is the increased risk of lymphomas, as reported in various cross-sectional studies. A strong evidence for such a relationship arises from a recent Taiwanese cohort study of about 11,000 individuals with HCV infection and about 50,000 matched uninfected controls followed for 8 years.[16] The investigators demonstrated that the incidence rates of any lymphoid neoplasms, and especially of non-Hodgkin lymphoma, were significantly greater in HCV-infected compared with uninfected individuals, reporting, after adjusting for confounders, a hazard ratio of 2.30 and 2, respectively.[16] Similar results were recently reported in a US study in a large cohort of Veterans.[17] Consistent with these data, a recent meta-analysis pooling available evidence from 16 studies estimated a risk of lymphoid neoplasm 1.6-fold higher in patients with HCV infection compared with uninfected individuals.[18] Further, indirect evidence about the link between HCV infection and lymphoid neoplasms arises from studies assessing the impact of antiviral therapy on cancer risk. Preliminary evidence was available following IFN-based therapies where Kawamura and colleagues[19] in 2007 showed that in a cohort of 501 never treated and 2708 IFN-treated HCV-infected patients, the risk of developing malignant lymphoma was 0% in patients achieving SVR and progressively higher in those treated with IFN but without SVR and further in those untreated. Similarly, a recent study in a large cohort of 24,133 patients with HCV reported a lower incidence of lymphoma in patients treated with pegylated (PEG)-IFN and ribavirin compared with those untreated, the beneficial effect being mainly observed in patients younger than 60 years and especially for non-Hodgkin lymphoma.[20] Consistent with these data, a meta-analysis of 5 studies reported a significant effect of SVR achievement on objective responses in lymphoproliferative diseases.[18] All these data suggested a role of virological eradication in reducing risk of lymphoma in patients with HCV, even if a possible impact of IFN as immunomodulating agent could not be excluded. The role of SVR in reducing the risk of lymphoid neoplasms in patients with HCV has been further investigated in the context of DAA therapy. Arcaini and colleagues[21] reported that in 46 patients with indolent B-cell non-Hodgkin lymphomas or chronic lymphocytic leukemia and HCV infection treated with DAA (98% achieving SVR) the lymphoproliferative disease response was 67%—and mainly observed in patients with marginal zone lymphoma—including 12 patients (26%) with a complete response. Similarly, another study evaluated the safety and efficacy of DAA along with the use of chemotherapy in patients with diffuse large B-cell lymphomas comparing clinical outcomes with a comparable historical retrospective cohort of patients not treated with antiviral therapy.[22] Notably the investigators found a trend for a better overall survival and a significantly higher disease-free survival in patients treated with DAA, further supporting a positive impact of HCV virological eradication on lymphoid neoplasms.[22] All the above-quoted evidence supports treating with DAA patients with HCV and lymphoid neoplasms because viral eradication can safely improve outcomes of the hematological disease.

Other studies have also documented an association between HCV infection and other immune-mediated disorders such as lichen planus, Sjogren syndrome, porphyria cutanea tarda syndrome, and arthritis.[18]

HEPATITIS C VIRUS INFECTION AND NEUROPSYCHIATRIC DISORDERS

A recent European consensus highlighted how HCV-infected subjects compared with the general noninfected population have a higher prevalence of major depression, anxiety disorders, bipolar disorders, and schizophrenia as well as risk factors for such disorders such as substance use and alcohol abuse.[23] Along this line, other studies have documented a high prevalence of asthenia in patients with HCV infection as well as a worsening of cognitive function such as concentration activity and speed of memory processes.[24] To explain these associations, different studies, by using proton magnetic resonance spectroscopy, demonstrated that HCV-infected patients even without advanced liver disease have altered cerebral metabolism in terms of elevated levels of choline in some brain regions (basal ganglia, white matter, occipital gray matter), reduced levels of N-acetylaspartate, and elevated myoinositol/creatine ratios in the white matter.[25–27] Further indirect evidence for a direct effect of HCV infection in causing neuropsychiatric disorders arises from recent studies that reported virological eradication by DAA to lead to a significant improvement in "patient-reported outcomes" (PROS) after only 2 weeks from starting treatment, with a main effect on fatigue and emotional profile.[28] Notably, effects of virological eradication on PROS were further confirmed by assessing PROS changes in patients treated with DAA compared with those treated with placebo: this kind of analysis highlighted a PROS improvement only in DAA-treated patients, suggesting a direct role of SVR in improving neuropsychiatric profile of patients.[29] Finally, available evidence supported a PROS improvement in patients with both mild and advanced liver disease.[30] The mechanisms by which HCV infection could contribute to the pathogenesis of neuropsychiatric disorders increase the possibility of induction of chronic systemic inflammation and the direct interaction between HCV and glial cells, events able of interfering with cerebral neurotransmission systems by inducing immune neuroinflammation.[23] Specifically, some studies suggested that serotonin, lactate dehydrogenase, IL-10, and granulocyte colony-stimulating factor increased, whereas PGDF and tryptophan significantly decreased during treatment and at follow-up in HCV-infected patients treated with DAA.[7]

HEPATITS C VIRUS INFECTION, INSULIN RESISTANCE, DIABETES, AND LIPID METABOLISM

Human clinical studies showed that patients with hepatitis C have significantly higher HOMA values (expression of IR) relative to uninfected controls[31] or HBV-infected individuals[32] and this evidence, being confirmed by using the euglycemichyperinsulinemic clamp method, shows an association between HCV infection and both hepatic[33–35] and extrahepatic[34] IR. Consistent with these data, evidence are also available about the association between HCV infection and type 2 diabetes. In 2000, Mehta and colleagues,[36] using US data from the "Third National Health and Nutrition Examination Survey 1988 to 1994," reported that in a cohort of more than 9000 individuals, and especially in those older than 40 years, the prevalence of diabetes in subjects with HCV infection was significantly higher than in noninfected individuals. In a subgroup without diabetes at baseline and stratified according to age and body mass index and at high or low risk of diabetes, they observed that the presence of HCV infection increased the risk of developing diabetes of about 11 times in high-risk subjects but not in the low-risk population.[37] The higher risk of developing diabetes in HCV-infected individuals was also shown in a large Taiwanese population of about 21,000 individuals.[38] Consistent with all these data a recent meta-analysis reported that patients with HCV infection, when compared with uninfected individuals, have a 1.5 higher risk of diabetes.[18] Various studies have explored the pathogenic mechanisms linking HCV infection to IR and diabetes and most highlighted the ability of the virus to indirectly, by inducing chronic inflammation and tumor necrosis factor alfa production, and directly interfere with the insulin signaling.[7] In experimental models, HCV can modulate insulin signaling by several mechanisms,[39] including interaction with the protein kinase B or Akt.[40]

The link between HCV infection and IR/diabetes has been further indirectly confirmed by studies assessing the impact of virological eradication on glucose and insulin homeostasis. Evidence arising from a cohort of HCV-infected patients treated with IFN-based therapies showed that virological eradication is able to improve IR and reduce the risk of developing diabetes,[41] even if biased by the selection of populations eligible for IFN treatment and by the potential effect of IFN on insulin signaling. However, these potential concerns were overcome by data arising from cohorts of patients treated with DAA. Specifically, clinical studies reported an improvement in insulin sensitivity in patients with HCV who achieve SVR after DAA, these results being confirmed when measuring IR both as HOMA and during oral glucose tolerance test.[42,43] Notably the beneficial effect of SVR on global (hepatic and adipose) tissue insulin sensitivity was also proved by using the gold standard euglycaemic clamp.[44] Consistent with these data, in a cohort of 2435 Veteran diabetic patients with HCV infection and treated with DAA, it has been demonstrated that SVR led to a significant drop in HbA1c, as well as a decrease in antidiabetic drug use.[45] Similarly, other studies reported an improvement in blood glucose serum levels and in the risk of developing diabetes in cohorts of patients achieving SVR by DAA.[46] Finally, a clinical positive impact of SVR by DAA on blood glucose homeostasis was also reported in the setting of liver transplantation where eradication of HCV has been associated with a lower risk of developing posttransplant diabetes and with glucose serum levels reduction in transplant recipients with a previous diagnosis of impaired fasting blood glucose.[47,48]

The relationship between HCV infection and metabolic comorbidities is further enriched by the evidence that the infection is associated with changes in lipid profile and by a greater prevalence of hepatic steatosis.[7] When looking at lipid profile, HCV-infected individuals are characterized by lower low-density lipoprotein and serum cholesterol levels than uninfected individuals, this issue being expression of the ability of the virus to interact with the intracellular systems that regulate lipid metabolism and that are necessary for virus entry into the cells, circulation in the blood, replication, and assembly.[49] Consistently, old studies demonstrated that ApoB and cholesterol serum levels significantly increased from baseline to follow-up only in responders but not in relapsers and in nonresponders to IFN-based regimens.[50] Similarly, recent reports in HCV-infected patients who underwent DAA-based antiviral therapies reported an increase in serum cholesterol levels occurring in parallel to HCV viral suppression.[51] HCV infection has been also linked to a higher prevalence of hepatic steatosis compared with uninfected individuals and that in turn can amplify the risk for IR and diabetes. Specifically, HCV can lead to fatty liver infiltration by indirect mechanism, that is, IR mostly observed in non-genotype 3 (G3) infections, and by direct mechanisms, typical of genotype 3, and related to the ability of the virus to increase de novo hepatic lipogenesis, and to reduced lipid export from the liver and decreased fatty acid beta oxidation.[52] The strong link between HCV infection and fatty liver infiltration has been further proved by studies assessing the impact of virological eradication on steatosis. Data arising from patients who underwent IFN-based therapies and pre- and posttherapy liver biopsy clearly reported an improvement in hepatic fat only in G3 but not in G1 patients, this issue being probably due to the main effect of G3 HCV on lipogenic pathways.[53] However, a recent study performed in a small cohort of patients with G1 HCV who underwent DAA-based therapy and had availability of paired liver biopsy showed in these patients a reduction after SVR in liver expression of genes involved in hepatic lipid metabolism such as APOC3, APOL3, LEPR, MTTP, and SREBF1.[51]

HEPATITS C VIRUS INFECTION AND KIDNEY INJURY

Several studies have reported an association between chronic HCV infection and kidney damage. Currently, available evidence suggest that HCV can induce kidney damage in a variety of manners, the most frequent being cryoglobulinemic nephropathy, followed by membranoproliferative glomerulonephritis and by membranous nephropathy.[54] However, it is possible to hypothesize that HCV infection may further contribute to the risk of renal damage by increasing, as thus far demonstrated, metabolic disorders such as IR, diabetes, and vascular damage that are well-known risk factors for kidney disease.

In 2007, in a large study in a cohort of nearly 500,000 Veterans, 10% of them with HCV infection, and with a median follow-up of 3.6 years, reported a decline in estimated glomerular filtration rate (eGFR) of 1.73 mL/m^2 per year in HCV-infected patients, while also demonstrating a 1.7 adjusted higher risk of developing end-stage kidney disease in HCV-infected compared with uninfected individuals.[55] Along this line, a more recent study, in about 1,000,000 individuals, confirmed that HCV infection, after correction for cardiometabolic risk factors, was associated with a risk of about 1.5 times and 3 times of reducing the creatinine clearance less than 60 mL/min and of developing end-stage renal disease, respectively.[3] Similar results were reported in a large Taiwanese cohort where the investigators confirmed

HCV infection as an independent risk factor for predicting the occurrence of end-stage kidney disease and identifying high HCV viral load and HCV genotype 1 as additional risk factors.[56] Consistent with all these data, a recent meta-analysis pooling data from 14 studies estimated a risk of chronic kidney disease of 1.2 times higher in patients with HCV infection relative to those without infection.[18] Finally, HCV seropositivity has been associated with increased risk for all-cause and cardiovascular mortality in patients on dialysis, as well as to reduced patient and graft survival after kidney transplantation.[57] Additional evidence to support an association between kidney damage and HCV infection stems from the assessment of HCV eradication on kidney function. A Taiwanese cohort study showed a reduction in the risk of developing end-stage kidney disease in HCV-infected subjects treated with IFN-based therapeutic regimens,[58] whereas a Swedish nationwide study reported improved survival in HCV-infected dialysis patients who received IFN-based antiviral treatment compared with those untreated.[57] When moving from IFN- to DAA-based antiviral regimens other evidence is available, although it is necessary to remember that all available DAA-based therapies can be used in patients with eGFR greater than 30 mL/min, whereas SOF-based regimens are not recommended in patients with eGFR less than 30 mL/min because of the renal excretion of sofosbuvir and potential concerns about toxicity by the accumulation of its metabolites.[8] In these patients, however, other combinations can be safely and effectively used also in the setting of patients on hemodialysis.[8] When looking at the effect of SVR by DAA in HCV-infected patients with chronic kidney disease only short-term outcomes are available. These studies showed contrasting results ranging from no effect on eGFR, to improvement in kidney function, and thus long-term follow-up is needed to obtain conclusive results.[59,60]

HEPATITIS C VIRUS INFECTION AND CARDIOVASCULAR DISEASE

In the past few years studies have investigated the potential association between HCV infection and cardiovascular damage, showing a higher prevalence/incidence of HCV infection in several cardiovascular disorders including atherosclerosis, stroke, myocardial infarction, coronary artery disease, peripheral arterial disease, myocarditis, and heart failure.[61]

When looking at carotid atherosclerosis, in 2003 an Asian study in a large cohort of 1992 individuals first observed a significant link between HCV infection and carotid atherosclerosis, this association being confirmed after adjusting for cardiometabolic confounders.[62] This association has been also validated in 3 independent Italian studies also reporting a higher intima-media thickness and a higher risk of carotid thickening according to HCV viral load, severity of liver fibrosis, and presence of hepatic steatosis.[63-65] Consistent with these data, other evidence from both Western and Asian cohorts, and in both HCV monoinfected or HCV-HIV coinfected patients, reported a higher risk of carotid atherosclerosis in patients with HCV relative to uninfected controls.[61] Other evidence reported an association between HCV infection and both coronary artery disease (CAD) and myocardial infarction. Butt and colleagues[66] demonstrated that HCV infection was associated with a 1.25 higher risk of CAD in a cohort of 82,083 HCV-infected patients (ERCHIVES) compared with 89,582 HCV-negative controls patients. Consistent with these data, in a large cohort study, including 13,983 HCV-infected patients and 55,932 HCV-negative controls, the incidence of acute coronary syndrome was significantly higher in infected patients even after adjusting for cardiometabolic risk factors.[67] Different case-control or cohort studies also investigated the potential association between HCV infection and ischemic stroke. Large Asian, US, and European longitudinal population cohort studies demonstrated a significantly higher incidence of stroke in HCV-infected patients,[68] also highlighting a link with inflammatory markers and HCV RNA levels.[69] Along this line other studies found a significant association between HCV infection and peripheral artery disease,[70] heart dysfunction,[71] and, most importantly, cardiovascular mortality.[72] Nevertheless, although all the above-quoted studies were positive, some negative evidence also exist. To that end, a recent meta-analysis pooling available data showed that HCV-infected patients, compared with uninfected subjects, had about twice higher risk of carotid plaques, 1.3 higher risk of cerebro-cardiovascular events, and 1.5 higher risk of cardiovascular mortality.[73] However, this meta-analysis confirmed the heterogeneity of the studies, suggesting that the effect of HCV on cardiovascular risk could be greater in populations with cardiovascular risk factors.[73] From a pathophysiologic point of view, it is possible to speculate that HCV infection can cause cardiovascular alterations by inducing metabolic comorbidities such as diabetes and IR, by leading to a proinflammatory and profibrogenic environment and by a potential direct viral mechanism.[61] Further indirect evidence on the role of HCV on cardiovascular risk arises from studies showing the impact of virological eradication. When looking at studies on cohort of patients who underwent IFN-based therapies, a proof of concept study in HCV-infected individuals reported an improvement in myocardial damage in patients who achieved an SVR, whereas not in nonresponders.[74] Along this line, a large Taiwanese cohort study reported a significant reduction in the development of both acute coronary syndrome and stroke, in patients treated with PEG-IFN–based antiviral therapy compared with those untreated,[58] and similar results were observed in other western studies. However, all these evidence raise the doubt that the observed results could be due to IFN per se or due to the selection bias of treating with IFN only those individuals without atherosclerotic and cardiovascular comorbidites. These concerns have been overcome by recent evidence obtained by using DAA. The authors demonstrated that in patients with advanced chronic liver disease due to HCV infection, virological eradication led to an improvement in intima-media thickness, and this has been largely observed in those with cardiometabolic risk factors.[75] Similarly, the achievement of SVR by DAA has been associated with improvement in endothelial function by flow-mediated dilation, reductions in levels of endothelium-derived cytokines, and improvement of tricuspid annular plane systolic excursion and lateral E' velocity compared with baseline.[76,77] Consistent with these data, large cohort studies in HCV-infected patients who underwent antiviral therapy with both PEG-IFN– and DAA-based therapies noted that SVR reduced the risk of overall cardiovascular or major cardiovascular events.[78]

SUMMARY

Available evidence strongly suggests that HCV infection leads to a systemic disease that can directly and indirectly affect different organs (other than the liver), leading to an increase in both immune-related, neuropsychiatric and cardiometabolic diseases. These manifestations, in an era where safe and effective DAA are available, represent a further indication to eradicate all HCV-infections independent of the severity of liver injury and fibrosis. Consistently, there have been observations on the beneficial effect of virological eradication on single extrahepatic outcomes, whereas recent evidence on large cohort of individuals with HCV infection and treated with DAA indicates that HCV clearance is responsible for a significant decrease in extrahepatic and all cause mortality.[79]

REFERENCES

1. Polaris Observatory HCV Collaborators. Global prevalence and genotype distribution of hepatitis C virus infection in 2015: a modelling study. LancetGastroenterolHepatol 2017;2(3):161–76.
2. Rein DB, Borton J, Liffmann DK, et al. The burden of hepatitis C to the United States Medicare system in 2009: Descriptive and economic characteristics. Hepatology 2016;63(4):1135–44.
3. Molnar MZ, Alhourani HM, Wall BM, et al. Association of hepatitis C viral infection with incidence and progression of chronic kidney disease in a large cohort of US veterans. Hepatology 2015;61(5):1495–502.
4. Macaluso FS, Maida M, Minissale MG, et al. Metabolic factors and chronic hepatitis C: a complex interplay. Biomed Res Int 2013;2013:564645.
5. Jepsen P, Vilstrup H, Lash TL. Development and validation of a comorbidity scoring system for patients with cirrhosis. Gastroenterology 2014;146(1):147–56.
6. Amin J, Law MG, Bartlett M, et al. Causes of death after diagnosis of hepatitis B or hepatitis C infection: a large community-based linkage study. Lancet 2006; 368(9539):938–45.
7. Negro F, Forton D, Craxì A, et al. Extrahepatic morbidity and mortality of chronic hepatitis C. Gastroenterology 2015;149(6):1345–60.
8. European Association for Study of Liver. EASL recommendations on treatment of hepatitis C 2015. J Hepatol 2015. https://doi.org/10.1016/j.jhep.2015.03.025.
9. Zignego AL, Pawlotsky JM, Bondin M, et al. Expert opinion on managing chronic HCV in patients with mixed cryoglobulinaemiavasculitis. AntivirTher 2018; 23(Suppl 2):1–9.
10. Gragnani L, Fognani E, Piluso A, et al, MaSVE Study Group. Long-term effect of HCV eradication in patients with mixed cryoglobulinemia: a prospective, controlled, open-label, cohort study. Hepatology 2015;61(4):1145–53.
11. Gragnani L, Visentini M, Fognani E, et al. Prospective study of guideline-tailored therapy with direct-acting antivirals for hepatitis C virus-associated mixed cryoglobulinemia. Hepatology 2016;64(5):1473–82.
12. Cacoub P, Si Ahmed SN, Ferfar Y, et al. Long-term Efficacy of Interferon-Free Antiviral Treatment Regimens in Patients With Hepatitis C Virus-Associated CryoglobulinemiaVasculitis. ClinGastroenterolHepatol 2019;17(3):518–26.
13. Del Padre M, Todi L, Mitrevski M, et al. Reversion of anergy signatures in clonal CD21(low) B cells of mixed cryoglobulinemia after clearance of HCV viremia. Blood 2017;130(1):35–8.
14. Saadoun D, Pol S, Ferfar Y, et al. Efficacy and Safety of Sofosbuvir Plus Daclatasvir for Treatment of HCV-Associated CryoglobulinemiaVasculitis. Gastroenterology 2017;153(1):49–52.e5.
15. Comarmond C, Garrido M, Pol S, et al. Direct-Acting Antiviral Therapy Restores Immune Tolerance to Patients With Hepatitis C Virus-Induced CryoglobulinemiaVasculitis. Gastroenterology 2017;152(8):2052–62.e2.
16. Su TH, Liu CJ, Tseng TC, et al. Hepatitis C viral infection increases the risk of lymphoid-neoplasms: A population-based cohort study. Hepatology 2016;63(3): 721–30.
17. Mahale P, Engels EA, Li R, et al. The effect of sustained virological response on the risk of extrahepatic manifestations of hepatitis C virus infection. Gut 2018; 67(3):553–61.

18. Younossi Z, Park H, Henry L, et al. Extrahepatic Manifestations of Hepatitis C: A Meta-analysis of Prevalence, Quality of Life, and Economic Burden. Gastroenterology 2016;150(7):1599–608.

19. Kawamura Y, Ikeda K, Arase Y, et al. Viral elimination reduces incidence of malignant lymphoma in patients with hepatitis C. Am J Med 2007;120(12):1034–41 [Erratum appears in Am J Med. 2008;121(12)].

20. Su TH, Liu CJ, Tseng TC, et al. Early antiviral therapy reduces the risk of lymphoma in patients with chronic hepatitis C infection. Aliment PharmacolTher 2019;49(3):331–9.

21. Arcaini L, Besson C, Frigeni M, et al. Interferon-free antiviral treatment in B-cell lymphoproliferative disorders associated with hepatitis C virus infection. Blood 2016;128(21):2527–32.

22. Persico M, Aglitti A, Caruso R, et al. Efficacy and safety of new direct antiviral agents in hepatitis C virus-infected patients with diffuse large B-cell non-Hodgkin's lymphoma. Hepatology 2018;67(1):48–55.

23. Schaefer M, Capuron L, Friebe A, et al. Hepatitis C infection, antiviral treatment and mental health: a European expert consensus statement. J Hepatol 2012; 57(6):1379–90.

24. Forton DM, Thomas HC, Murphy CA, et al. Hepatitis C and cognitive impairment in a cohort of patients with mild liver disease. Hepatology 2002;35(2):433–9.

25. Weissenborn K, Krause J, Bokemeyer M, et al. Hepatitis C virus infection affects the brain-evidence from psychometric studies and magnetic resonance spectroscopy. J Hepatol 2004;41:845–51.

26. Forton DM, Allsop JM, Main J, et al. Evidence for a cerebral effect of the hepatitis C virus. Lancet 2001;358:38–9.

27. Bokemeyer M, Ding XQ, Goldbecker A, et al. Evidence for neuroinflammation and neuroprotection in HCV infectionassociated encephalopathy. Gut 2011;60:370–7.

28. Younossi ZM, Stepanova M, Marcellin P, et al. Treatment with ledipasvir and sofosbuvir improves patient-reported outcomes: Results from the ION-1, -2, and -3 clinical trials. Hepatology 2015;61(6):1798–808.

29. Younossi ZM, Stepanova M, Feld J, et al. Sofosbuvir/velpatasvir improves patient-reported outcomes in HCV patients: Results from ASTRAL-1 placebo-controlled trial. JHepatol 2016;65(1):33–9.

30. Younossi ZM, Stepanova M, Afdhal N, et al. Improvement of health-related quality of life and work productivity in chronic hepatitis C patients with early and advanced fibrosis treated with ledipasvir and sofosbuvir. J Hepatol 2015;63(2): 337–45.

31. Hui JM, Sud A, Farrell GC, et al. Insulin resistance is associated with chronic hepatitis C virus infection and fibrosis progression. Gastroenterology 2003;125: 1695–704.

32. Moucari R, Asselah T, Cazals-Hatem D, et al. Insulin resistance in chronic hepatitis C: association with genotypes 1 and 4, serum HCV RNA level, and liver fibrosis. Gastroenterology 2008;134:416–23.

33. Mukhtar NA, Bacchetti P, Ayala CE, et al. Insulin sensitivity and variability in hepatitis C virus infection using direct measurement. Dig Dis Sci 2013;58:1141–8.

34. Vanni E, Abate ML, Gentilcore E, et al. Sites and mechanisms of insulin resistance in nonobese, nondiabetic patients with chronic hepatitis C. Hepatology 2009;50: 697–706.

35. Milner KL, van der Poorten D, Trenell M, et al. Chronic hepatitis C is associated with peripheral rather than hepatic insulin resistance. Gastroenterology 2010; 138:e931–3.

36. Mehta SH, Brancati FL, Sulkowski MS, et al. Prevalence of type 2 diabetes mellitus among persons with hepatitis C virus infection in the United States. Ann Intern Med 2000;133:592–9.
37. Mehta SH, Brancati FL, Strathdee SA, et al. Hepatitis C virus infection and incident type 2 diabetes. Hepatology 2003;38:50–6.
38. Lin YJ, Shaw TG, Yang HI, et al, R.E.V.E.A.L.-HCV Study Group. Chronic hepatitis C virus infection and the risk for diabetes: a community-based prospective study. Liver Int 2017;37(2):179–86.
39. Kaddai V, Negro F. Current understanding of insulin resistance in hepatitis C. Expert Rev GastroenterolHepatol 2011;5:503–16.
40. Aytug S, Reich D, Sapiro LE, et al. Impaired IRS-1/PI3- kinase signaling in patients with HCV: a mechanism for increased prevalence of type 2 diabetes. Hepatology 2003;38:1384–92.
41. Arase Y, Suzuki F, Suzuki Y, et al. Sustained virological response reduces incidence of onset of type 2 diabetes in chronic hepatitis C. Hepatology 2009; 49(3):739–44.
42. Adinolfi LE, Nevola R, Guerrera B, et al. Hepatitis C virus clearance by direct-acting antiviral treatments and impact on insulin resistance in chronic hepatitis C patients. J GastroenterolHepatol 2018;33(7):1379–82.
43. Gualerzi A, Bellan M, Smirne C, et al. Improvement of insulin sensitivity in diabetic and non diabetic patients with chronic hepatitis C treated with direct antiviral agents. PLoS One 2018;13(12):e0209216.
44. Lim TR, Hazlehurst JM, Oprescu AI, et al. Hepatitis C virus infection is associated with hepatic and adipose tissue insulin resistance that improves after viral cure. ClinEndocrinol (Oxf) 2019;90(3):440–8.
45. Hum J, Jou JH, Green PK, et al. Improvement in Glycemic Control of Type 2 Diabetes After Successful Treatment of Hepatitis C Virus. Diabetes Care 2017;40(9): 1173–80.
46. Li J, Zhang T, Gordon SC, et al, CHeCS Investigators. Impact of sustained virologic response on risk of type 2 diabetes among hepatitis C patients in the United States. J ViralHepat 2018;25(8):952–8.
47. Roccaro GA, Mitrani R, Hwang WT, et al. Sustained Virological Response Is Associated with a Decreased Risk of Posttransplant Diabetes Mellitus in Liver Transplant Recipients with Hepatitis C-Related Liver Disease. LiverTranspl 2018; 24(12):1665–72.
48. Saab S, Barnard A, Challita Y, et al. Impact of Sustained Viral Response With Direct-Acting Agents on Glycemic Control and Renal Function in Hepatitis C Liver Transplant Recipients. ExpClin Transplant 2018;16(4):419–24.
49. Filipe A, McLauchlan J. Hepatitis C virus and lipid droplets: finding a niche. TrendsMol Med 2015;21(1):34–42.
50. Hofer H, Bankl HC, Wrba F, et al. Hepatocellular fat accumulation and low serum cholesterol in patients infected with HCV-3a. Am J Gastroenterol 2002;97(11): 2880–5.
51. Meissner EG, Lee YJ, Osinusi A, et al. Effect of sofosbuvir and ribavirin treatment on peripheral and hepatic lipid metabolism in chronic hepatitis C virus, genotype 1-infected patients. Hepatology 2015;61(3):790–801.
52. Bugianesi E, Salamone F, Negro F. The interaction of metabolic factors with HCV infection: does it matter? J Hepatol 2012;56(Suppl 1):S56–65.
53. Kumar D, Farrell GC, Fung C, et al. Hepatitis C virus genotype 3 is cytopathic to hepatocytes: Reversal of hepatic steatosis after sustained therapeutic response. Hepatology 2002;36(5):1266–72.

54. Cacoub P, Desbois AC, Isnard-Bagnis C, et al. Hepatitis C virus infection and chronic kidney disease: Time for reappraisal. J Hepatol 2016;65(1 Suppl): S82–94.

55. Tsui JI, Vittinghoff E, Shlipak MG, et al. Association of hepatitis C seropositivity with increased risk for developing end-stage renal disease. Arch Intern Med 2007;167(12):1271–6.

56. Lai TS, Lee MH, Yang HI, et al, REVEAL-HCV Study Group. Hepatitis C viral load, genotype, and increased risk of developing end-stage renal disease: REVEAL-HCV study. Hepatology 2017;66(3):784–93.

57. Söderholm J, Millbourn C, Büsch K, et al. Higher risk of renal disease in chronic hepatitis C patients: Antiviral therapy survival benefit in patients on hemodialysis. J Hepatol 2018;68(5):904–11.

58. Hsu YC, Ho HJ, Huang YT, et al. Association between antiviral treatment and extrahepatic outcomes in patients with hepatitis C virus infection. Gut 2015; 64(3):495–503.

59. Mehta DA, Cohen E, Charafeddine M, et al. Effect of Hepatitis C Treatment with Ombitasvir/Paritaprevir/R + Dasabuvir on Renal, Cardiovascular and Metabolic Extrahepatic Manifestations: A Post-Hoc Analysis of Phase 3 Clinical Trials. Infect Dis Ther 2017;6(4):515–29.

60. Tran TT, Mehta D, Mensa F, et al. Pan-Genotypic Hepatitis C Treatment with Glecaprevir and Pibrentasvir for 8 Weeks Resulted in Improved Cardiovascular and Metabolic Outcomes and Stable Renal Function: A Post-Hoc Analysis of Phase 3 Clinical Trials. Infect Dis Ther 2018;7(4):473–84.

61. Petta S, Macaluso FS, Craxì A. Cardiovascular diseases and HCV infection: a simple association or more? Gut 2014;63(3):369–75.

62. Ishizaka Y, Ishizaka N, Takahashi E, et al. Association between hepatitis C virus core protein and carotid atherosclerosis. Circ J 2003;67(1):26–30.

63. Targher G, Bertolini L, Padovani R, et al. Differences and similarities in early atherosclerosis between patients with non-alcoholic steatohepatitis and chronic hepatitis B and C. J Hepatol 2007;46:1126–32.

64. Adinolfi LE, Restivo L, Zampino R, et al. Chronic HCV infection is a risk of atherosclerosis. Role of HCV and HCV-related steatosis. Atherosclerosis 2012;221: 496–502.

65. Petta S, Torres D, Fazio G, et al. Carotid atherosclerosis and chronic hepatitis C: a prospective study of risk associations. Hepatology 2012;55:1317–23.

66. Butt AA, Xiaoqiang W, Budoff M, et al. Hepatitis C virus infection and the risk of coronary disease. Clin Infect Dis 2009;49:225–32.

67. Tsai MS, Hsu YC, Yu PC, et al. Long-term risk of acute coronary syndrome in hepatitis C virus infected patients without antiviral treatment: A cohort study from an endemic area. Int J Cardiol 2015;181:27–9.

68. Adinolfi LE, Restivo L, Guerrera B, et al. Chronic HCV infection is a risk factor of ischemic stroke. Atherosclerosis 2013;231:22–6.

69. Lee MH, Yang HI, Wang CH, et al. Hepatitis C virus infection and increased risk of cerebrovascular disease. Stroke 2010;41:2894–900.

70. Hsu YH, Muo CH, Liu CY, et al. Hepatitis C virus infection increases the risk of developing peripheral arterial disease: a 9-year population-based cohort study. J Hepatol 2015;62(3):519–25.

71. Perticone M, Miceli S, Maio R, et al. Chronic HCV infection increases cardiac left ventricular mass index in normotensive patients. J Hepatol 2014;61(4):755–60.

72. Lee MH, Yang HI, Lu SN, et al, R.E.V.E.A.L.-HCV Study Group. Chronic hepatitis C virus infection increases mortality from hepatic and extrahepatic diseases: a community-based long-term prospective study. J Infect Dis 2012;206:469–77.

73. Petta S, Maida M, Macaluso FS, et al. Hepatitis C virus infection is associated with increased cardiovascular mortality: a meta-analysis of observational studies. Gastroenterology 2016;150(1):145–55.

74. Maruyama S, Koda M, Oyake N, et al. Myocardial injury in patients with chronic hepatitis C infection. J Hepatol 2013;58(1):11–5.

75. Petta S, Adinolfi LE, Fracanzani AL, et al. Hepatitis C virus eradication by direct-acting antiviral agents improves carotid atherosclerosis in patients with severe liver fibrosis. J Hepatol 2018;69(1):18–24.

76. Schmidt FP, Zimmermann T, Wenz T, et al. Interferon- and ribavirin-free therapy with new direct acting antivirals (DAA) for chronic hepatitis C improves vascular endothelial function. Int J Cardiol 2018;271:296–300.

77. Novo G, Macaione F, Giannitrapani L, et al. Subclinical cardiovascular damage in patients with HCV cirrhosis before and after treatment with direct antiviral agents: a prospective study. Aliment PharmacolTher 2018;48(7):740–9.

78. Cacoub P, Nahon P, Layese R, et al, ANRS CO12 CirVirGroup. Prognostic value of viral eradication for major adverse cardiovascular events in hepatitis C cirrhotic patients. Am Heart J 2018;198:4–17.

79. Carrat F, Fontaine H, Dorival C, et al, French ANRS CO22 Hepather cohort. Clinical outcomes in patients with chronic hepatitis C after direct-acting antiviral treatment: a prospective cohort study. Lancet 2019;393(10179):1453–64.

Pyogenic and Amebic Infections of the Liver

Rebecca Roediger, MD, Mauricio Lisker-Melman, MD*

KEYWORDS

- Pyogenic liver • Amebic liver • Liver abscess

KEY POINTS

- Pyogenic liver abscesses are localized collections of pus from a bacterial cause. Biliary disease is the most common cause of pyogenic liver abscess.
- Amebic liver abscess is caused by *Entamoeba histolytica*, which is acquired by fecal-oral transmission and in rare cases becomes invasive. Liver abscesses are the most common extraintestinal manifestation of *E histolytica*.
- Both pyogenic and amebic liver abscesses are diagnosed based on imaging, either computed tomography or ultrasonography.
- The treatment of pyogenic liver abscess is antibiotics to target the causative organism along with drainage either by percutaneous catheter or aspiration.
- Amebic liver abscesses are treated with metronidazole and only 15% of cases require percutaneous drainage.

INTRODUCTION

A hepatic abscess is defined by the Merriam-Webster dictionary as "a localized collection of pus surrounded by inflammatory tissue." Others defined it as a mass caused by invasion of microorganisms into healthy liver parenchyma.[1–3] Causes include bacterial, parasitic, and fungal.[1,4] In pyogenic liver abscess, bacteria are the invasive microorganisms and the abscess contains pus. In amebic liver abscess, the mass is created by parenchymal invasion of amebas, usually *Entamoeba histolytica*. This article focuses on pyogenic and amebic liver abscesses.

PYOGENIC LIVER ABSCESS
General Principles

Classification
Liver abscesses are usually classified by the causative bacteria of the abscess. Knowing which bacterium is the infective agent points to the underlying reason for

Division of Gastroenterology, Hepatology Program, Washington University School of Medicine, 660 S. Euclid Avenue, St. Louis, MO 63110, USA
* Corresponding author. Department of Gastroenterology, VA Medical Center, 915 North Grand Boulevard, St. Louis, MO 63106, USA
E-mail addresses: mlisker@wustl.edu; mauricio.lisker@VA.gov

Gastroenterol Clin N Am 49 (2020) 361–377
https://doi.org/10.1016/j.gtc.2020.01.013
0889-8553/20/© 2020 Elsevier Inc. All rights reserved.

abscess formation, predicts potential complications, and dictates treatment options.[1,2,5,6] The most common causative bacteria are *Escherichia coli*, *Streptococcus* species, *Klebsiella pneumoniae*, or *Enterococcus* species,[7–9] and up to 16% of abscesses are polymicrobial.[10] Usually the bacteria originate from the gastrointestinal (GI) tract flora, but hematogenous spread should be suspected when *Streptococcus* or *Staphylococcus* species are the causative bacteria.[6] *Staphylococcus* species are also associated with trauma-induced liver abscesses.[11] *Yersinia enterocolitica* is associated with pyogenic abscesses in hemochromatosis.[12]

Anaerobic bacteria are rare causes of liver abscesses and probably arise from opportunistic infections; they only cause abscesses when natural barriers are broken down. The most common anaerobes found in pyogenic liver abscesses are *Bacteroides* and Fusobacteria.[13] Fusobacteria are normal bacteria of the GI, oropharyngeal, and female genital tracts. Fusobacteria liver abscesses typically occur in immunocompetent hosts only with recent periodontal disease or pharyngitis.[14,15]

Epidemiology

Incidence of pyogenic liver abscess Pyogenic liver abscesses are rare and their incidence varies depending on the region of the world. In the United States, bacterial causes account for more than 80% of all liver abscesses.[16] There have been multiple US studies of the incidence of pyogenic liver abscess, estimating the incidence as high as 20 per 100,000 from 1973 to 1993.[8] A recent US study estimated the incidence at 4.1 per 100,000.[7] Other Western countries have reported similar low incidence rates. The incidence rate of Canada, the United Kingdom, and Denmark is 1.1 to 2.3 per 100,000 in population-based studies.[10,17,18] Southeast Asia has a high incidence of pyogenic liver abscesses; the incidence in mainland China is 5.6 per 100,000,[19] and the incidence in Taiwan has been estimated at 17.6 per 100,000.[20]

The incidence of pyogenic liver abscess increases in patients with comorbid conditions such as diabetes mellitus, malnutrition, and immunosuppression.[1] Pyogenic liver abscesses are more prevalent in men than in women,[3,7,16,17] with an odds ratio of 1.85[7] and a ratio of 1.5 to 2.5 men affected to every 1 female.[16] Incidence also increases with increasing age.[7,17] The odds ratio of developing pyogenic liver abscess is 11.9 in persons aged 65 to 84 years compared with those aged 18 to 34 years.[7]

Incidence of bacterial causes Epidemiologic studies have found an increasing incidence of *K pneumoniae*–induced hepatic abscesses, especially in Southeast Asia, where it has become the most common bacterial cause of pyogenic liver abscesses.[3,4,9,21,22] In Taiwan, *Klebsiella* accounts for 82% of pyogenic liver abscesses.[20] A meta-analysis of Chinese cases of pyogenic liver abscess found that *Klebsiella* accounted for most of the abscesses (54%) caused by gram-negative bacteria. *E coli* (29%) was the next most prevalent bacterium, followed by *Enterobacter* species (9%), *Proteus* species (6%), and *Pseudomonas* species (5%).[23] In the United States, *E coli* remains the most common bacterium to cause liver abscesses; over the course of the twentieth century, the incidence of *E coli* infections has decreased, whereas the incidence of *Klebsiella* infections increased.[8,16] One study found an increasing prevalence of *Klebsiella* liver abscesses over the years 1994 to 2005, increasing up to 41% of all cases; this study was performed in New York City and had a large proportion of Asian patients.[16]

Diabetes mellitus has been found to be an especially important risk factor for *Klebsiella* abscesses.[3,4,19,21] In one Asian study, the prevalence of diabetes in *Klebsiella* abscess was 61%, whereas the prevalence of diabetes in other pyogenic liver abscess was 51.4%.[24] It is proposed that poor glycemic control impairs neutrophil phagocytosis of *Klebsiella* K1/K2 capsules, preventing a robust immune response to the bacteria.[24]

Causes of pyogenic liver abscess

In the early decades of the twentieth century, the predominant cause of pyogenic liver abscess was pylephlebitis (infectious thrombophlebitis of the portal vein or any of its branches) from appendicitis.[8] During the mid–twentieth century, the most common cause changed to biliary disease (benign and malignant). This change is attributed to the ease of diagnosis and treatment of appendicitis as well as an increasing prevalence of hepatobiliary disease.[7] By the end of the twentieth century, malignant biliary strictures emerged as the most common cause of pyogenic liver abscess[8] (**Box 1**).

Biliary infections Intra-abdominal biliary infections currently account for most pyogenic liver abscesses (50%–60%).[1,8,15,25] The incidence of biliary infection causing liver abscesses has increased over the past century as the population has aged and biliary disease has become more prevalent.[7,8] The underlying causes of biliary abscesses are malignant obstruction, instrumentation of the biliary ducts, choledocholithiasis, primary sclerosing cholangitis, Caroli disease, and (rarely) obstruction from parasites such as *Ascaris lumbricoides*.[11,12]

Intra-abdominal infections Before the increasing incidence of biliary disease, seeding of the portal vein from an intra-abdominal infection was the most common cause of pyogenic liver abscess.[16] The intra-abdominal infections are usually appendicitis or diverticulitis, but infected GI tumors and inflammatory bowel disease can also lead to liver abscess formation. Now intra-abdominal infections account for 10% to 20% of all bacterial liver abscesses.[26] Most liver abscesses are found in the right hepatic lobe because of the preferential portal vein flow.[2,9]

Direct extension Direct extension from cholecystitis, perinephric abscess, and subphrenic abscess can cause pyogenic liver abscesses. Microbes invade the liver via contiguous spread from the gallbladder or nearby abscess.[11]

Hematogenous spread Blood stream bacteria enter the liver via the hepatic artery. Cases of bacteremia from endocarditis, severe sepsis, central line–associated blood stream infections,[11] and periodontal disease[14,15] have been shown to cause pyogenic liver abscess.

Trauma Liver trauma, whether iatrogenic (eg, radiofrequency ablation [RFA], chemoembolization, surgery) or as direct blunt trauma, can cause pyogenic liver abscess.[12] Necrosis is the main risk factor for abscess formation; severe trauma or severe arterial compromise have higher odds of causing a pyogenic liver abscess.[6] Interestingly, trauma-induced bilomas are rarely infected (one case series, 7% of bilomas became infected).[1]

Other risk factors for trauma-related abscesses are alterations to the liver anatomy that allow bacterial colonization, such as in choledochoenterostomy, biliary sphincterotomy, or biliary drainage.[1] Abscesses occur in 5% of patients undergoing chemoembolization and less than 1% undergoing RFA.[27,28] Abscesses after chemoembolization are more frequent in cases related to neuroendocrine tumors because they are surrounded by healthy tissue that develops necrosis after treatment.[27]

Posttraumatic abscesses have a higher incidence of anaerobic infection. Anaerobic bacteria can cause abscesses more quickly than aerobic bacteria; for instance, *Clostridium* abscesses may form as soon as 24 to 48 hours after trauma.[29]

Box 1
Causes of pyogenic liver abscess

Biliary infections
- Malignant obstruction
- Biliary instrumentation (eg, stenting)
- Choledocholithiasis
- Primary sclerosing cholangitis
- Malformations (eg, Caroli disease)

Intra-abdominal infections
- Appendicitis
- Diverticulitis

Direct extension
- Cholecystitis
- Perinephric abscess
- Subphrenic abscess

Hematogenous spread
- Endocarditis
- Central line–associated blood stream infection
- Periodontal disease
- Bacteremia from any source of sepsis (eg, urinary tract infection or pneumonia)
- Translocation of GI bacteria
  - GI tumors
  - Inflammatory bowel disease

Trauma
- Radiofrequency ablation
- Chemoembolization
- Surgery
- Blunt trauma

Postoperative complications
- Hepatic artery stenosis
- Stricture of choledochoenterostomy
- Biliary reflux
  - Short Roux limb
  - Stricture of jejunojejunostomy
  - Liver transplant

Cryptogenic

Superinfection
- Existing cyst
- Necrotic metastasis

Foreign body

Postoperative complications Postoperative stenosis of the hepatic artery after pancreaticoduodenectomy produces biliary ischemia and necrosis, allowing pyogenic abscess formation.[6] Mortality reaches as high as 80% in cases of hepatic artery stenosis.[30] Strictures of choledochoenterostomies, which occur in about 5% of patients after a pancreaticoduodenectomy, can also cause liver abscess.[31] However, unlike stenosis of the hepatic artery, the prognosis is better in these cases as long as the complication is identified early and treated promptly.[31]

Cryptogenic No cause for the liver abscess is found in about 35% of cases of pyogenic liver abscess.[13,25] *Klebsiella* abscesses are usually cryptogenic and present without any biliary disease[9]; however colonization of the GI tract by *Klebsiella* is a predisposing factor for liver abscess.[4,21]

Superinfection Pyogenic liver abscess can occur when there is a bacterial infection on an existing liver lesion, which occurs in less than 2% of patients with liver cysts and in association with cysts larger than 5 cm. Superinfection can also occur in necrotic metastasis, but occurs rarely in hepatocellular carcinomas.[32]

In the developing world, pyogenic liver abscess is associated with concomitant infection with parasites, such as in schistosomiasis and toxocariasis. It is thought that the parasites incite liver necrosis, which can then be colonized by bacteria, or that the parasites cause alterations in immunity making infected patients more susceptible to developing pyogenic abscess.[33]

Foreign body There are 65 case reports in the literature of ingested foreign bodies (predominantly chicken and fish bones, and tooth picks) perforating through the stomach or duodenum, causing pyogenic liver abscesses. These abscesses are usually recurrent after antibiotic treatment and drainage. The abscess only fully resolves once the foreign body is surgically removed.[34]

Diagnosis

The diagnosis of liver abscess is mainly based on imaging findings and microbiological culture results because the clinical presentation and blood laboratory results are nonspecific.[1,13]

Clinical presentation
The clinical presentation is usually a compilation of nonspecific symptoms that indicate abdominal infection. The most common presenting complaints are fever (90%), abdominal pain (50%–75%), and chills (69%).[1,16,21] Rarer complaints are nausea, vomiting, weight loss, anorexia, headache, myalgia, and diarrhea.[16]

Physical examination can reveal fever, tachycardia, hypotension, and jaundice. Hepatomegaly or a palpable mass can been found on abdominal examination.[2,12,33,35] *Klebsiella* liver abscesses can also have extrahepatic manifestations, including septic emboli to the eye, meninges, or brain. Symptoms of these organ systems, such as vision impairment or altered mental status, can be present on initial evaluation.[2,9]

Laboratory
The abnormal laboratory values in pyogenic liver abscess are nonspecific but frequently useful to indicate liver involvement.[1,5] Complete blood count with differential, complete metabolic profile, C-reactive protein, erythrocyte sedimentation rate, and blood cultures are recommended. The most common laboratory abnormalities are hypoalbuminemia (70%) and leukocytosis (68%).[11,16] Aspartate aminotransferase, alanine aminotransferase, and alkaline phosphatase levels are nonspecifically increased in around 50% of cases.[16,25] C-reactive protein level was increased in 100% of cases in 2 case series.[13,36]

Depending on the underlying cause of the pyogenic liver abscess, other laboratory results can be abnormal. When biliary tract disease leads to pyogenic liver abscess, alkaline phosphatase level is increased in 67% to 90% of patients and total bilirubin level is increased in 53%.[16] Blood cultures are positive in ~50% of all cases; they are more often positive when the cause of the abscess is hematogenous spread.[1,12,17] Cultures from abscess aspiration are helpful to guide diagnosis and treatment but should be sent from aspirated fluid during the initial placement of the drainage catheters; catheters subsequently become contaminated with skin flora and do not provide useful culture data after placement.[2,37] Up to 30% of cultures can be negative if antibiotics are started before drawing the abscess cultures.[4,6]

Radiology

The diagnosis of liver abscess relies on imaging. Most pyogenic liver abscesses are solitary lesions in the right lobe of the liver, are less than10 mm in diameter, and have septations.[21,25,36] Klebsiella abscesses can have gas within the abscess on imaging. Gas formation in Klebsiella abscess occurs more frequently in diabetic patients (32.9% v 13.5%), likely because of Klebsiella producing more carbon dioxide from glucose fermentation in the setting of hyperglycemia.[21,24]

Plain radiographs were the mainstay of diagnosis before ultrasonography (US), computed tomography (CT) scanning, and MRI; and in resource-limited settings they remain useful.[8] Abdominal radiographs can show extraluminal free air in a minority (7%) of cases of pyogenic liver abscess, and rarely show air-fluid level or portal venous gas.[7,21] Chest radiographs can show an increased right hemidiaphragm or pleural effusion in ~25% of patients.[8,16,21]

At present, US and CT scanning diagnose more than 90% of cases of pyogenic liver abscess.[16,25,36] The sensitivity of CT scanning is superior to US. Although US has a 94% sensitivity, it is not able to pick up smaller abscesses.[38] CT scanning sensitivity approaches 100% and is more accurate in differentiating abscess from tumor.[38]

On US, pyogenic liver abscess appears as either a hyperechoic or hypoechoic lesion and can have internal debris or septations.[1,11] CT scanning appearance varies according to the stage of the abscess. In a presuppurative stage, it appears as a heterogeneous, hypodense lesion with poorly defined irregular contours.[1] In this stage, the abscesses simulate the appearance of a tumor. When the abscess is in the suppurative stage, it appears hypoechoic or anechoic with clearly delineated rounded contours that enhance with contrast showing a ring sign[24,26] (**Fig. 1**).

MRI can be performed for diagnosis; it shows an abscess as a T1-hypointense and T2-hyperintense lesion.[32,39] However, MRI is not performed as often as US or CT scanning because it takes more time to perform and is not a suitable modality for drainage guidance.

At present, there is a limited role for nuclear scans; they have lower sensitivity for pyogenic liver abscess than CT scanning. Technetium is 80% sensitive, gallium 50% to 80% sensitive, and indium 90% sensitive.[10,40]

Treatment

The mainstay of treatment is antibiotics in conjunction with drainage, and, when indicated, treatment of the underlying cause. Treatment is considered effective if there is normalization of the temperature, white blood cell count, and C-reactive protein level, and disappearance of pain. Laboratory values and inflammatory markers should normalize within several days of initiating antibiotics and drainage. Imaging resolution of the abscess occurs later than the clinical resolution.[36,37] Imaging follow-up is recommended. US is the modality of choice for most surveillance imaging given its sensitivity and does not need radiation. However, CT scanning allows assessment for underlying malignancy once the abscess has resolved[12] (**Fig. 2**).

Medical

Empiric antibiotics should be started promptly when a pyogenic liver abscess is suspected and after initial blood cultures have been drawn.[3,36,41] Antibiotics should be tailored to cover all possible bacteria: gram-negative rods, gram-positive cocci, and anaerobes. Empiric antibiotic regimens can include amoxicillin-clavulanic

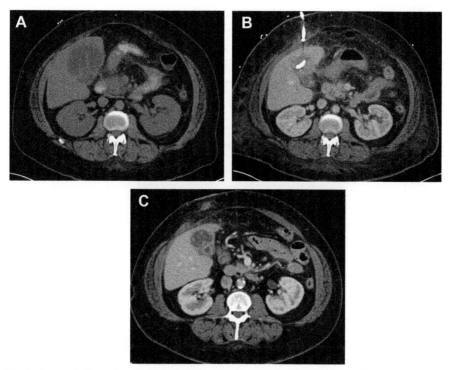

Fig. 1. Pyogenic liver abscess. A) Early pyogenic liver abscess characterized by ill-defined hypodensity with a focus of hemorrhage and adjacent fat stranding. B) Pyogenic liver abscess decreased in size with a percutaneous drain in place. C) residual well enhancing fluid collection in the gallbladder fossa status post removal of percutaneous drainage catheter.

acid, third-generation cephalosporins combined with an aminoglycoside, or piperacillin/tazobactam.[4,5,21,42] In cases of penicillin allergy or antibiotic resistance, fluoroquinolones or carbapenems can be used.[11] Metronidazole should be added if the chosen antibiotic regimen does not have anaerobic coverage.[5,37] Anaerobes are difficult to culture so should be covered in all treatment regimens.[12] Narrowing of the antibiotic regimen is based on culture and sensitivity data obtained from the aspiration specimen[2,19] (**Box 2**).

Duration for antibiotics varies in studies and case series, with most recommending therapy for 2 to 6 weeks.[17,36,43] The recommended antibiotic treatment is administered intravenously for around 2 weeks before transitioning to oral antibiotics for the duration of the course.[12] Risk factors for failure of antibiotic therapy are presence of malignancy, septic shock, older age, biochemical derangements (specifically anemia, azotemia, hyperbilirubinemia), and an APACHE (Acute Physiology and Chronic Health Evaluation) score greater than 15.[14] Prolonged antibiotic regimens should be given in patients with these risk factors.

Glycemic control is recommended alongside antibiotics for all *Klebsiella* infections, to reduce the chance of extrahepatic infections.[21]

Drainage
Percutaneous drainage should become a treatment consideration in all patients who remain febrile 48 to 72 hours after initiation of antibiotics, have an abscess greater than 6 cm, or have signs of impending rupture on imaging.[21] Small abscesses (<3 cm in

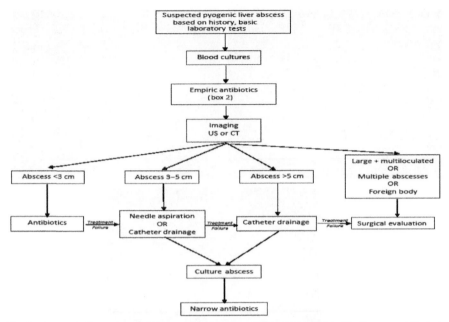

Fig. 2. Pyogenic liver abscess treatment algorithm. (*Data from* Webb GJ, Chapman TP, Cadman PJ, Gorard DA. Pyogenic liver abscess. *Frontline Gastroenterol*. 2014;5:60-67.)

diameter) can be treated solely with antibiotics. One case series reported a 100% success rate in treating abscess less than 3 cm with antibiotics only.[41] However, there are no clear guidelines on the need for draining abscesses 3 to 6 cm in diameter. In a review of pyogenic liver abscesses treated only with antibiotics, abscesses greater than 5 cm had a 61% response rate to antibiotics and the median course duration on antibiotics was 42 days.[42]

Image-guided needle puncture and catheter drainage is the first-line treatment of large abscesses; this provides a specimen for culture and allows the evacuation of the purulent collection.[8,44] In a randomized trial, catheter placement for prolonged drainage has a better success than aspiration alone (100% vs 60%).[45] However, a more recent randomized trial comparing repeat aspiration and catheter drainage

---

Box 2
Antibiotic regimens for pyogenic liver abscess

- Amoxicillin-clavulanic acid + metronidazole

- Third-generation cephalosporin + metronidazole

- Piperacillin/tazobactam

If penicillin/cephalosporin allergy
- Fluoroquinolone + metronidazole ± aminoglycoside
- Carbapenem + metronidazole

Data from Tian LT, Yao K, Zhang XY, et al. Liver abscesses in adult patients with and without diabetes mellitus: An analysis of the clinical characteristics, features of the causative pathogens, outcomes and predictors of fatality: A report based on a large population, retrospective study in China. *Clin Microbiol Infect*. 2012;18:E314-E330; and Akhondi H, Sabih DE. Liver Abscess. *StatPearls*. 2019:1-7.

showed equivalent response to treatment; 60% of patients getting a needle aspiration required at least 1 repeat aspiration.[37] A randomized trial compared needle aspiration and catheter drainage. It found success rates of 67% with needle aspiration, but 40% required repeat aspirations, whereas 100% of patients receiving catheter drainage were cured.[44] The investigators concluded that abscesses less than 5 cm can be managed with needle aspiration, but patients may need repeated procedures. However, in abscesses greater than 5 cm, percutaneous drainage was recommended.[44]

If a drainage catheter is placed, it should be flushed with saline 3 times a day and removed once its output decreases to less than 10 mL/d.[46] If the pyogenic abscess is from a biliary cause, dedicated biliary imaging should be undertaken and relief of obstruction with endoscopic retrograde cholangiopancreatography (ERCP) or percutaneous transhepatic cholangiography should be performed.[12]

If the abscess culture grows *Klebsiella* or is polymicrobial, patients should undergo a colonoscopy. *Klebsiella* has a high association with colon cancer, and polymicrobial abscesses are suggestive of a colonic disorder such as tumor, diverticulitis, appendicitis, or inflammatory bowel disease.[1,6,40]

Surgery

Surgery was the preferred treatment method until the 1980s when percutaneous drainage was found to be safe and efficacious.[16] Surgery is rarely indicated in countries with radiologic-guided drainage capabilities; currently more than 90% of liver abscesses are treated without a surgical intervention.[7] There is a role for surgical treatment if attempts at percutaneous drainage fail, if the patient has ongoing sepsis after antibiotics and percutaneous drainage, or in difficult-to-access sites such as the liver dome.[37] Surgery is also indicated if the abscess is not amenable to percutaneous drainage, such as multiloculated abscesses or thick purulent material that cannot be aspirated.[13,41] In one case series, surgical drainage of large (>5 cm) multiloculated abscesses was associated with higher treatment success rate, fewer repeat procedures, and a shorter hospital stay.[35] In patients with multiple liver abscesses, surgery is the preferred treatment modality. Surgery is necessary when the abscess has ruptured and when the underlying cause requires surgical removal, such as in cases with foreign bodies.[2,21]

Surgery can be performed either with laparoscopy or with exploratory laparotomy.[5] If the abscess is superficial, fenestration and drainage is an option. In patients with deep abscesses, intraoperative Doppler-guided drainage or limited hepatic resections are performed.[41]

Overall outcomes of surgical treatment are worse than for percutaneous drainage but there is likely a selection bias of severe and complicated abscesses requiring surgery.[38]

Complications

If pyogenic liver abscesses are not treated, they can rupture causing peritonitis, bacteremia, septic shock, and death.[11] There is a higher risk of spontaneous abscess rupture in *Klebsiella* abscesses than in other bacterial abscesses. Risk factors for rupture include diabetes, large abscess size, thin abscess wall, and abscess with gas formation.[21] One case series found a 33% complication rate in abscesses after treatment with percutaneous drainage, including rupture, hemorrhage, and complications from septic shock such as renal failure.[13] Bacteremia, septic shock, acute renal failure, and acute respiratory failure are all more prevalent in *Klebsiella* liver abscess compared with other pyogenic liver abscesses.[21]

Klebsiella liver abscesses are also potentially complicated by endophthalmitis or meningitis in 10% to 45% of patients. Diabetic patients and those with *Klebsiella* abscesses greater than 5 cm are at especially high risk for extrahepatic involvement. Patients with endophthalmitis develop severe vision loss that does not improve despite appropriate intravenous and intravitreous antibiotic treatment.[21]

Rhabdomyolysis is a rare complication of pyogenic liver abscess.[22]

Outcome and Prognosis

The mean hospital stay for pyogenic liver abscess is 13.6 days, and the average duration of antibiotics is 35 days.[43] In a cross-sectional study that examined the trends of pyogenic abscess over two 20-year periods, the mortality decreased over time from 65% (1952–1972) to 31% (1973–1992).[8] Part of this downward trend is attributable to the ability to perform image-guided percutaneous drainage. This study found that the mortality was 100% with antibiotic treatment alone in the earlier time period (1952–1972). In the later time period (1973–1992), patients were treated with antibiotics plus drainage, contributing to a downward mortality trend.[8]

In more recent studies, the in-hospital mortality for pyogenic liver abscess ranges from 2.5% to 19% and varies by region.[2] In an US series, the in-hospital mortality was 5.6%,[7] in a French series 8.7%,[47] and in 2 British series it varied from 2.3%[48] to 11%.[49] In a Taiwanese study, hospitalization for pyogenic liver abscess was associated with a 15% case fatality rate.[50]

The mortality is higher in immunocompromised and elderly patient populations. Studies have found that patients presenting with bacteremia, septic shock, cirrhosis, renal failure, or cancer also have a higher mortality.[12] Multiple abscesses, associated malignancy, jaundice, hypoalbuminemia, leukocytosis, bacteremia, and any significant complications are associated with increased mortality.[8]

Recurrence of liver abscess is more frequent and the mortality is higher in patients with abscesses of biliary origin compared with other causes.[2] Mortality is increased in *Klebsiella* liver abscesses complicated by extrahepatic infectious spread (mortality without infectious spread is 0%–1.1% and 16%–17%[21] in cases with extrahepatic manifestations).

AMEBIC LIVER ABSCESS
General Principles

Classification
The causative microorganism for amebic liver abscess is *E histolytica*, which is spread fecal-orally. The protozoa first cause colitis, which allows invasion into the blood stream and then spreading to the liver via the portal vein.[51]

Epidemiology
Incidence Although in Western countries around 80% of hepatic abscesses are bacterial, in other parts of the world amebic liver abscesses are more common than bacterial.[1] The World Health Organization estimates that amebic liver abscess accounts for 50 million infections and 100,000 deaths worldwide.[51] The regions with the highest prevalence are India, Mexico, and countries in Central/South America and Africa.[1] Amebic liver abscess is the most frequent extraintestinal complication of *E histolytica* and can occur years after initial enteric infection.[52] Only about 2% to 5% of patients with intestinal amebiasis develop liver abscesses.[53]

The incidence of amebic liver abscesses is highest among men aged 18 to 50 years. Although *E histolytica* infection is more common in women and children, it remains as either asymptomatic colonization or enteric amebiasis causing diarrhea. In contrast, GI infections with *E histolytica* are less common in adult men, but amebic liver abscesses are more likely to form in men. Amebic liver abscesses are 10 times more prevalent in men (male to female ratio of 21:1 in one series).[54] The gender difference is hypothesized to be caused by hormonal effects and/or increased alcohol (fermented drinks) use in men. In one mouse model, testosterone increased host susceptibility to E histolytica by reducing secretion of interferon gamma by natural killer cells.[55] Many studies have found a close relationship between alcohol and development of amebic liver abscess. In an Indian case series, 72% of patients with amebic liver abscess were alcoholics. In the same series, alcoholics were more likely to have larger abscesses, more complications, and delayed resolution of abscess.[54] The correlation of amebic liver abscess in alcoholics is thought to be multifactorial. It is likely that locally, contaminated brewed beverages deliver large infective doses of E histolytica. In addition, alcohol induces liver dysfunction and can suppress the immune system both as a direct effect of alcohol and as a source of malnutrition.[54]

Pathophysiology

For amebic liver abscess, the causative parasite is E histolytica, which is spread via fecal-oral transmission.[52,53] There are 2 stages in the life cycle of E histolytica: the cyst and the trophozoite. The cystic stage is the infective state and the trophozoite stage is the invasive state.[56] The cysts are ingested when the host drinks contaminated water and they travel into the small intestine where they undergo excystation (Fig. 3). They then become motile trophozoites, which can invade the intestinal mucosa. In 90% of infections, E histolytica colonizes the lumen and causes asymptomatic, noninvasive disease. In the other 10% of cases, the trophozoite invades the GI tract, causing diarrhea, colitis, or rarely liver abscesses.[51]

Most E histolytica ingestion results in asymptomatic colonization, in which the trophozoite remains in the intestinal mucin layer and feeds on resident bacteria. However, in invasive E histolytica, the trophozoite adheres to the colonic epithelium and lyses intestinal cells, causing mucosal ulcerations and microabscesses. Most cases of invasive E histolytica remain diarrheal illnesses from colonic inflammation.[33,56]

Extraintestinal amebiasis occurs after E histolytica has invaded the intestinal mucosa and subsequently enters the bloodstream. The usual sites of extraintestinal amebiasis are the liver and brain.[56] E histolytica travels through the portal vasculature to the liver, where the protozoa cause inflammation and subsequently leukocyte and macrophage lysis. This process then leads to liver necrosis and amebic abscess formation.[51] Creating chronic liver inflammation is key to the formation of amebic liver abscesses. In one study, leukopenic hamsters without inflammatory cells were inoculated with E histolytica trophozoites and the amebas were cleared from the parenchyma without producing liver abscesses.[57]

It is not clear why some E histolytica cyst ingestions lead to asymptomatic colonization, whereas in other hosts it can cause invasive diarrhea, and in still others amebic liver abscess. The spectrum of infection is likely caused by an interplay of parasite virulence factors and host factors. The parasite factors that seem to be related to virulence are the surface lectins that bind intestinal mucin, the pore-forming peptides that allow the killing of host cells, and proteases that lyse host extracellular matrix.[51,56] The most likely host factors that contribute to invasive E histolytica infections involve polymorphisms in leptin receptor; malnutrition; and the host microbiota, which interacts with the E histolytica in the GI tract and likely affects the host immunity.[56]

Risk factors

The main risk factor for amebic liver disease is poor sanitation, because the ameba is usually ingested via contaminated food or water. It can be transmitted by oral and anal

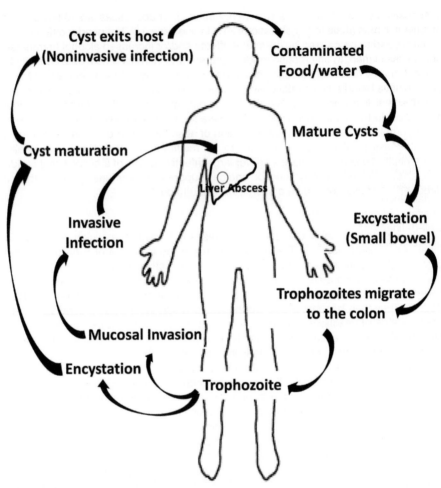

Fig. 3. Life cycle of *E histolytica*.

sex, so *E histolytica* infection is also seen in men who have sex with men.[53] Invasive amebiasis predominantly affects men, which is thought to be related to gender-associated hormones and/or the effect of X chromosome genes on the host immune system.[57]

Diagnosis

Clinical presentation

For patients with amebic liver abscess, 80% develop symptoms of fever and right upper quadrant pain within 2 to 4 weeks of abscess formation and 10% to 35% experience concomitant GI symptoms such as diarrhea.[53] Amebic liver abscess can develop years after infection with *E histolytica* infection, so searching thoroughly for a travel history is important, in particular if the patient is not living in an endemic region.[53] Physical examination reveals right upper quadrant pain, hepatomegaly, and fever. When there is pleuropulmonary involvement, amebic liver abscesses can be associated with cough, right lower lung dullness, or crackles in the right lung.[5] Occasionally patients are jaundiced, depending on the location of abscess.[1]

Laboratory

In amebic liver abscess, serologic testing for *E histolytica* can be performed, although antibody levels remain high for years after infection. Serologies are only helpful in regions where *E histolytica* is not endemic.[11,43] Serum antigen detection has a sensitivity of more than 95%. Indirect hemagglutination carries a sensitivity of 70% to 80% in acute disease and 90% in the chronic, convalescent state. The serology can be falsely negative in the first week of infection. Stool microscopy has a low sensitivity (10%–40%).[53]

Radiology

The diagnosis of amebic abscess relies on imaging because the clinical presentation and laboratories are nonspecific. For amebic liver disease, US is the best modality for diagnosis. Sonographic features include a rounded, homogeneous, hypoechoic lesion usually located near the liver capsule.[11] CT imaging is better in the initial phases of abscess formation but can be equivocal in later phases.[1] CT shows a rounded, well-defined hypodense lesion and is often difficult to distinguish from pyogenic liver abscess radiographically[11] (**Fig. 4**). MRI can also be used.[11]

Treatment

Medical

Amebic liver abscess should be treated with metronidazole 500 mg to 750 mg by mouth 3 times a day for 7 to 10 days.[5] Tinidazole and ornidazole are alternative medications of the same class that can also be used. Patients with amebic liver abscesses continue to have amebas in the intestinal lumen in 40% to 60% of cases, so it is recommended to treat any patient with amebic liver abscess for enteric amebiasis. Treatment regimens include paromomycin 500 mg 3 times a day for 7 days, iodoquinol 650 mg 3 times a day for 20 days, or tiliquinol-tilbroquinol 2 capsules twice a day for 10 days.[5]

Drainage

Up to 15% of amebic liver abscesses fail medical treatment with antibiotics alone. Catheter drainage should be performed if there is no clinical improvement after 5 to 7 days of metronidazole treatment. Percutaneous drainage is also indicated if the abscess is larger than 10 cm, subcapsular, close to rupture, or superinfected with

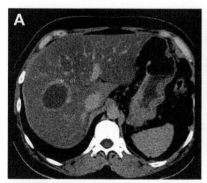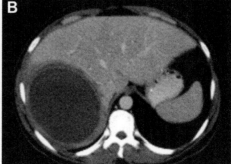

Fig. 4. Amebic liver abscess A) Amebic liver abscess in segment 8 with a thick, hypervascular capsule and diffuse increase in density in the adjacent parenchyma. B) Amebic liver abscess in segment 7 and 8 with a thick capsule and a hypodense halo. (*Courtesy of* Jorge Patricio Campos Lara, MD, Puebla, México; with permission.)

bacteria.[52] Abscesses greater than 5 cm in the left lobe should be drained because they can rupture into the pericardium.[5,52] Percutaneous catheter drainage is superior to aspiration, with higher success rate and quicker resolution.[39]

Surgical

There is a limited role, if any, for surgical management of amebic abscesses because they respond well to imidazoles and in most cases resolve without need for further intervention. Surgery would only be indicated to treat a complication of amebic abscess, such as in the case of an abscess rupture.[1,5]

Complications

Amebic liver abscesses, if untreated, rupture to nearby organs, such as the pleura, peritoneum, pericardium, biliary tract, or bronchus, causing infection of those organ systems.[1,11] Bacterial superinfection of amebic abscess occurs in 0% to 4% of cases.[33]

Outcome/Prognosis

For amebic abscesses, the prognosis is excellent.[5,52,53] Amebic liver abscesses are very sensitive to antimicrobial medical therapy. Only complicated cases require drainage for resolution. In one cross-sectional study of hospital admissions with amebic liver abscesses, the mean hospital stay was 7.7 days and the patients were on antibiotics for average of 11.8 days. All patients in this series were cured.[43] Because of the effectiveness of medical treatment of amebic liver abscesses, the mortality is as low as 1% to 3%.[52]

DISCLOSURE

The authors have nothing to disclose.

REFERENCES

1. Lardière-Deguelte S, Ragot E, Amroun K, et al. Hepatic abscess: Diagnosis and management. J Visc Surg 2015;152(4):231–43.
2. Akhondi H, Sabih DE. Liver abscess. StatPearls; 2019. p. 1–7.
3. Liu L, Chen W, Lu X, et al. Pyogenic liver abscess: a retrospective study of 105 cases in an Emergency Department from East China. J Emerg Med 2017; 52(4):409–16.
4. Kong H, Yu F, Zhang W, et al. Clinical and microbiological characteristics of pyogenic liver abscess in a tertiary hospital in East China. Medicine (Baltimore) 2017; 96(37):1–5, e8050.
5. Lübbert C, Wieggand J, Karlas T. Therapy of Liver Abscesses. Vizeralmedizin 2014;30:334–41.
6. Cerwenka H. Pyogenic liver abscess: differences in etiology and treatment in Southeast Asia and central Europe. World J Gastroenterol 2010;16(20):2458–62.
7. Meddings L, Myers RP, Hubbard J, et al. A population-based study of pyogenic liver abscesses in the united states: Incidence, mortality, and temporal trends. Am J Gastroenterol 2010;105(1):117–24.
8. Huang CJ, Pitt HA, Lipsett PA, et al. Pyogenic hepatic abscess: changing trends over 42 years. Ann Surg 1996;223(5):600–9.
9. Qian Y, Wong CC, Lai S, et al. A retrospective study of pyogenic liver abscess focusing on Klebsiella pneumoniae as a primary pathogen in China from 1994 to 2015. Sci Rep 2016;6:1–12.

10. Mohsen AH, Green ST, Read RC, et al. Liver abscess in adults: Ten years experience in a UK centre. QJM 2002;95(12):797–802.
11. Kurland JE, Brann OS. Pyogenic and amebic liver abscesses. Curr Gastroenterol Rep 2004;6(4):273–9.
12. Webb GJ, Chapman TP, Cadman PJ, et al. Pyogenic liver abscess. Frontline Gastroenterol 2014;5:60–7.
13. Pang TCY, Fung T, Samra J, et al. Pyogenic liver abscess: an audit of 10 years' experience. World J Gastroenterol 2011;17(12):1622–30.
14. Jayasimhan D, Wu L, Huggan P. Fusobacterial liver abscess: a case report and review of the literature. BMC Infect Dis 2017;17(1):1–9.
15. Kajiya T, Uemura T, Kajiya M, et al. Pyogenic liver abscess related to dental disease in an immunocompetent host. Intern Med 2008;47(7):675–8.
16. Rahimian J, Wilson T, Oram V, et al. Pyogenic liver abscess: recent trends in etiology and mortality. Clin Infect Dis 2004;39(11):1654–9.
17. Kaplan GG, Gregson DB, Laupland KB. Population-based study of the epidemiology of and the risk factors for pyogenic liver abscess. Clin Gastroenterol Hepatol 2004;2(11):1032–8.
18. Jepsen P, Vilstrup H, Schønheyder HC, et al. A nationwide study of the incidence and 30-day mortality rate of pyogenic liver abscess in Denmark, 1977-2002. Aliment Pharmacol Ther 2005;21:1185–8.
19. Tian LT, Yao K, Zhang XY, et al. Liver abscesses in adult patients with and without diabetes mellitus: an analysis of the clinical characteristics, features of the causative pathogens, outcomes and predictors of fatality: a report based on a large population, retrospective study in China. Clin Microbiol Infect 2012;18:E314–30.
20. Tsai FC, Huang YT, Chang LY, et al. Pyogenic liver abscess as endemic disease, Taiwan. Emerg Infect Dis 2008;14(10):1592–600.
21. Liu Y, Wang J, Jiang W. An increasing prominent disease of klebsiella pneumoniae liver abscess: etiology, diagnosis, and treatment. Gastroenterol Res Pract 2013;2013:1–12.
22. Deng L, Jia R, Li W, et al. A Klebsiella pneumoniae liver abscess presenting with myasthenia and tea-colored urine. Medicine (Baltimore) 2017;96(51):1–4.
23. Luo M, Yang XX, Tan B, et al. Distribution of common pathogens in patients with pyogenic liver abscess in China: a meta-analysis. Eur J Clin Microbiol Infect Dis 2016;35(10):1557–65.
24. Lee NK, Kim S, Lee JW, et al. CT differentiation of pyogenic liver abscesses caused by Klebsiella pneumoniae vs non-Klebsiella pneumoniae. Br J Radiol 2011;84(1002):518–25.
25. Zhu X, Wang S, Jacob R, et al. A 10-year retrospective analysis of clinical profiles, laboratory characteristics and management of pyogenic liver abscesses in a Chinese hospital. Gut Liver 2011;5(2):221–7.
26. Mazza OM, de Santibanes M, De Santibañes E. Pyogenic liver abscess. In: Blumgart's surgery of the liver, biliary tract and pancreas. 2017.
27. Woo S, Chung JW, Hur S, et al. Liver abscess after transarterial chemoembolization in patients with bilioenteric anastomosis: Frequency and risk factors. Am J Roentgenol 2013;200(6):1370–7.
28. Livraghi T, Solbiati L, Meloni MF, et al. Treatment of focal liver tumors with percutaneous radio-frequency ablation: complications encountered in a multicenter study. Radiology 2003;226(2):441–51.
29. Hsieh C-H, Chen R-J, Fang J-F, et al. Liver abscess after non-operative management of blunt liver injury. Langenbecks Arch Surg 2003;387(9–10):343–7.

30. Gaujoux S, Sauvanet A, Vullierme MP, et al. Ischemic complications after pancreaticoduodenectomy: Incidence, prevention, and management. Ann Surg 2009;249(1):111–7.
31. Yeo CJ, Cameron JL, Sohn TA, et al. Six Hundred Fifty Consecutive Pancreaticoduodenectomies in the 1990s. Ann Surg 1997;226(3):248–60.
32. Reid-Lombardo KM, Khan S, Sclabas G. Hepatic cysts and liver abscess. Surg Clin North Am 2010;90(4):679–97.
33. Lambertucci JR, Rayes AA, Serufo JC, et al. Pyogenic abscesses and parasitic diseases. Rev Inst Med Trop Sao Paulo 2001;43(2):67–74.
34. Santos SA, Alberto SCF, Cruz E, et al. Hepatic abscess induced by foreign body: case report and literature review. World J Gastroenterol 2007;13(9):1466–70.
35. Chung YFA, Tan YM, Lui HF, et al. Management of pyogenic liver abscesses-percutaneous or open drainage? Singapore Med J 2007;48(12):1158–65.
36. Heneghan HM, Healy NA, Martin ST, et al. Modern management of pyogenic hepatic abscess: a case series and review of the literature. BMC Res Notes 2011; 4(80):1–8.
37. Yu SCH, Ho SSM, Lau WY, et al. Treatment of pyogenic liver abscess: prospective randomized comparison of catheter drainage and needle aspiration. Hepatology 2004;39(4):932–8.
38. Alvarez Pérez JA, González JJ, Baldonedo RF, et al. Clinical course, treatment, and multivariate analysis of risk factors for pyogenic liver abscess. Am J Surg 2001;181(2):177–86.
39. Waghmare M, Shah H, Tiwari C, et al. Management of liver abscess in children: our experience. Euroasian J Hepatogastroenterol 2017;7(1):23–6.
40. Qu K, Liu C, Wang ZX, et al. Pyogenic liver abscesses associated with nonmetastatic colorectal cancers: an increasing problem in Eastern Asia. World J Gastroenterol 2012;18(23):2948–55.
41. Hope WW, Vrochides DV, Newcomb WL, et al. Optimal treatment of hepatic abscess. Am Surg 2008;74(2):178–82.
42. Bamberger DM. Outcome of medical treatment of bacterial abscesses without therapeutic drainage: review of cases reported in the literature. Clin Infect Dis 1996;23(3):592–603.
43. Abbas MT, Khan FY, Muhsin SA, et al. Epidemiology, clinical features and outcome of liver abscess: a single reference center experience in Qatar. Oman Med J 2014;29(4):260–3.
44. Zerem E, Hadzic A. Sonographically guided percutaneous catheter drainage versus needle aspiration in the management of pyogenic liver abscess. Am J Roentgenol 2007;189:138–42.
45. Rajak C, Gupta S, Jain S, et al. Percutaneous treatment of liver abscesses: needle aspiration versus catheter drainage. Am J Roentgenol 1998;170:1035–9.
46. Andersson R, Bengmark S, Forsberg L, et al. Percutaneous management of pyogenic hepatic abscesses. HPB Surg 1990;2:185–8.
47. Alkofer B, Dufay C, Parienti JJ, et al. Are pyogenic liver abscesses still a surgical concern? a western experience. HPB Surg 2012;2012:1–7.
48. Pearce NW, Knight R, Irving H, et al. Non-operative management of pyogenic liver abscess. HPB (Oxford) 2003;5(2):91–5.
49. Bosanko NC, Chauhan A, Brookes M, et al. Presentations of pyogenic liver abscess in one UK centre over a 15-year period. J R Coll Physicians Edinb 2011; 41(1):13–7.

50. Kuo SH, Lee YT, Li CR, et al. Mortality in Emergency Department Sepsis score as a prognostic indicator in patients with pyogenic liver abscess. Am J Emerg Med 2013;31(6):916–21.
51. Begum S, Quach J, Chadee K. Immune evasion mechanisms of Entamoeba histolytica: Progression to disease. Front Microbiol 2015;6:1–8.
52. Stanley S. Amoebiasis. Lancet 2003;361:1025–34.
53. Prakash V, Oliver T. Amebic liver abscess (ALA). StatPearls; 2019.
54. Kumanan T, Sujanitha V, Balakumar S, et al. Amoebic liver abscess and indigenous alcoholic beverages in the tropics. J Trop Med 2018;2018:1–6.
55. Lotter H, Helk E, Bernin H, et al. Testosterone increases susceptibility to amebic liver abscess in mice and mediates inhibition of IFNγ secretion in natural killer T cells. PLoS One 2013;8(2):1–10.
56. Burgess SL, Petri WA. The intestinal bacterial microbiome and E. histolytica infection. Curr Trop Med Rep 2016;3:71–4.
57. Campos-Rodríguez R, Gutiérrez-Meza M, Jarillo-Luna RA, et al. A review of the proposed role of neutrophils in rodent amebic liver abscess models. Parasite 2016;23:1–14.

Fungal and Parasitic Infections of the Liver

Sirina Ekpanyapong, MD[a], K. Rajender Reddy, MD[b],*

KEYWORDS

• Fungi • Parasites • Protozoa • Helminths • Immunocompromised

KEY POINTS

- Hepatosplenic candidiasis and other fungal infections of the liver are not common in healthy individuals; however, high index of suspicion is essential in immunocompromised patients with prolonged fever.
- Parasitic infections of the liver include both protozoan and helminthic infections. The distribution and epidemiology of the infections is variable among different geographic regions of the world.
- Clonorchiasis, opisthorchiasis, fascioliasis, and ascariasis are helminthic infections that commonly involve the biliary systems. Signs and symptoms of cholangitis require prompt management with endoscopic retrograde cholangiopancreatography to relieve biliary obstruction and the addition of antihelminthic agents is essential.
- Parasitic infections of the liver are mostly transmitted to humans by fecally contaminated food and water. Proper hand and food sanitation measures are essential in preventing disease transmission.

INTRODUCTION

Nonviral infections of the liver can have a variety of clinical presentations that include asymptomatic hepatic biochemical test abnormalities, symptomatic hepatitis, and space-occupying lesions. Fungal infections predominantly occur in immunocompromised patients and commonly present with disseminated patterns,[1] whereas parasitic infections can infect healthy individuals depending on sanitary conditions and the prevalence of such infections in various geographic regions of the world. Biliary parasites may cause symptoms of biliary obstruction, cholecystitis, cholangitis, and pancreatitis.[2] Diagnosis requires a high index of suspicion

---

[a] Department of Medicine, Division of Gastroenterology and Hepatology, University of Pennsylvania, Philadelphia, PA, USA; [b] Department of Medicine, Division of Gastroenterology and Hepatology, University of Pennsylvania, 2 Dulles, 3400 Spruce Street, HUP, Philadelphia, PA 19104, USA
* Corresponding author.
E-mail address: reddyr@pennmedicine.upenn.edu

Gastroenterol Clin N Am 49 (2020) 379–410
https://doi.org/10.1016/j.gtc.2020.01.009
0889-8553/20/© 2020 Elsevier Inc. All rights reserved.

Table 1
Fungal infections of the liver

Etiology	Risk Factors	Pathophysiology	Manifestations	Treatment
Hepatosplenic candidiasis				
Candida albicans, Candida tropicalis, Candida parapsilosis, Candida glabrata, and *Candida krusei*	• Neutropenic patients • Patients receiving immunosuppressive agents and corticosteroids • Patients in intensive care units (ICUs) • AIDS	*Candida* that colonizes in the gastrointestinal tract (also skin and genitourinary tract) can access the bloodstream, especially in a neutropenic host with gut mucosa disruption due to chemotherapy. Via hematogenous spread, it can produce microabscesses in many organs, including liver and spleen.	• High-spiking fever • Right upper quadrant abdominal pain, nausea, vomiting • CT/MRI imaging shows multiple microabscesses in the liver and spleen	• Lipid formulation amphotericin B (3–5 mg/kg IV daily) or • Echinocandin, such as caspofungin (70 mg loading dose then 50 mg IV daily), anidulafungin (200 mg loading dose then 100 mg IV daily), or micafungin (100 mg IV daily) for several weeks • Followed by a step-down with oral fluconazole 400 mg daily (patients with fluconazole-resistant strains or those with *C glabrata* or *C krusei*, a recommendation is either of voriconazole or posaconazole).

Disseminated cryptococcosis

| Cryptococcus neoformans | • Opportunistic infection in patients with AIDS
• Organ transplant patients
• Patients receiving corticosteroid treatment
• Elderly, diabetes mellitus, renal failure | • Inhaled organism can be localized in the lungs in normal host, but can cause pulmonary infection and disseminate to other organs in immunosuppressed host | • Meningoencephalitis is the most common presentation
• Pulmonary infection
• Skin lesions
• Hepatomegaly | HIV with meningoencephalitis
• *Induction therapy:* amphotericin B deoxycholate (0.7–1.0 mg/kg/d) plus flucytosine (100 mg/kg/d) for 2 wk or amphotericin B deoxycholate (0.7–1.0 mg/kg/d) or liposomal amphotericin B (3–4 mg/kg/d) or amphotericin B lipid complex (5 mg/kg/d) for 4–6 wk
• *Consolidation therapy:* fluconazole (400 mg/d) 8 wk
• *Maintenance therapy:* fluconazole (200 mg/d) ≥1 y
Non-HIV with meningoencephalitis
• *Induction therapy:* amphotericin B deoxycholate (0.7–1.0 mg/kg/d) plus flucytosine (100 mg/kg/d) ≥4 wk or amphotericin B deoxycholate (0.7–1.0 mg/kg/d) ≥6 wk
• *Consolidation therapy:* fluconazole (400–800 mg/d) 8 wk |

(continued on next page)

Table 1
(continued)

Etiology	Risk Factors	Pathophysiology	Manifestations	Treatment
				Maintenance therapy: fluconazole (200 mg/d) 6–12 mo Nonmeningeal cryptococcosis • Fluconazole 400 mg/d for 6–12 mo in nonsevere patients
Disseminated histoplasmosis				
Histoplasma capsulatum	• Opportunistic infection in patients with AIDS • Patients with hematologic malignancy • Organ transplant patients • Patients receiving corticosteroid treatment or tumor necrosis factor antagonists • Elderly	• Infected patients inhale organism into lungs (most cases are subclinical) • In immunosuppressed host, this can cause disseminated infection to other organs	• Hepatosplenomegaly • High-grade fever and lymphadenopathy • Pulmonary infection • Weight loss • Skin lesions	Progressive disseminated histoplasmosis Moderately severe to severe: • Liposomal amphotericin B (3.0 mg/kg/d), amphotericin B lipid complex (5.0 mg/kg/d), or deoxycholate amphotericin B (0.7–1.0 mg/kg/d) for 1–2 wk • Followed by oral itraconazole (200 mg twice daily for ≥12 mo) Mild to moderate: • Oral itraconazole (200 mg twice daily for ≥12 mo)

Abbreviations: CT, computed tomography; HIV, human immunodeficiency virus; IV, intravenous.
Data from Refs.[4,8,105,106]

Table 2
Parasitic infections of the liver

Etiology	Risk Factors	Pathophysiology	Endemic Areas	Manifestations	Diagnosis	Treatment
Protozoa						
Amebiasis (*Entamoeba histolytica*)	Male gender, alcohol intake, HLA-DR3, oral and anal sex, and poor sanitation	Ingested cysts develop into invasive trophozoites that colonize in colon and can spread to the liver by the portal system	Worldwide	Fever, RUQ pain, leukocytosis without eosinophilia, liver abscess formation	• Imaging • Serology (eg, ELISA, IHA) • Stool antigen test	• Metronidazole (500–750 mg PO TID × 7–10 d) or tinidazole (2 g daily × 3 d) • Followed by Iodoquinol (650 mg PO TID × 20 d) or paromomycin (25–30 mg/kg PO daily in 3 divided doses × 7 d) or diloxanide furoate (500 mg PO TID × 10 d) to eradicate intestinal colonization
Toxoplasmosis (*Toxoplasma gondii*)	Ingestion of undercooked meat or contact with contaminated soil	• Ingestion of oocysts in contaminated soil or water or in infected meat • Systemic spread of tachyzoites in the circulation • Replication in the liver leads to inflammation	Worldwide	• Immuno-competent: asymptomatic or hepatomegaly or mild hepatic biochemical test elevations • Immuno-compromised: occasional overt hepatitis	• Serology (IFA, ELISA) • Isolation from tissue organism	• Pyrimethamine 100 mg loading then 25–50 mg/d plus • Sulfadiazine 2–4 g/d in 4 divided doses or clindamycin 300 mg 4 times daily, plus • Folinic acid 10–25 mg daily for 2–4 wk

(continued on next page)

Table 2
(continued)

Etiology	Risk Factors	Pathophysiology	Endemic Areas	Manifestations	Diagnosis	Treatment
Leishmaniasis *(Leishmania donovani)*	Children and immuno-compromised adults who have contact with sand flies	Sand fly bite transmits promastigotes and they proliferate in the RE system	Worldwide	• Fever, weight loss • Hepatospl-enomegaly months to years after infection • Skin lesions	• Amasti-gotes seen in the spleen, l iver, bone marrow by histopa-thology and culture • Molecular techniques by PCR • Serology (IFA, ELISA)	• Pentavalent antimonial 20 mg/kg/d × 28 d; or liposomal amphotericin B (IV) 3 mg/kg/d on days 1–5, 14, and 21; or miltefosine 2.5 mg/kg/d × 28 d • Alternative drugs: paromomycin, pentamidine isethionate

| Malaria (Plasmodium species) | Mosquito (Anopheles) bites | Mosquito (Anopheles) bite transmits sporozoites | Africa, Asia, South America | Proliferation in hepatocytes causes hepatomegaly, hepatic biochemical test elevations, and jaundice | Identification of the parasite on a blood smear | • *Plasmodium falciparum:* *Chloroquine-resistant* Atovaquone-proguanil, artemether-lumefantrine, quinine sulfate plus doxycycline or tetracycline or clindamycin, mefloquine *Chloroquine-sensitive* Chloroquine phosphate, hydroxychloroquine
• *Plasmodium malariae, Plasmodium knowlesi:* Chloroquine phosphate or hydroxychloroquine
• *Plasmodium vivax, Plasmodium ovale:* Chloroquine phosphate or hydroxychloroquine plus primaquine phosphate
• *P vivax:* *Chloroquine-resistant* Quinine sulfate plus either doxycycline or tetracycline plus primaquine phosphate, artemether-lumefantrine plus primaquine phosphate, atovaquone-proguanil plus primaquine phosphate, mefloquine plus primaquine phosphate |

(continued on next page)

Table 2
(continued)

Etiology	Risk Factors	Pathophysiology	Endemic Areas	Manifestations	Diagnosis	Treatment
Cryptosporidiosis and Microsporidiosis	AIDS	Ingested cysts develop into trophozoites in intestinal mucosa	Worldwide	• Biliary tract obstruction and cholangitis • Diarrhea	Cryptosporidiosis: • Modified AFB, PCR, EIA, serology (ELISA, IFA) in stool, duodenal aspirate, bile secretion, biopsy specimens Microsporidiosis: • Modified trichrome stain, electron microscopy, PCR, serology (IFA) in stool, body fluid, tissue specimens	Cryptosporidiosis: • Nitazoxanide 500–1000 mg bid for 2–8 wk • HAART therapy Microsporidiosis: • Albendazole 400 mg bid for 14–28 d or until CD4>200 cells/μL for >6 mo • HAART therapy

Disease	Risk factors/Exposure	Transmission/Life cycle	Geographic distribution	Clinical features	Diagnosis	Treatment
Babesiosis (Babesia microti)	• Asplenia is a risk factor for hepatic failure • Exposure to deer tick	Tick bite transmits the agent, which infect red blood cells	Europe, America, Asia	• Fever • Elevated hepatic biochemical tests • Hemolysis, anemia • Diarrhea • Hepatosplenomegaly	Identification of the parasite from blood smear, PCR, serology	• Azithromycin 500–1000 mg orally on day 1, then 250–1000 mg daily and atovaquone 750 mg BID × 7–10 d • Alternative drugs: clindamycin 600 mg orally every 8 h and quinine 650 mg orally every 8 h × 7–10 d
Helminths: Nematodes						
Ascariasis (Ascaris lumbricoides)	Consumption of eggs that are fecally contaminated in food or water	• Ingested eggs develop into larvae • Larvae migrate to the lungs and are coughed then swallowed and develop into roundworms in the small intestine • Adult worms can invade into bile ducts	Global distribution with high prevalence in tropical countries	• Pulmonary phase presents with asthma-like symptoms, chest pain, or hemoptysis • Intestinal phase presents with nutritional impairment, hepatomegaly, cholangitis, or obstructive jaundice	• Stool examination • Imaging: "bull's-eye" appearance on cross-sectional imaging • ERCP: adult worms in the common bile duct	Albendazole 400 mg orally single dose
Toxocariasis (Toxocara canis, Toxocara cati)	Consumption of eggs in soil-contaminated food	After ingestion of soil contaminated with dog or cat feces, larvae disseminate throughout the body and to the liver causing visceral larva migrans	Highest prevalence in southeastern United States	• Asymptomatic • Hepatomegaly • Granuloma formation with eosinophilia	• Serology: ELISA • Imaging studies • Larvae in tissue	• Albendazole 400 mg orally twice daily × 5 d or • Mebendazole 100–200 mg orally twice daily × 5 d

(continued on next page)

Table 2
(continued)

Etiology	Risk Factors	Pathophysiology	Endemic Areas	Manifestations	Diagnosis	Treatment
Hepatic capillariasis (*Capillaria hepatica*)	Ingestion of food contaminated with rodent feces	• Ingested eggs develop into larvae in the intestinal mucosa • Larvae migrate to the liver by portal blood flow	Human infection is rare	• Fever, eosinophilia, and hepatomegaly • Foci of liver fibrosis, granulomas, and calcification	• Adult worms or eggs in the liver biopsy specimen • Serology: ELISA, IFA	• Mebendazole 200 mg orally twice daily × 20 d or • Albendazole 400 mg orally once daily × 10 d
Strongyloidiasis (*Strongyloides stercoralis*)	Ingestion of food contaminated with soil-containing eggs, in immunocompromised individuals	• Ingested eggs develop into larvae that invade the hepatic vasculature, lymphatics, and biliary tract	Tropical and subtropical areas especially in Southeast America, Southern and Eastern Europe	• Hepatomegaly, jaundice, abdominal pain • Diarrhea, cough • Eosinophilia is uncommon	• Larvae in the stool or duodenal aspirate • Serology: ELISA, IFA	• Ivermectin 200 µg/kg/d orally × 2 d or • Albendazole 400 mg orally twice daily × 7 d

Helminths: Trematodes

| Schistosomiasis (Schistosoma mansoni, Schistosoma japonicum, Schistosoma mekongi, Schistosoma haematobium) | Contact with fresh water containing cercaria of schistosomes | • Cercaria in fresh water penetrate the skin, migrate by the circulation to portal vein
• Host immune response to eggs in the portal vein | • S mansoni found in South America, Africa, and Middle East
• S haematobium found in Africa, and Middle East
• S japonicum found in East Asia
• S mekongi found along the Mekong River in Laos and Cambodia | • Acute: itching, fever, chills, myalgia
• Chronic: presinusoidal portal hypertension, ruptured esophageal varices, periportal fibrosis, splenomegaly | • Eosinophilia is common
• Imaging: extensive calcification, "turtleback" appearance along portal tracts
• Microscopic examination of ova in the stool
• Serology: seroconversion occurs within 4–6 wk (ELISA, IHA, RIA)
• Antigen detection in blood, urine, stool
• Molecular test: PCR in stool, urine, serum
• Rectal or liver biopsy | • S. haematobium, S. mansoni: Praziquantel 40 mg/kg/d orally in 2 divided doses for 1 day
• S. japonicum, S. mekongi: Praziquantel 60 mg/kg/d orally in 3 divided doses for 1 day
• Repeated dose at 2–4 wk later if necessary |

(continued on next page)

Table 2
(continued)

Etiology	Risk Factors	Pathophysiology	Endemic Areas	Manifestations	Diagnosis	Treatment
Fascioliasis (*Fasciola hepatica*)	Ingestion of contaminated freshwater or aquatic plants	• Ingested cysts • The leaf-shaped fluke excysts in the duodenum, migrates through the bowel wall into peritoneal cavity, burrows into the liver, and then penetrates into the bile ducts • Adult flukes live in the large bile ducts	Worldwide	• Acute: fever, abdominal pain, eosinophilia, jaundice • Chronic: symptomatic biliary obstruction, hepatomegaly • Often leukocytosis, hypergammaglobulinemia	• Ova in the stool, duodenal aspirates, or bile specimens • Serology: IHA, complement fixation, ELISA, CIE, IFA • Imaging: CT hypodense nodules or tortuous tracks, thickening of liver capsule, or parenchymal calcifications may be seen • ERCP: Adult flukes in the bile ducts	Triclabendazole 10 mg/kg orally once or twice

| Opistho-rchiasis and Clonorchiasis (Opisthorchis viverrini, Clonorchis sinensis) | Ingestion of contaminated raw freshwater fish | • Ingested cysts
• The fluke excysts in the duodenum, migrates into the bile ducts via ampulla
• Adult flukes deposit eggs in the bile ducts | • Opisthorchis sp: Southeast Asia, Central and Eastern Europe
• C sinensis: China, Japan, Korea | • Abdominal pain, fever, hepatomegaly, diarrhea, common eosinophilia
• Intermittent biliary obstruction, intrahepatic pigment stones formation, secondary sclerosing cholangitis, cholangioc-arcinoma | • Ova in the stool, duodenal aspirates, or bile specimens
• Serology: ELISA
• ERCP: Adult flukes in the bile ducts | Praziquantel 75 mg/kg/d orally in 3 divided doses per day × 2 d |

(continued on next page)

Table 2
(continued)

Helminths: Cestodes

Etiology	Risk Factors	Pathophysiology	Endemic Areas	Manifestations	Diagnosis	Treatment
Echinococcosis (*Echinococcus granulosus, Echinococcus multilocularis*)	Ingestion of food or water with fecally contaminated eggs from cattle, sheepdogs, foxes	Ingested eggs produce larval oncospheres that migrate to the liver and form cysts in humans (hydatid cysts)	Worldwide	RUQ abdominal pain, hepatomegaly, fever, eosinophilia, occasional cyst rupture, episodes of pruritus	• Imaging showing daughter cysts or peripheral focal calcification • Serology (ELISA, IHA) or antigen assays	• Percutaneous drainage (PAIR) • Albendazole 400 mg PO bid × 1–6 mo • Surgical resection in complicated cysts

Abbreviations: AFB, acid-fast bacilli; AIDS, acquired immune deficiency syndrome; BID, twice a day; CD4, cluster of differentiation 4; CIE, counterimmunoelectrophoresis; CT, computed tomography; EIA, enzyme immunoassay; ELISA, enzyme-linked immunosorbent assay; ERCP, endoscopic retrograde cholangiopancreatography; HAART, highly active antiretroviral therapy; HLA-DR, Human Leukocyte Antigen–DR isotype; IFA, immunofluorescence assay; IHA, indirect hemagglutination; IV, intravenous; LFT, liver function test; PAIR, puncture-aspiration-injection-reaspiration; PCR, polymerase chain reaction; PO, by mouth; RE, reticuloendothelial; RIA, radioimmunoassay; RUQ, right upper quadrant; TID, three times a day.

Data from Centers for Disease Control and Prevention. https://www.cdc.gov/. Accessed March 18th, 2019 *and Reddy KR. Bacterial, Parasitic, Fungal, and Granulomatous Liver Diseases, Goldman-Cecil Medicine. 25th edition. Elsevier Health Sciences, 2019.*

and consideration of endemicity in a particular area. Newer serologic and molecular diagnostic techniques can be helpful for early diagnosis and thereafter initiation of therapy.[3,4]

FUNGAL INFECTIONS OF THE LIVER
Hepatosplenic Candidiasis

Hepatosplenic candidiasis (or chronic disseminated candidiasis) is typically caused by *Candida albicans*, but other species, such as *Candida tropicalis, Candida parapsilosis, Candida glabrata*, and *Candida krusei,* have occasionally been reported.[1,5] It is commonly seen in patients with an immunocompromised state, especially in those with leukemia and undergoing high-dose chemotherapy and have neutropenia or just recovered from severe neutropenia. The pathogenesis is presumably due to translocation of *Candida* species from the gastrointestinal tract into the bloodstream and due to prolonged neutropenia and loss of mucosal integrity. Nowadays, hepatosplenic candidiasis is seen less frequently because of the prophylactic use of antifungal agents and early initiation of antifungal treatment in high-risk neutropenic patients with high-grade fever.

Clinical manifestations

Common manifestations of hepatosplenic candidiasis include persistently high-spiking fevers in a patient who was previously neutropenic.[1] Associated symptoms include right upper quadrant abdominal pain, nausea, vomiting, or anorexia. Patients typically have elevated serum alkaline phosphatase levels, and may have mild elevation of aminotransferases and bilirubin.[6] Contrast-enhanced computed tomography (CT) scan is a sensitive imaging modality for diagnosis and frequently reveals multiple micro abscesses in the liver, spleen, and sometimes in the kidneys[1,7,8] (**Fig. 1**). However, if CT scan does not show typical lesions but there is still a high suspicion for hepatosplenic candidiasis, MRI should be performed because MRI has very high sensitivity at 100% and specificity at 96%.[9] A definitive diagnosis can be made by a liver biopsy, which typically shows multiple granulomas. A negative tissue culture does not rule out the diagnosis. However, liver biopsy is not always performed because of the high risk presented by thrombocytopenia; thus, the diagnosis is often based on clinical suspicion and typical imaging studies.

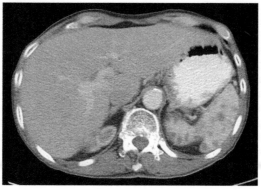

Fig. 1. CT scan of splenic candidiasis. (*Courtesy of* Seksan Chitwiset, MD, Bangkok, Thailand; with permission.)

Therapy

The initial recommendation for antifungal therapy is a lipid formulation of amphotericin B (3–5 mg/kg intravenous [IV] daily) or an echinocandin, such as caspofungin (70 mg loading dose then 50 mg IV daily), anidulafungin (200 mg loading dose then 100 mg IV daily), or micafungin (100 mg IV daily) for several weeks, and followed by a step-down with oral fluconazole at 400 mg daily.[8] The duration of therapy is recommended for it to be continued until the resolution of the lesions on imaging, and it mostly occurs within 6 months.[10] In patients with fluconazole-resistant strains or in those experiencing candidemia due to C glabrata or C krusei, a recommendation for step-down therapy is either voriconazole or posaconazole.[8] Treatment should be continued until the lesions resolve on a follow-up imaging study, after approximately 6 months of treatment. It is advised that high-risk patients (eg, receiving chemotherapy or hematopoietic stem cell transplantation) who have a history of hepatosplenic candidiasis be treated prophylactically with oral fluconazole (400 mg daily) to prevent relapse.

Other Fungi

There are some fungal infections that predominantly infect immunocompromised patients. Hepatic Cryptococcus neoformans is an opportunistic infection in patients with AIDS that usually presents with hepatomegaly. In patients not infected with human immunodeficiency virus (HIV), disseminated cryptococcosis can cause focal granulomatous hepatitis and secondary sclerosing cholangitis.[4] Hepatic histoplasmosis, which is due to Histoplasma capsulatum, is also another opportunistic infection in patients with AIDS. Patients can present with hepatosplenomegaly, high-grade fever, and lymphadenopathy. The liver histology of hepatic histoplasmosis may demonstrate diffuse hepatic granulomas and portal lymphohistiocytic infiltrate.[4] Treatment options include amphotericin B, fluconazole, or itraconazole. Paracoccidioides brasiliensis, which commonly infects male adults, may present with jaundice or hepatomegaly. Hepatic biochemical tests may demonstrate elevated aminotransferase and alkaline phosphatase levels. Liver pathology ranges from small granuloma lesions to diffuse fibrosis and with bile duct involvement (**Table 1**).[4]

PROTOZOAN INFECTION OF THE LIVER
Malaria

Malaria is an infection caused by a protozoa of the genus Plasmodium.[11–13] The disease is transmitted by bites from infected Anopheles mosquitoes, which are frequently found in tropical countries. Sporozoites migrate to the liver via the bloodstream and mature into schizonts. Hypnozoites are as a quiescent stage in the liver, which exist only in Plasmodium vivax and Plasmodium ovale infections. The hepatic schizonts rupture and release merozoites into circulation and infect red blood cells. Within red blood cells, ring forms mature into trophozoites and blood-stage schizonts (erythrocytic stage). Release of merozoites from infected red cells causes fever and the other malarial manifestations. Some parasites differentiate into sexual erythrocytic stages (gametocytes), which are then ingested by an Anopheles mosquito and subsequently transform into zygotes and oocysts and thus completing the malaria life cycle.[11]

Plasmodium falciparum is the most common cause of severe malaria. P vivax is another common species with less disease severity. P ovale and Plasmodium malariae are much less common and generally do not cause severe illness. P vivax and P ovale often have a relapse because they have hypnozoite phase (dormant stage in the liver that may cause relapse weeks to years after initial infection).[14] The recently discovered, Plasmodium knowlesi, a zoonosis from macaque monkeys with symptoms resembling *P malariae*, can be transmitted to humans and especially has been noted in Southeast Asia.[11]

Clinical manifestations

The typical presentations include fever and chills, and symptoms also can be nonspecific, such as malaise, anorexia, nausea and vomiting, myalgia, and diarrhea. Symptoms usually develop 30 to 60 days after exposure. Jaundice can be caused by hemolysis following heavy parasitemia of *P falciparum* infection. Severe malaria is defined when any of the following symptoms related to organ dysfunction occur: impaired consciousness, convulsions, metabolic acidosis, hypoglycemia, severe anemia, bleeding, coagulopathy, renal failure, jaundice, hepatic failure, acute respiratory distress syndrome, shock, or hyperparasitemia (mostly from *P falciparum* and is >10%).[15] *P falciparum* and *P malariae* have no hypnozoite phase and thus do not cause relapse, whereas *P vivax* and *P ovale* may cause relapse months after the primary infection is treated. Diagnosis is often made by detection of parasites by Giemsa-stained blood smears under light microscopy, which can be prepared by both thin or thick smear methods.[16] Thin smears allow for both species identification and parasite density. Thick smears can provide information on parasite density and allow for screening for the presence of parasites.[11] Nowadays, rapid diagnostic tests that detect malaria antigen or antibody can be alternative methods when microscopy is not available in resource-limited endemic settings.[11]

Therapy

Treatment for uncomplicated *P falciparum* malaria is based on whether infection was acquired in an area with chloroquine sensitivity or resistance. In chloroquine-sensitive areas, chloroquine or hydroxychloroquine can be used as the primary regimen. In a chloroquine-resistant area, artemisinin combination therapy, atovaquone-proguanil, quinine plus doxycycline or tetracycline or clindamycin, and mefloquine are therapeutic regimens of choice.[11] For uncomplicated non-falciparum malaria, treatment of *P vivax* and *P ovale* requires eradication of hypnozoites to prevent relapse. Therapy of choice consists of chloroquine or an artemisinin combination therapy, and primaquine is used for prevention of relapse.[15]

Treatment of severe malaria requires parenteral therapy. IV quinine or quinidine has been a standard therapy; however, IV artesunate has demonstrated better efficacy and with less toxicity.[15,17] Prompt therapy and appropriate supportive care are necessary. After an acute illness, parenteral quinine, quinidine, or artesunate should be followed by long-acting oral agents such as doxycycline, clindamycin, mefloquine, or a full course of an oral artemisinin-based combination therapy.[15]

Leishmaniasis

The disease is caused by protozoan parasites of the genus *Leishmania* that are transmitted to mammalian hosts by female sand fly bites. There are many species of *Leishmania*, which are distributed widely in Europe, Asia, Africa, and America. Clinical presentations are varied from cutaneous lesions to multiorgan involvement, and as such are classified into cutaneous leishmaniasis (CLs) and visceral leishmaniasis (VLs). VL is primarily caused by 2 related species: *Leishmania donovani* and *Leishmania infantum*. Example species that cause CLs are *Leishmania major*, *Leishmania tropica*, *Leishmania aethiopica*, *Leishmania mexicana*, *Leishmania (Viannia) braziliensis*, and *Leishmania (Viannia) guyanensis*.[12]

Clinical manifestations

Many leishmaniasis infections are asymptomatic, reflecting the effectiveness of host immune systems. The most important clinical manifestation of VL is "Kala-azar" or "black fever" syndrome. Symptoms are often insidious in onset and with slow progression characterized by weight loss, fever, malaise, and splenomegaly.[18] Hepatomegaly is less remarkable, but lymphadenopathy may be observed. Kala-azar refers to darkening of the skin, which is a common symptom in South Asia.[19] Advanced disease may present with cachexia, hypoalbuminemia, edema, hepatic dysfunction, jaundice, and hemorrhagic manifestations. Symptomatic CL may cause a spectrum of clinical manifestations, including localized CL, diffuse CL, mucosal leishmaniasis, and leishmania recidivans. Diagnosis is made by demonstration of parasite by needle aspiration or biopsy of the affected organ and requires identification of amastigotes, and culture can be performed in Novy-McNeal-Nicolle media.[20] Serologic testing, such as indirect fluorescent antibody or enzyme-linked immunosorbent assay (ELISA) also can be used in endemic regions with limited laboratory resources. Molecular technique by polymerase chain reaction (PCR) has higher sensitivity than smear and culture, but the result can be variable depending on the tissue used.[21]

Therapy

Therapeutic drug of choice for VL is IV liposomal amphotericin B. Miltefosine is an oral agent that has been approved by the Food and Drug Administration for treatment of VL caused by *L donovani* in adults. Pentavalent antimonial compounds (sodium stibogluconate and meglumine antimoniate) remain another widely used antileishmanial agents and with unknown mechanism. Paromomycin is an aminoglycoside antibiotic that has activity against *Leishmania*, as it binds the 30S ribosomal subunit causing parasite protein synthesis impairment, but is not currently available in the United States.[12] Local wound care and topical forms (eg, paromomycin ointment) have been used as the main approach for the treatment of uncomplicated CL. Oral systemic therapy, such as azole antifungal agents and/or parenteral systemic therapy, is considered when treating complicated CL.[12]

Cryptosporidiosis

Cryptosporidiosis is the disease caused by protozoan parasites of the genus *Cryptosporidium*. *Cryptosporidium parvum* and *Cryptosporidium hominis* are the main species that cause clinical disease in humans.[22] Transmission occurs when fecally contaminated food with the *Cryptosporidium* oocysts is ingested by humans. Excystation releases sporozoites within the lumen of small intestine where they grow into trophozoites and merozoites. Merozoites further develop into male and female forms that can then be fertilized to form zygotes. Zygotes then develop into thin-walled autoinfectious oocysts in approximately 20%, and then 80% become thick-walled oocysts that are subsequently excreted into stool.[13]

Clinical manifestations

Clinical presentations include an asymptomatic state, mild diarrheal disease, severe enteritis, and/or biliary tract involvement, depending on immunocompetent or immunocompromised states of patients. Patients with diarrhea may have associated symptoms, such as malaise, anorexia, abdominal cramping, and fever. The diarrhea can be acute or chronic, or have scant or voluminous watery stools. Fecal blood and leukocytes are rarely found. The infection can spontaneously resolve within 10 to 14 days and without any specific treatment in healthy individuals. In an immunocompromised host (eg, HIV infection), the illness is often more severe especially when CD4 count is <100 cells/μL. Other manifestations also have been described in patients with

AIDS, such as acalculous cholecystitis, sclerosing cholangitis, and pancreatitis. Diagnosis is generally made by microscopy. The organism can be detected in a stool specimen, duodenal aspirate, biliary secretion, or in biopsy specimens of affected intestinal tissues. Modified acid-fast stains are frequently used to identify the pink-stained 4-µm to 6-µm oocysts. Other diagnostic methods that are more sensitive than routine light microscopy include PCR,[23] monoclonal antibodies, and enzyme immunoassays[24]; however, the diagnostic kits remain expensive.

Therapy
Most patients usually have mild to moderate symptoms that may resolve without additional treatment. However, patients with severe and prolonged symptoms may need supportive care for repletion of electrolyte losses and antimicrobial therapy. Nitazoxanide 500 mg oral twice daily is the preferred agent, which is well tolerated. In areas where nitazoxanide is not available, paromomycin can be an alternative drug of choice.[25] In HIV-infected patients, antiretroviral therapy is recommended to restore immune function in addition to supportive care.[26] Antimicrobial therapy is to be administered in HIV-infected patients with persistent diarrhea and slow CD4 recovery; however, the response appears to be less effective compared with immunocompetent hosts. In patients with biliary complications, such as cholangitis associated with papillary stenosis, endoscopic retrograde cholangiopancreatography (ERCP) with biliary sphincterotomy should be performed to relieve symptoms.[27]

HELMINTHIC INFECTIONS OF THE LIVER
Nematodes

Ascariasis
Ascaris lumbricoides is the largest intestinal nematode living in human intestine. The infection is prevalent worldwide; however, it is most prevalent in tropical countries.[28,29] Humans are infected by ingesting contaminated food or water with the parasite's eggs. The eggs hatch into larvae in the small intestine; the larvae can then migrate through the mucosa from the proximal colon to the liver via portal system and also to the lungs, which are then regurgitated and re-swallowed within its cycle.[30] The adult worms can grow in the small intestine up to a length of 20 to 30 cm with a life span of 10 to 24 months, and can accidently migrate into the biliary tract causing biliary obstruction. Both adult worms and eggs can be passed in the stool.

Clinical manifestations Most patients experience an asymptomatic infection. However, in patients with high worm burden, symptoms can occur during 2 phases: the early-phase larval migration stage (pulmonary manifestation) and the late-phase adult worm intestinal stage (intestinal, hepatobiliary, or pancreatic manifestations).[31] During the first 2 weeks of early-phase, patients may experience transient respiratory tract symptoms and pulmonary eosinophilia (Loeffler syndrome)[32] and may relate dry cough, fever, dyspnea, chest discomfort, and wheezing, which can be self-limited. Chronic infection may manifest as intermittent periumbilical pain. In heavy *Ascaris* infection, adult worms can obstruct bowel lumen, causing acute intestinal obstruction,[33] and also can cause other manifestations, such as volvulus, ileocecal intussusception, intestinal gangrene, and perforation.[31] Notably, adult worms also can migrate into the bile ducts, causing obstructive jaundice, ascending cholangitis, and liver abscesses.[34,35] Retained worm fragments can become a nidus for biliary stone formation, causing recurrent pyogenic cholangitis. Pancreatitis can result as well, if adult worms obstruct the pancreatic duct.[31,36] Chronic ascariasis can lead to malnutrition, especially in children.[37] Diagnosis is made by identification of eggs in the stool specimen under microscopy by concentration methods. Larvae can be detected in sputum and gastric lavage, but this is rarely possible. Eosinophilia is occasionally found in the early-phase. In patients suspected to have complications such as intestinal obstruction, plain radiography and CT scan can be adjunctive tools. In patients with biliary ascariasis, magnetic resonance cholangiopancreatography or ERCP should be performed for the diagnosis, and ERCP additionally allows treatment by removal of the worms from the biliary tract[38] (**Fig. 2**).

Therapy The following treatment regimens can be used:

1. Albendazole 400 mg orally as a single dose.
2. Mebendazole 500 mg orally single dose or 100 mg twice daily for 3 days.
3. Pyrantel pamoate (especially in pregnant women) 11 mg/kg up to 1 g as a single dose.

According to the systematic reviews and meta-analysis, the average cure rates from these treatment regimens have been 96%, 96%, and 93%, respectively.[39] Other alternative drugs, such as ivermectin and nitazoxanide, also can be used with comparable cure rates. Patients who have complications of biliary obstruction or intestinal obstruction may require further endoscopic treatment (eg, ERCP), or surgical intervention, respectively.

Strongyloidiasis

Strongyloidiasis, an infection caused by *Strongyloides stercoralis,* is endemic in tropical and subtropical regions of sub-Saharan Africa, Asia, Latin America, and Eastern and Southern Europe.[40] In the United States, the highest prevalence is among refugees and military personnel.[41] The infectious cycle begins when filariform larvae, which are contaminated in soil, penetrate through human skin. The filariform larvae then migrate via the bloodstream and lymphatic system to the lungs and alveoli, and then ascend the tracheobronchial tree and are coughed/regurgitated and then swallowed. Adult worms reside in the mucosa of the duodenum and jejunum for many years. Female adults produce eggs that hatch into rhabditiform larvae and are generally passed into feces and then they develop into the infective filariform stage, completing the cycle.[40] *S stercoralis* can complete its life cycle within the human

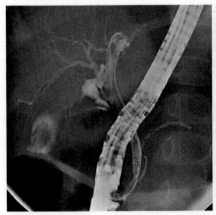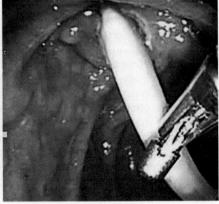

Fig. 2. Endoscopic and ERCP findings of biliary ascariasis showing tubular structure filling defect in the common bile duct while a worm is also being extracted. (*Courtesy of* Worapot Rojsanga, MD and Nisa Netinatsunton MD, Songkla, Thailand; with permission.)

host by autoinfection, whereas the rhabditiform larvae also can mature into filariform larvae within the gastrointestinal tract and penetrate colonic mucosa or perianal skin to complete their cycle of autoinfection.[40]

Clinical manifestations S stercoralis infection in immunocompetent hosts can be asymptomatic or cause mild gastrointestinal symptoms, such as abdominal pain, nausea, vomiting, and diarrhea. Skin reactions may be present when larvae penetrate the skin. Once larvae migrate, an evanescent track, the so-called "larva currens," develops, indicating pathognomonic strongyloidiasis.[42] Autoinfection can lead to a hyperinfection syndrome that results from massive dissemination of filariform larvae to the lungs, liver, heart, endocrine glands, and central nervous system. Immunosuppressed patients are at high risk for fatal hyperinfection with disseminated disease.[43] Symptoms of hyperinfection include fever, dyspnea, cough, wheezing, hemoptysis, and diarrhea, and this can further lead to secondary gram-negative bacteremia and associated high mortality rates.[44,45] The diagnosis is made by detection of rhabditiform larvae in concentrated stool specimens (**Fig. 3**) or by serologic methods. In disseminated strongyloidiasis, filariform larvae can be found in stool, sputum, bronchoalveolar lavage fluid, and pleural or peritoneal fluid.[46,47] Serologic testing by ELISA for detecting S stercoralis immunoglobulin G to filariform larvae demonstrated high sensitivity (83%–89%) and high specificity (97.2%) for intestinal strongyloidiasis.[48]

Therapy Treatment of choice for uncomplicated strongyloidiasis is ivermectin (200 µg/kg per dose for 2 consecutive days and may be repeated 2 weeks apart).[49] Albendazole (400 mg twice daily for 3–7 days) is an alternative drug.[50] In disseminated disease/hyperinfection syndrome, the optimal treatment data are limited. It is suggested that ivermectin be continued until clinical improvement and daily stool examinations have been negative for at least 2 weeks.[51] Additional hemoculture should be obtained in the setting of hyperinfection syndrome, and broad-spectrum antibiotics should be empirically administered for enteric gram-negative bacterial coverage.

Trematodes

Schistosomiasis
Schistosomiasis is a parasitic infection that can result in periportal fibrosis and liver cirrhosis that is initiated by egg deposition in the terminal portal venules causing a

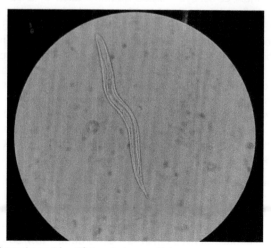

Fig. 3. Fresh stool specimen identifying S stercoralis larvae.

granulomatous reaction. There are 5 schistosome species that can infect humans. *Schistosoma mansoni* is commonly found in parts of South America and Africa; *Schistosoma haematobium* is found in Africa and the Middle East; *Schistosoma intercalatum* is primarily in West and Central Africa; and *Schistosoma mekongi* and *Schistosoma japonicum* are found in the Far East. Humans are infected by contact with water that contains the cercariae. After penetration of the skin, the cercariae shed their tails and become schistosomulae, which then migrate to the liver and develop into adults within 2 to 4 weeks. Adult worms migrate via the portal system to the mesenteric venules (except for *S haematobium,* which migrates to the vesical venous plexus). After a few months, the female worms deposit eggs in the terminal venules of the mesenteric system where they can enter the portal vein and become lodged in the terminal branches of the portal venules, causing a granulomatous inflammation, and the lesions heal by periportal fibrosis. The eggs are eliminated in feces or urine (in *S haematobium*). Excreted eggs hatch in water and become miracidia, which penetrate the snail as an intermediate host, and the snail produces cercariae that are released into water and reinfect humans as a complete cycle.[52,53]

Clinical manifestations Initial skin penetration by cercariae is often unnoticed, but can also manifest as itching and localized dermatitis, so-called "swimmer's itch."[54] Acute schistosomiasis syndrome (Katayama fever) is a hypersensitivity reaction due to the host immune response to schistosome antigens, which occurs approximately 4 to 6 weeks after exposure. Manifestations include headache, fever, chills, urticaria, diarrhea, myalgias, tender hepatomegaly, and eosinophilia, which can then spontaneously resolve within days to weeks.[55–57] Untreated chronic infection (5–15 years later) is due to inflammation from eggs that are lodged in portal venules, resulting in periportal fibrosis (pipe stem fibrosis), presinusoidal occlusion with presinusoidal portal hypertension, and splenomegaly.[58,59] At this stage, patients generally have preserved hepatic function, but present with hematemesis from ruptured gastroesophageal varices. Gold standard for the diagnosis of schistosomiasis is from the identification of schistosome eggs detected on microscopic examination of stool or urine specimens. Specific diagnosis on each species can be made by different egg morphology. Other direct assays include demonstration of schistosome antigen or DNA in the blood/urine/stool. Indirect assays include demonstration of antibodies in blood.[53] Seroconversion usually occurs within 6 to 12 weeks of infection[60]; however, serologic testing using ELISA technique cannot distinguish an active infection from previous exposure. A newer diagnostic method of PCR technique for detection of schistosome DNA in blood, stool, or urine has its potential for diagnosing schistosomiasis in all disease stages,[61–63] but mostly still remains a research tool. Rectal biopsy can be useful for the diagnosis of intestinal schistosomiasis if other diagnostic tools are unhelpful.[64] Imaging study using CT or MRI may show extensive calcification along the portal tracts with the typical "turtle-back" appearance reflecting the calcified eggs along the portal triads. In chronic infection, liver biopsy histopathology may demonstrate granulomatous change along with schistosome eggs in the portal tract causing typical pipe stem fibrosis.

Therapy Praziquantel (a single dose of 40 mg/kg for *S haematobium, S mansoni,* or *S intercalatum* infections,[65] or 2 divided doses of 60 mg/kg for *S japonicum, S mekongi* infections)[66,67] is the therapeutic drug of choice. Presence of viable eggs in the stool after 6 to 12 weeks of initial treatment warrants repeat treatment with the same dose of praziquantel.   In   acute   schistosomiasis   syndrome,   low-dose   short-course corticosteroid therapy (prednisolone 20–40 mg/d for 5 days) may be needed to suppress inflammatory reactions.[68–70] Despite treatment, 5% to 20% of patients develop significant hepatic fibrosis.[71]

Fascioliasis

The 2 main species of fascioliasis are *Fasciola hepatica*, which can be found worldwide, and *Fasciola gigantica*, which is more prevalent in tropical countries.[72] The common definitive hosts are sheep and cattle, with snails as intermediate hosts. Humans, as incidental hosts, can become infected by ingestion of contaminated water or vegetables containing metacercariae, which then become excysted and migrate through the intestinal wall, to the peritoneal cavity, and enter liver parenchyma causing parenchymal injury and necrosis before tracking into bile ducts. The adult flukes lodge in the large bile ducts, which can result in partial biliary obstruction. They release eggs in the stool which hatch and become miracidia in water. Miracidia penetrate the snail and grow in several stages. The snails release free-cercariae back to the environment and encyst as metacercariae in infected water, completing the cycle.[73]

Clinical manifestations The acute phase, when excysted metacercariae migrate through the liver, can present with fever and tender hepatomegaly, including other signs and symptoms, such as jaundice, myalgia, and urticaria. Disease severity depends on the fluke burden.[74] Peripheral eosinophilia is common. With this phase, symptoms usually resolve within 6 weeks. Patients with chronic phase, beginning at 6 months after infection, usually are asymptomatic.[75] The chronic phase is when adult flukes migrate to the bile ducts and cause common bile duct obstruction, biliary pain, cholangitis, cholelithiasis, and secondary pancreatitis.[76,77] Heavy infection also can cause secondary sclerosing cholangitis and biliary cirrhosis. Extrahepatic manifestations may occur if the parasites migrate hematogenously to other organs or through soft tissues.[78] Diagnosis can be made by egg identification in the stool, duodenal aspirate, or bile specimens. Occasionally, adult flukes can be seen via endoscopy done in case of biliary obstruction. Serologic testing, such as ELISA-based technique, has good sensitivity and specificity.[79] Imaging, such as CT or MRI, can be an adjunctive useful tool for diagnosis by demonstrating hypodense nodules and tortuous tracks due to parasitic migration in the liver (**Fig. 4**). Subcapsular hematoma, thickening of liver capsule, and parenchymal calcification also can be detected.[80] Adult flukes can sometimes be seen by ERCP or cholangiography techniques as leaflike flukes in the bile ducts and gall bladder, together with stones.[81]

Therapy Triclabendazole is a therapy of choice for fascioliasis, in a dosage of 10 mg/kg orally for 1 to 2 days.[82] Alternative agents, such as nitazoxanide 500 mg twice daily for 7 days, can be considered, although with limited evidence.[83] Patients with ascending cholangitis require prompt antibiotics and therapeutic ERCP to relieve biliary obstruction.[84]

Clonorchiasis and opisthorchiasis

Clonorchis sinensis and *Opisthorchis* species are major liver trematodes found in humans. *C sinensis* is particularly endemic in the Far East. Opisthorchiasis is usually caused by *Opisthorchis viverrini* and *Opisthorchis felineus* (*O felineus* is commonly found in Southeast Asia, and Central and Eastern Europe).[85] *O viverrini* is more prevalent in Thailand, Vietnam, Cambodia, and Laos, where the risk of cholangiocarcinoma is also increased.[86] They are liver flukes of cats, dogs, and fish-eating mammals. Humans are incidental hosts and serve as reservoirs. The cycle begins

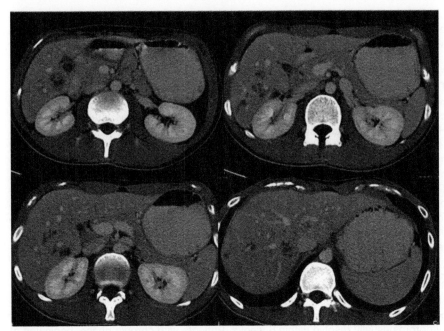

Fig. 4. CT scan of tortuous tracks of hepatic fascioliasis. (*Courtesy of* Chalermrat Bunchorn-tavakul, MD, Bangkok, Thailand; with permission.)

with adult flukes passing eggs into the bile ducts and into the stool. Eggs are ingested by a snail (first intermediate host) where miracidia are released and develop into cercariae. The cercariae can penetrate the freshwater fish (second intermediate host) and become encysted as metacercariae. By ingesting the raw and under-cooked fish, animals (definitive hosts) or humans (incidental hosts) acquire this infection. The metacercariae excyst in the duodenum and travel into the bile ducts where they become mature. Adult flukes usually reside in the small to medium-sized bile ducts.[87]

Clinical manifestations Most patients are asymptomatic. Symptomatic disease depends on intensity and duration of infection. Peripheral eosinophilia can be found in 10% to 20%. In patients with heavy infection, acute infection can result in right upper quadrant abdominal pain, fever, anorexia, flatulence, diarrhea, and fatigue, which are nonspecific symptoms and usually last approximately 2 to 4 weeks.[75,88] Chronic complications from clonorchiasis and opisthorchiasis are as a consequence of adult flukes causing bile duct obstruction. An elevated alkaline phosphatase can be observed. Dead parasites can become a nidus for stone formation in the bile ducts, causing obstructive jaundice, ascending cholangitis, pancreatitis, and liver abscesses. A long-term complication includes cholangiocarcinoma where the risk appears to be highest in O viverrini-infected individuals in the northern part of Thailand.[2,89,90] The diagnosis is made by demonstrating eggs in the stool, duodenal aspirates, or bile specimens. Serologic testing, such as ELISA, is not widely available, and cannot distinguish between current and past infection.[91,92] Imaging studies, including ultrasonography, CT, MRI, and ERCP, are useful additional tools for diagnosis. Adult flukes can occasionally be demonstrated by ERCP, with filling defects ranging from a few millimeters to a few centimeters in size (**Fig. 5**).

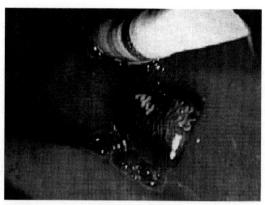

Fig. 5. Endoscopic finding of *O viverrini* during ERCP with parasite removal from bile duct. (*Courtesy of* Aroon Siripun, MD, Bangkok, Thailand; with permission.)

Therapy Standard treatment for clonorchiasis and opisthorchiasis is praziquantel 25 mg/kg per dose orally 3 times daily for 1 to 2 days.[93] Alternative drugs include albendazole (10 mg/kg orally for 7 days) or mebendazole (30 mg/kg orally for 20–30 days).[2,94] Patients with heavy parasitic infection and biliary tract complications may need additional interventions; for example, patients with ascending cholangitis may require antibiotics and ERCP for biliary drainage. Patients who have already developed cholangiocarcinoma usually have poor prognosis and should be treated according to the cancer staging. Prevention should be motivated through adequate cooking of freshwater fish, and sanitary conditions need improvement to reduce water contamination.

Cestodes

Echinococcosis

There are 4 species of *Echinococcus* that can infect humans: *Echinococcus granulosus* and *Echinococcus multilocularis* are the major 2 species, causing cystic echinococcosis and alveolar echinococcosis, respectively. The 2 other species are *Echinococcus vogeli* and *Echinococcus oligarthrus*, causing polycystic echinococcosis, and are rarely seen in humans. Cystic echinococcosis is a zoonosis caused by *E granulosus* and is often called "hydatid cyst disease" due to its typical characteristic of fluid-filled cyst infection. The disease is more prevalent in the sheep-raising areas worldwide, including Africa, the Middle East, and Eastern Mediterranean, Asia, South America, Australia, and New Zealand.

E granulosus: Dogs are the definitive hosts and sheep are the major intermediate hosts, whereas goats, camels, horses, and cattle are other relevant intermediate hosts. Humans are the accidental hosts. The adult tapeworm infects the small intestine of the dogs. Each adult worm can produce eggs and release in the stool where they can infect an intermediate host and humans as accidental host by ingesting fecally contaminated food. In the intermediate host, the oncospheres hatch from the eggs, which then penetrate intestinal mucosa and travel in the bloodstream to the liver or other organs and develop into hydatid cysts. Inside these cysts are protoscolices. When the definitive hosts ingest the intermediate host organs containing hydatid cysts, the protoscolices are then released and they subsequently develop into adult worms, completing their life cycles.[95]

E multilocularis: Foxes are typical definitive hosts and rodents are the major intermediate hosts. Humans are the accidental hosts who ingest fecally contaminated eggs from definitive hosts. The oncospheres hatch from the eggs in the small intestine and travel to the liver where they form multilocular hydatid cysts. Unlike E granulosus, protoscolices are rarely observed in humans, and the infection usually leads to mass formation in the liver, which then resembles a malignancy because they can extensively invade the surrounding tissue by exogenous budding. The mortality rates are high, reaching 90% if left untreated.[95,96]

Clinical manifestations The initial phase of infection is asymptomatic. Clinical symptoms depend on the sites of the infected cysts and their sizes. When the hydatid cysts grow overtime, they can cause signs and symptoms due to mass effect (eg, abdominal pain, hepatomegaly, or palpable mass), obstruction of blood flow, or complications such as secondary bacterial infections and rupture. In some cases, cysts may rupture into the bile ducts and cause cholestatic jaundice or cholangitis. Ruptured cysts into the peritoneum can lead to the development of extrahepatic cysts that may induce allergic reactions resulting in eosinophilia, pruritic urticaria, and systemic anaphylaxis, which can be a life-threatening condition. Diagnosis can be made by an imaging study and serology. Ultrasonography, contrast-enhanced CT, or MRI may demonstrate a cyst with rim calcification (eggshell appearance), detachment of the germinal layer from the cyst wall ("water lily" sign), intracystic septations, and daughter cyst formation.[97,98] Serologic testing by ELISA technique is another useful method for diagnosis and follow-up after treatment.[99] However, negative serology does not rule out the diagnosis, whereas approximately 85% to 95% of liver cysts have positive results.[100]

Therapy The primary antiparasitic drug of choice is albendazole (15 mg/kg per day, divided into 2 doses, to a maximum of 400 mg orally twice daily) for 1 to 3 months and depending on the clinical severity, up to 6 months of use has also been pursued. However, treatment with albendazole alone may not be effective for a cyst with a diameter larger than 5 cm, that has multiple compartments, or that has daughter cysts that may need further adjunctive therapy.[101] Unilocular cysts without daughter cysts can be drained percutaneously by puncture; aspiration; injection of scolicidal solutions, such as chlorhexidine, hydrogen peroxide, 80% alcohol, or 0.5% cetrimide; and re-aspiration (PAIR). In those with daughter cysts, it is preferred to use either modified catheterization technique (use of large-bore catheters and cutting devices with subsequent aspiration) or surgery to remove the entire daughter cysts while the patients have been treated with albendazole. Patients with a complicated cyst, such as a ruptured cyst into the peritoneum or a cyst with biliary communication, typically require surgery, as the PAIR technique can lead to spillage of cyst contents into the peritoneum or carry a risk of secondary sclerosing cholangitis, respectively; thus PAIR technique is contraindicated.[102–104] Albendazole is administered 1 week before surgery and continued for at least 4 weeks after surgery to minimize the risk of secondary echinococcosis in the event of spillage (**Table 2**).

SUMMARY

As a consequence of unique dual (portal vein and hepatic artery) blood supply of the liver, this organ may be relatively more susceptible to a variety of infections, particularly those that use the gastrointestinal tract as a pathway. Fungal infections commonly occur in immunocompromised patients and are often seen as an opportunistic infection in those infected with HIV. Prevalence of parasitic infections of the liver can vary among the various endemic areas of the world, and present with a variety of clinical features ranging from asymptomatic state, hepatic granuloma, and liver abscess. Further, some parasites may migrate to the pancreatico-biliary system and result in complications, such as biliary obstruction, cholangitis, and pancreatitis. Prompt endoscopic therapeutic intervention is required, in such cases, in addition to the use of antiparasitic agents. Adequate dosage and duration of the various therapeutic agents should be considered in treating parasitic infections, and broad sanitation strategies are essential to minimize disease transmission.

DISCLOSURE

Nothing to disclose.

REFERENCES

1. Thaler M, Pastakia B, Shawker TH, et al. Hepatic candidiasis in cancer patients: the evolving picture of the syndrome. Ann Intern Med 1988;108(1):88–100.
2. Mahanty S, Maclean JD, Cross JH. Liver, Lung, and Intestinal Fluke Infections. In: Guerrant RL, Walker DH, Weller PF, editors. Tropical Infectious Diseases: Principles, Pathogens and Practice. 3rd ed. Philadelphia: Saunders Elsevier; 2011. p. 854.
3. Centers for Disease Control and Prevention. Available at: https://www.cdc.gov/. Accessed March 18, 2019.
4. Reddy KR. Bacterial, Parasitic, Fungal, and Granulomatous Liver Diseases, Goldman-Cecil Medicine. 26th edition. Philadelphia, PA: Elsevier Health Sciences; 2019.
5. Messer SA, Jones RN, Fritsche TR. International surveillance of Candida spp. and Aspergillus spp.: report from the SENTRY Antimicrobial Surveillance Program (2003). J Clin Microbiol 2006;44(5):1782–7.
6. Kontoyiannis DP, Luna MA, Samuels BI, et al. Hepatosplenic candidiasis. A manifestation of chronic disseminated candidiasis. Infect Dis Clin North Am 2000;14(3):721–39.
7. Anttila VJ, Lamminen AE, Bondestam S, et al. Magnetic resonance imaging is superior to computed tomography and ultrasonography in imaging infectious liver foci in acute leukaemia. Eur J Haematol 1996;56(1–2):82–7.
8. Pappas PG, Kauffman CA, Andes DR, et al. Clinical practice guideline for the management of candidiasis: 2016 update by the Infectious Diseases Society of America. Clin Infect Dis 2016;62(4):e1–50.
9. Masood A, Sallah S. Chronic disseminated candidiasis in patients with acute leukemia: emphasis on diagnostic definition and treatment. Leuk Res 2005; 29(5):493–501.
10. Anaissie E, Bodey GP, Kantarjian H, et al. Fluconazole therapy for chronic disseminated candidiasis in patients with leukemia and prior amphotericin B therapy. Am J Med 1991;91(2):142–50.
11. Malaria. Available at: https://www.cdc.gov/dpdx/malaria/index.html. Accessed March 7, 2019.
12. Leishmaniasis. Available at: https://www.cdc.gov/dpdx/leishmaniasis/index. html. Accessed March 8, 2019.
13. Cryptosporidiosis. Available at: https://www.cdc.gov/dpdx/cryptosporidiosis/ index.html. Accessed November 8, 2017.
14. White NJ, Imwong M. Relapse. Adv Parasitol 2012;80:113–50.
15. World Health Organization. Guidelines for the treatment of malaria, 3rd edition. WHO, Geneva (Switzerland) 2015. Available at: https://www.who.int/malaria/ publications/atoz/9789241549127/en/. Accessed March 7, 2019.

16. Abanyie FA, Arguin PM, Gutman J. State of malaria diagnostic testing at clinical laboratories in the United States, 2010: a nationwide survey. Malar J 2011; 10:340.

17. Dondorp AM, Fanello CI, Hendriksen IC, et al. Artesunate versus quinine in the treatment of severe falciparum malaria in African children (AQUAMAT): an open-label, randomised trial. Lancet 2010;376(9753):1647–57.

18. Jeronimo SMB, de Queiroz Sousa A, Pearson RD. In: Guerrant RL, Walker DH, Weller PF, editors. Leishmaniasis. Tropical infectious diseases: principles, pathogens and practice. 3rd edition. Philadelphia: Saunders Elsevier; 2011. p. 696.

19. Magill AJ. Visceral leishmaniasis (kala-azar). In: Strickland GT, editor. Hunter's tropical medicine and emerging infectious diseases. 8th edition. Philadelphia: W.B. Saunders Company; 2000. p. 670.

20. Sundar S, Rai M. Laboratory diagnosis of visceral leishmaniasis. Clin Diagn Lab Immunol 2002;9(5):951–8.

21. Antinori S, Calattini S, Longhi E, et al. Clinical use of polymerase chain reaction performed on peripheral blood and bone marrow samples for the diagnosis and monitoring of visceral leishmaniasis in HIV-infected and HIV-uninfected patients: a single-center, 8-year experience in Italy and review of the literature. Clin Infect Dis 2007;44(12):1602–10.

22. Morgan-Ryan UM, Fall A, Ward LA, et al. *Cryptosporidium hominis* n. sp. (Apicomplexa: Cryptosporidiidae) from *Homo sapiens*. J Eukaryot Microbiol 2002; 49(6):433–40.

23. Van Lint P, Rossen JW, Vermeiren S, et al. Detection of *Giardia lamblia*, *Cryptosporidium* spp. and *Entamoeba histolytica* in clinical stool samples by using multiplex real-time PCR after automated DNA isolation. Acta Clin Belg 2013; 68(3):188–92.

24. Garcia LS, Brewer TC, Bruckner DA. Fluorescence detection of *Cryptosporidium* oocysts in human fecal specimens by using monoclonal antibodies. J Clin Microbiol 1987;25(1):119–21.

25. Hussien SM, Abdella OH, Abu-Hashim AH, et al. Comparative study between the effect of nitazoxanide and paromomycine in treatment of cryptosporidiosis in hospitalized children. J Egypt Soc Parasitol 2013;43(2):463–70.

26. Guidelines for the prevention and treatment of opportunistic infections in HIV-infected adults and adolescents: recommendations from the Centers for Disease Control and Prevention, the National Institutes of Health, and the HIV Medicine Association of the Infectious Diseases Society of America. Available at: https://aidsinfo.nih.gov/contentfiles/lvguidelines/adult_oi.pdf. Accessed March 7, 2019.

27. Cello JP, Chan MF. Long-term follow-up of endoscopic retrograde cholangio-pancreatography sphincterotomy for patients with acquired immune deficiency syndrome papillary stenosis. Am J Med 1995;99(6):600–3.

28. Jourdan PM, Lamberton PHL, Fenwick A, et al. Soil-transmitted helminth infections. Lancet 2018;391(10117):252–65.

29. Pullan RL, Smith JL, Jasrasaria R, et al. Global numbers of infection and disease burden of soil transmitted helminth infections in 2010. Parasit Vectors 2014;7:37.

30. Murrell KD, Eriksen L, Nansen P, et al. *Ascaris suum*: a revision of its early migratory path and implications for human ascariasis. J Parasitol 1997;83(2):255–60.

31. Khuroo MS. Ascariasis. Gastroenterol Clin North Am 1996;25(3):553–77.

32. Spillmann RK. Pulmonary ascariasis in tropical communities. Am J Trop Med Hyg 1975;24(5):791–800.

33. de Silva NR, Guyatt HL, Bundy DA. Morbidity and mortality due to *Ascaris*-induced intestinal obstruction. Trans R Soc Trop Med Hyg 1997;91(1):31–6.
34. Javid G, Wani NA, Gulzar GM, et al. *Ascaris*-induced liver abscess. World J Surg 1999;23(11):1191–4.
35. al-Karawi M, Sanai FM, Yasawy MI, et al. Biliary strictures and cholangitis secondary to ascariasis: endoscopic management. Gastrointest Endosc 1999; 50(5):695–7.
36. Khuroo MS. Hepatobiliary and pancreatic ascariasis. Indian J Gastroenterol 2001;20(Suppl 1):C28–32.
37. Hlaing T. Ascariasis and childhood malnutrition. Parasitology 1993;107(Suppl): S125–36.
38. Rana SS, Bhasin DK, Nanda M, et al. Parasitic infestations of the biliary tract. Curr Gastroenterol Rep 2007;9(2):156–64.
39. Moser W, Schindler C, Keiser J. Efficacy of recommended drugs against soil transmitted helminths: systematic review and network meta-analysis. BMJ 2017;358:j4307.
40. Strongyloidiasis. Available at: https://www.cdc.gov/parasites/strongyloides/biology.html. Accessed January 10, 2019.
41. Posey DL, Blackburn BG, Weinberg M, et al. High prevalence and presumptive treatment of schistosomiasis and strongyloidiasis among African refugees. Clin Infect Dis 2007;45(10):1310–5.
42. Arthur RP, Shelley WB. Larva currens; a distinctive variant of cutaneous larva migrans due to *Strongyloides stercoralis*. AMA Arch Dermatol 1958;78(2):186–90.
43. Keiser PB, Nutman TB. *Strongyloides stercoralis* in the immunocompromised population. Clin Microbiol Rev 2004;17(1):208–17.
44. Woodring JH, Halfhill H 2nd, Reed JC. Pulmonary strongyloidiasis: clinical and imaging features. AJR Am J Roentgenol 1994;162(3):537–42.
45. Lam CS, Tong MK, Chan KM, et al. Disseminated strongyloidiasis: a retrospective study of clinical course and outcome. Eur J Clin Microbiol Infect Dis 2006; 25(1):14–8.
46. Williams J, Nunley D, Dralle W, et al. Diagnosis of pulmonary strongyloidiasis by bronchoalveolar lavage. Chest 1988;94(3):643–4.
47. Eveland LK, Kenney M, Yermakov V. Laboratory diagnosis of autoinfection in strongyloidiasis. Am J Clin Pathol 1975;63(3):421–5.
48. van Doorn HR, Koelewijn R, Hofwegen H, et al. Use of enzyme-linked immunosorbent assay and dipstick assay for detection of *Strongyloides stercoralis* infection in humans. J Clin Microbiol 2007;45(2):438–42.
49. Zaha O, Hirata T, Kinjo F, et al. Efficacy of ivermectin for chronic strongyloidiasis: two single doses given 2 weeks apart. J Infect Chemother 2002;8(1):94–8.
50. Archibald LK, Beeching NJ, Gill GV, et al. Albendazole is effective treatment for chronic strongyloidiasis. Q J Med 1993;86(3):191–5.
51. Segarra-Newnham M. Manifestations, diagnosis, and treatment of *Strongyloides stercoralis* infection. Ann Pharmacother 2007;41(12):1992–2001.
52. Schistosomiasis Infection. Available at: https://www.cdc.gov/dpdx/schistosomiasis/. Accessed January 18, 2019.
53. Gryseels B, Polman K, Clerinx J, et al. Human schistosomiasis. Lancet 2006; 368(9541):1106–18.
54. Bouree P, Caumes E. Cercarial dermatitis. Presse Med 2004;33(7):490–3 [in French].
55. Lambertucci JR. Acute schistosomiasis: clinical, diagnostic and therapeutic features. Rev Inst Med Trop Sao Paulo 1993;35(5):399–404.

56. Leshem E, Maor Y, Meltzer E, et al. Acute schistosomiasis outbreak: clinical features and economic impact. Clin Infect Dis 2008;47(12):1499–506.

57. Rocha MO, Pedroso ER, Lambertucci JR, et al. Gastro-intestinal manifestations of the initial phase of schistosomiasis mansoni. Ann Trop Med Parasitol 1995; 89(3):271–8.

58. Homeida M, Abdel-Gadir AF, Cheever AW, et al. Diagnosis of pathologically confirmed Symmers' periportal fibrosis by ultrasonography: a prospective blinded study. Am J Trop Med Hyg 1988;38(1):86–91.

59. Dessein A, Arnaud V, He H, et al. Genetic analysis of human predisposition to hepatosplenic disease caused by schistosomes reveals the crucial role of connective tissue growth factor in rapid progression to severe hepatic fibrosis. Pathol Biol 2013;61(1):3–10.

60. Jones ME, Mitchell RG, Leen CL. Long seronegative window in schistosoma infection. Lancet 1992;340(8834–8835):1549–50.

61. Lier T, Simonsen GS, Wang T, et al. Real-time polymerase chain reaction for detection of low-intensity *Schistosoma japonicum* infections in China. Am J Trop Med Hyg 2009;81(3):428–32.

62. Sandoval N, Siles-Lucas M, Perez-Arellano JL, et al. A new PCR-based approach for the specific amplification of DNA from different *Schistosoma* species applicable to human urine samples. Parasitology 2006;133(Pt 5):581–7.

63. Cnops L, Soentjens P, Clerinx J, et al. A *Schistosoma haematobium*-specific real-time PCR for diagnosis of urogenital schistosomiasis in serum samples of international travelers and migrants. PLoS Negl Trop Dis 2013;7(8):e2413.

64. Harries AD, Fryatt R, Walker J, et al. Schistosomiasis in expatriates returning to Britain from the tropics: a controlled study. Lancet 1986;1(8472):86–8.

65. Kramer CV, Zhang F, Sinclair D, et al. Drugs for treating urinary schistosomiasis. Cochrane Database Syst Rev 2014;(8):CD000053.

66. Guisse F, Polman K, Stelma FF, et al. Therapeutic evaluation of two different dose regimens of praziquantel in a recent *Schistosoma mansoni* focus in Northern Senegal. Am J Trop Med Hyg 1997;56(5):511–4.

67. Utzinger J, N'Goran EK, N'Dri A, et al. Efficacy of praziquantel against *Schistosoma mansoni* with particular consideration for intensity of infection. Trop Med Int Health 2000;5(11):771–8.

68. Ross AG, Vickers D, Olds GR, et al. Katayama syndrome. Lancet Infect Dis 2007;7(3):218–24.

69. Chapman PJ, Wilkinson PR, Davidson RN. Acute schistosomiasis (Katayama fever) among British air crew. BMJ 1988;297(6656):1101.

70. Harries AD, Cook GC. Acute schistosomiasis (Katayama fever): clinical deterioration after chemotherapy. J Infect 1987;14(2):159–61.

71. Olveda DU, Inobaya M, Olveda RM, et al. Diagnosing schistosomiasis-induced liver morbidity: implications for global control. Int J Infect Dis 2017;54:138–44.

72. Mas-Coma S. Epidemiology of fascioliasis in human endemic areas. J Helminthol 2005;79(3):207–16.

73. Fasciola. Available at: https://www.cdc.gov/parasites/fasciola/biology.html. Accessed January 18, 2019.

74. Chan CW, Lam SK. Diseases caused by liver flukes and cholangiocarcinoma. Baillieres Clin Gastroenterol 1987;1(2):297–318.

75. Marcos LA, Terashima A, Gotuzzo E. Update on hepatobiliary flukes: fascioliasis, opisthorchiasis and clonorchiasis. Curr Opin Infect Dis 2008;21(5):523–30.

76. Sezgin O, Altintas E, Tombak A, et al. Fasciola hepatica-induced acute pancreatitis: report of two cases and review of the literature. Turk J Gastroenterol 2010; 21(2):183–7.

77. Kaya M, Bestas R, Cetin S. Clinical presentation and management of *Fasciola hepatica* infection: single-center experience. World J Gastroenterol 2011; 17(44):4899–904.

78. Xuan le T, Hung NT, Waikagul J. Cutaneous fascioliasis: a case report in Vietnam. Am J Trop Med Hyg 2005;72(5):508–9.

79. Gonzales Santana B, Dalton JP, Vasquez Camargo F, et al. The diagnosis of human fascioliasis by enzyme-linked immunosorbent assay (ELISA) using recombinant cathepsin L protease. PLoS Negl Trop Dis 2013;7(9):e2414.

80. Van Beers B, Pringot J, Geubel A, et al. Hepatobiliary fascioliasis: noninvasive imaging findings. Radiology 1990;174(3 Pt 1):809–10.

81. Sezgin O, Altintas E, Disibeyaz S, et al. Hepatobiliary fascioliasis: clinical and radiologic features and endoscopic management. J Clin Gastroenterol 2004; 38(3):285–91.

82. el-Karaksy H, Hassanein B, Okasha S, et al. Human fascioliasis in Egyptian children: successful treatment with triclabendazole. J Trop Pediatr 1999;45(3): 135–8.

83. Favennec L, Jave Ortiz J, Gargala G, et al. Double-blind, randomized, placebo-controlled study of nitazoxanide in the treatment of fascioliasis in adults and children from northern Peru. Aliment Pharmacol Ther 2003;17(2):265–70.

84. Danilewitz M, Kotfila R, Jensen P. Endoscopic diagnosis and management of *Fasciola hepatica* causing biliary obstruction. Am J Gastroenterol 1996; 91(12):2620–1.

85. Pakharukova MY, Mordvinov VA. The liver fluke *Opisthorchis felineus*: biology, epidemiology and carcinogenic potential. Trans R Soc Trop Med Hyg 2016; 110(1):28–36.

86. Aung WPP, Htoon TT, Tin HH, et al. First report and molecular identification of *Opisthorchis viverrini* infection in human communities from Lower Myanmar. PLoS One 2017;12(5):e0177130.

87. Clonorchiasis. Available at: https://www.cdc.gov/dpdx/clonorchiasis/index.html. Accessed January 18, 2019.

88. Keiser J, Utzinger J. Food-borne trematodiases. Clin Microbiol Rev 2009;22(3): 466–83.

89. Surapaitoon A, Suttiprapa S, Mairiang E, et al. Subsets of inflammatory cytokine gene polymorphisms are associated with risk of carcinogenic liver fluke opisthorchis viverrini-associated advanced periductal fibrosis and cholangiocarcinoma. Korean J Parasitol 2017;55(3):295–304.

90. Mairiang E, Haswell-Elkins MR, Mairiang P, et al. Reversal of biliary tract abnormalities associated with *Opisthorchis viverrini* infection following praziquantel treatment. Trans R Soc Trop Med Hyg 1993;87(2):194–7.

91. Akai PS, Pungpak S, Chaicumpa W, et al. Serum antibody responses in opisthorchiasis. Int J Parasitol 1995;25(8):971–3.

92. Lin YL, Chen ER, Yen CM. Antibodies in serum of patients with clonorchiasis before and after treatment. Southeast Asian J Trop Med Public Health 1995; 26(1):114–9.

93. Abramowicz M. Handbook of Antimicrobial Therapy. 20th ed. NY: The Medical Letter, New Rochelle; 2015.

94. Jaroonvesama N, Charoenlarp K, Cross JH. Treatment of *Opisthorchis viverrini* with mebendazole. Southeast Asian J Trop Med Public Health 1981;12(4): 595–7.

95. Echinococcosis. Available at: https://www.cdc.gov/parasites/echinococcosis/biology.html. Accessed January 18, 2019.

96. Ammann RW, Eckert J. Cestodes. Echinococcus. Gastroenterol Clin North Am 1996;25(3):655–89.

97. Salama H, Farid Abdel-Wahab M, Strickland GT. Diagnosis and treatment of hepatic hydatid cysts with the aid of echo-guided percutaneous cyst puncture. Clin Infect Dis 1995;21(6):1372–6.

98. Suwan Z. Sonographic findings in hydatid disease of the liver: comparison with other imaging methods. Ann Trop Med Parasitol 1995;89(3):261–9.

99. McManus DP, Zhang W, Li J, et al. Echinococcosis. Lancet 2003;362(9392): 1295–304.

100. Biava MF, Dao A, Fortier B. Laboratory diagnosis of cystic hydatic disease. World J Surg 2001;25(1):10–4.

101. Guidelines for treatment of cystic and alveolar echinococcosis in humans. WHO Informal Working Group on Echinococcosis. Bull World Health Organ 1996; 74(3):231–42.

102. Junghanss T, da Silva AM, Horton J, et al. Clinical management of cystic echinococcosis: state of the art, problems, and perspectives. Am J Trop Med Hyg 2008;79(3):301–11.

103. Brunetti E, Kern P, Vuitton DA. Expert consensus for the diagnosis and treatment of cystic and alveolar echinococcosis in humans. Acta Trop 2010;114(1):1–16.

104. Yagci G, Ustunsoz B, Kaymakcioglu N, et al. Results of surgical, laparoscopic, and percutaneous treatment for hydatid disease of the liver: 10 years experience with 355 patients. World J Surg 2005;29(12):1670–9.

105. Perfect JR, Dismukes WE, Dromer F, et al. Clinical practice guidelines for the management of cryptococcal disease: 2010 update by the Infectious Diseases Society of America. Clin Infect Dis 2010;50(3):291–322.

106. Wheat LJ, Freifeld AG, Kleiman MB, et al. Clinical practice guidelines for the management of patients with histoplasmosis: 2007 update by the Infectious Diseases Society of America. Clin Infect Dis 2007;45(7):807–25.

Moving?

Make sure your subscription moves with you!

To notify us of your new address, find your **Clinics Account Number** (located on your mailing label above your name), and contact customer service at:

Email: **journalscustomerservice-usa@elsevier.com**

800-654-2452 (subscribers in the U.S. & Canada)
314-447-8871 (subscribers outside of the U.S. & Canada)

Fax number: **314-447-8029**

Elsevier Health Sciences Division
Subscription Customer Service
3251 Riverport Lane
Maryland Heights, MO 63043

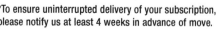

*To ensure uninterrupted delivery of your subscription, please notify us at least 4 weeks in advance of move.

Printed and bound by CPI Group (UK) Ltd, Croydon, CR0 4YY

03/10/2024

01040408-0005